HUMAN BIOLOGY FOR SOCIAL WORKERS

Development, Ecology, Genetics, and Health

LEON GINSBERG

University of South Carolina

LARRY NACKERUD

University of Georgia

CHRISTOPHER R. LARRISON

University of Illinois

PEARSON

Boston ■ New York ■ San Francisco
Mexico City ■ Montreal ■ Toronto ■ London ■ Madrid ■ Munich ■ Paris
Hong Kong ■ Singapore ■ Tokyo ■ Cape Town ■ Sydney

Series Editor: *Patricia Quinlin*
Series Editorial Assistant: *Annemarie Kennedy*
Marketing Manager: *Taryn Wahlquist*
Production Administrator: *Michael Granger*
Editorial-Production Service: *Omegatype Typography, Inc.*
Composition and Prepress Buyer: *Linda Cox*
Manufacturing Buyer: *JoAnne Sweeney*
Cover Administrator: *Kristina Mose-Libon*
Electronic Composition: *Omegatype Typography, Inc.*

For related titles and support materials, visit our online catalog at www.ablongman.com.

Between the time Website information is gathered and then published, it is not unusual for some sites to have closed. Also, the transcription of URLs can result in typographical errors. The publisher would appreciate notification where these errors occur so that they may be corrected in subsequent editions.

Library of Congress Cataloging-in-Publication Data

Ginsberg, Leon H.
  Human biology for social workers : development, ecology, genetics, and health / Leon Ginsberg, Larry Nackerud, Christopher Larrison.
    p. cm.
  Includes bibliographical references and index.
  ISBN 0-205-34405-4 (alk. paper)
  1. Human biology. 2. Social workers. 3. Social medicine. I. Nackerud, Larry G. (Larry Glenn) II. Larrison, Christopher R. III. Title.
QP34.5.G567 2004
612—dc21

2002043765

Printed in the United States of America

10   9   8   7   6   5   4   3   2   1   08   07   06   05   04   03

*To my grandchildren, Avery Appalachian Mooney-Cantey
and Corey, Lizzie, and Max Ginsberg—part of the world's future.
—Leon Ginsberg*

*To Michelle with thanks for your love and dedication.
—Larry Nackerud*

*To David and Joyce Larrison, my parents,
and Tim Larrison, my brother.
—Chris Larrison*

CONTENTS

CHAPTER THREE

Determinism, Biology, Culture, and the Ecological Perspective   42

PREFACE

Before anyone can effectively practice any kind of social work, he or she must understand the basics of human biology. Although the problems with which social workers deal with people often surround issues such as a client's social needs or physical or mental health, a community's social problems, or the need to establish a service designed to overcome a personal or social concern, the biology of human beings is always a part of the equation. Poverty, which is the overriding problem faced by those who receive services from social workers, is often a product of a client or client system's physical illness. The crossover between such problems as mental or physical disability and unemployment is so great that it is almost impossible to distinguish between the problem and the poverty.

Many communities face social problems such as pollution and other matters in the ecology. Many social and personal problems result from the use, especially the misuse, of substances such as alcohol, drugs, and tobacco.

Social workers, especially social work educators and public health social workers, frequently encounter clients whose health conditions are a result of or are being treated with pseudoscientific treatments that can delay the use of proper treatment or that can leave the patient without effective treatment throughout the course of the disease.

And social workers, no matter what their specific assignment at a given time, are often faced with clients or client family members who are suffering from diseases such as cancer, heart disease, or epidemic conditions such as AIDS and other illnesses. Social workers often need to know about those conditions or about the places they may search to find out more about them.

As a backdrop to their work, social workers also need to know about the concepts of evolution and the growingly important science of genetics and the human genome. Ignorance of such matters is unbefitting a professionally educated helping person, who may be called on, at any time, to know something about such matters.

Increasingly, mental illness and developmental disabilities are understood, at least in part, as products of human biology. At an earlier time, knowledge of cognitive psychology might be all that would be expected as a knowledge base, especially for mental illness. However, more and more information is becoming available that suggests that some forms of mental illness have some biological bases.

How people learn and develop intellectually is increasingly being viewed as, at least in part, a product of physical or biological forces. Understanding the points of view about the human intellect's reliance on biology is, again, crucial for dealing with clients.

So, for all these reasons, a comprehension of human biology is critical for social workers as well as others who deliver human services in the professional context.

This book covers, in easy-to-understand language, with appropriate applications to social work and the human services, all the subjects discussed above and more. It traces the human lifespan from conception through death (a subject that had once been the basis for human behavior courses in social work), with special attention to the first year of life and the biology of aging. It describes human biology from all the relevant perspectives such as physiology and anatomy as well as details the physical systems such as the skeletal, neurological (with special emphasis on the brain), and circulatory. A full chapter is devoted to understanding the biological components of the development of the human intellect.

The book discusses the major disease systems such as heart disease, cancer, and viral conditions. Such special disease categories as AIDS and leprosy are also detailed. Alcoholism and other substance abuse are also discussed in detail in a separate chapter—not primarily from social perspectives but from the point of view of their impact on the biological systems and, especially, the ways in which the brain handles psychoactive substances.

As a backdrop to understanding the rest of the book, it includes details on the Human Genome Project, which is revolutionizing the comprehension of the physical human being. That chapter builds on the analyses of genetics and heredity, which are also discussed in detail.

A full chapter is devoted to critical thinking, a major issue in the development of social work curriculum, because critical thinking about biological issues is called for in better understanding the role of biology in human development and human problems.

Public health issues are discussed in a full chapter because many of the most important biological considerations are public health considerations. Issues such as air and water pollution, the relatively new threat of bioterrorism, and environmental matters of other kinds are detailed from the perspective of social work's connection to the field of public health.

These are issues that are being increasingly slated for coverage in social work and other human services education curricula. Education about modern human services that does not cover the biological and physical dimensions is incomplete and can, in reality, be misleading for students of the subject.

Ironically, human biology is not new subject matter for social work. In its earlier days and even in the 1950s and 1960s, typical graduate social work curricula included courses called by such names as "medical information," which covered many of the concepts that are detailed in this book. For several decades, however, the importance of psychological and, later, sociological material began to dominate social work education and material on the physical aspects of behavior were deemphasized.

As social work began to notice the lack of biology-related information in the social work curriculum, organizations such as the Council on Social Work Education Commission on Accreditation began adding requirements for information on human biology to their standards. Now, virtually all social work programs at the bachelor's and master's levels attempt to insure that their students are educated about human biology. However, until now there has been no text about human biology that is designed for social work students and practitioners. This book was designed and published to fill that gap. Standard biology texts are helpful in explaining the basics of the science but fall short, as might be expected, in applying that knowledge to social work. This book attempts to do both—to cover the basics of human biology and to show why and how it is important to those who are pursuing social work careers.

The three authors are experienced social work educators who have, in their courses over the years, taught about the biological components of human behavior. They are social workers rather than biologists—and their goal is to offer a bridge between biological facts and the ways in which social workers may use them. Of course, extensive research has gone into this book. Each of the authors knew a good bit of each of the topics they covered but none was completely well informed about all the diverse and complex subjects that the text covers, although they have learned a great deal from each other during the years they spent preparing the book.

The authors hope that this volume will be a source of important and useable information for those who read it. It was challenging to develop but more than a bit enjoyable. Breaking new ground in the production of texts has been the goal and the authors hope it meets the needs and wishes of those who read this book.

ACKNOWLEDGMENTS

The authors acknowledge the support and assistance of several individuals in the development and preparation of this book.

Peter Davis, Annemarie Kennedy, and Patricia Quinlin of Allyn and Bacon were especially encouraging and supportive. Their belief in the need for this book and their suggestions for its development have been especially helpful throughout the two years that the book was being written. Thanks also to Diana Neatrour and the team at Omegatype Typography, Inc.

At the University of South Carolina, Leon Ginsberg is grateful for the assistance of Kelly Gray, Christina Hutchinson, Barbara Kohn, Krista Lewis, Joyce Shaw, and Dena Sims in research and manuscript preparation. Leon also expresses his appreciation to his wife, Connie, for her support and suggestions throughout the preparation of the manuscript. At the University of Georgia, Larry Nackerud is grateful for the assistance of Sarah Chase and So-Young Lee. Chris Larrison thanks his wife Tara and his son Max for their love, support, and encouragement, and Marge Wood, his first mentor, for her inspiration.

The authors want to thank the reviewers who made helpful comments on the manuscript: Lynn Adkins of University of Pittsburgh, Scarlett A. Benjamin of Keuka College, Ronnie Martin of Methodist College, Gertrude R. Sanders of Yeshiva University, and Joseph Walsh of Virginia Commonwealth University.

PART I

THE BASICS OF
HUMAN BIOLOGY

The first part of this text introduces some basic concepts of human biology and makes the case for social workers to better understand biological phenomena as well as learning to understand human behavior and the social environment from biological as well as social and behavioral science perspectives.

The first chapter deals with the reasons for studying biology. It points out that biology has long been a part of the social work education curriculum and, at times, a much larger part of that curriculum than it has been in relatively recent years. The authors argue that understanding the physical aspects of human beings and human behavior is as central to understanding the ways in which people function as are the social and behavioral sciences such as psychology and sociology.

The second chapter discusses the basic concepts of the biological sciences. There is particular emphasis on human biological concepts as well as the study of human anatomy and physiology. Of course, anatomy and physiology are critical understandings for people who want to know more about the biology of human behavior and the social environment.

The ecology of human behavior is closely tied to understanding the biology of human beings. Knowing how people connect with the environment and understanding the ways in which behavioral systems relate to one another are central concepts in human ecology. Therefore, a whole chapter is devoted to the subject.

Chapter 4 discusses the biological development of the human being from conception to death. The stages of human life are discussed in detail and a reprinted article on the first year of life is included with the chapter. The understanding of the ways in which people grow and develop, particularly physiologically, is important to understanding human beings and human behavior. Some psychosocial material is included in the chapter because understanding the stages of physical development is closely tied to better understanding of the psychological and social development of the human being.

CHAPTER ONE

WHY STUDY BIOLOGY?

The sciences have developed in an order the reverse of what might have been expected. What was most remote from ourselves was first brought under the domain of law, and then, gradually, what was nearer: first the heavens, next the earth, then animal and vegetable life, then the human body, and last of all (as yet very imperfectly) the human mind.

—Bertrand Russell, 1935

Studying human biology is crucial for social workers. Although the professional interventions of social workers are generally in the areas of psychological and social situations, those are heavily affected by biology. The more people learn about biology, the more significant it appears to be in understanding all dimensions of human behavior and human problems. In many ways, the twenty-first century seems to be an era in which more and more is understood about the interplay between human biology and human behavior. Perhaps the twentieth-century achievements were more in the development of psychological and sociological understandings. As Bertrand Russell stated in the quotation that begins this chapter, all science, including biology, moved late in history toward understanding human beings and later still in understanding mental and emotional functioning, which are still only imperfectly comprehended. But social work and other human services, with their emphases on understanding and working with people, need as much up-to-date knowledge as they can acquire about human biology.

That is important because many human problems, whether they are thought of as social, psychological, or physical, are biologically based. Knowing about the biology of human conditions is so essential for effective social work that it is almost an ethical requirement for a practitioner to have some understanding of the biology of human behavior and the social environment. For example, although we may think of poverty as primarily a social or economic problem, many of the adult poor are unable to earn satisfactory incomes because of problems associated with biological phenomena. Chronic illness is a major example. Diseases such as cancer, diabetes, multiple sclerosis, cystic fibrosis, and many others require constant treatment and specific lifestyle adjustments. Serving those who face such conditions requires knowledge of the conditions and the biological phenomena associated with them. People with orthopedic disabilities are often unable to secure adequate employment because they cannot (or potential employers think they cannot) carry out the physical responsibilities of the available jobs. Advocacy groups for people who are deaf or hard of hearing and for people who are blind say that there is an enormous percentage of those they represent who are unemployed or significantly underemployed.

Social workers also need to understand how their own behavior and practice patterns require some sensitivity to human biology. For example, social workers need to understand the impact on their own health and the health of their clients of tobacco use. That does not mean constantly admonishing clients to avoid smoking but a sophisticated understanding of the health risks associated with tobacco use so they can be explained to clients, especially children, seems crucial for practitioners. Those social workers who smoke cigarettes and also deal with cancer patients need to be aware of the effects the odors of smoking may have on those patients, even though the smoking is usually not in the presence of the patients. Clearly, social workers should not contribute to the increased illness of the patients.

For much of its history, social work focused heavily on biological issues, including normal and abnormal physical development, wellness and illness, and such specialized areas of biology as human reproduction. However, in its mid-twentieth-century approaches, the profession began focusing, first, on psychological forces, especially the theories of Sigmund Freud, and, in a minority of social work schools and agencies, Otto Rank.

Later in its history, in the late 1950s and the 1960s, social work began turning a corner in its theoretical orientations. Because social workers dealt largely with issues facing disadvantaged people such as those eligible for assistance, people who are physically or mentally ill, families in conflict, and persons in difficulty with the law, many within and outside the profession demanded a lesser emphasis on personal and psychological issues and a greater emphasis on social forces as they affected the work of social workers and the social problems with which they deal. So social work students began studying social systems, social deprivation, and culture.

Some studies find that science knowledge is not as strong as it should be across the whole age range of the United States. According to Malcolm Ritter (2002), who reported on a National Science Foundation report, only 22 percent of Americans who were surveyed could define a molecule, which is the basic unit of a chemical compound. However, nearly half (45 percent) could define DNA, which is the substance that carries the inherited genetic code. Of course, having some understanding of chemical compounds and heredity is crucial for making sense of human biology.

In the late 1950s, when the most senior of the three authors of this text studied social work at Tulane University in New Orleans, the emphasis of the master's curriculum's human behavior courses was, in one semester, physical systems and, in another, mental processes and mental illness. The instructors in the first course were primarily physicians, whose work was coordinated by a social work educator. Pediatricians, public health specialists, and a physiologist taught the classes. In the second course, the instructors were primarily psychiatrists, coordinated by the same social work educator. That was not an unusual approach in social work education. However, in today's curriculum, the emphasis of education about human behavior and the social environment is on, in some programs, the human life cycle, especially the psychosocial dimensions of the life cycle, and on content dealing with social and cultural phenomena. There is a special emphasis, which makes sense for a variety of reasons, on ethnicity and ethnic groups, especially on ethnic groups of color. The name of the instruction also demonstrates the changed emphases. We now call that block of education Human Behavior and the Social Environment. Not only are individuals, families, and other targets of direct service discussed, but there is also emphasis on larger systems—organizations, institutions, and communities. The interactions of individuals and families with the social environment are a major emphasis in today's social work education.

However, in the 1980s the Curriculum Policy statements that are promulgated by the Council on Social Work Education, the profession's educational accrediting body, which governs the education program standards, agreed that the deemphasis on the physical went too far and that some greater emphasis on human biology needed to be included in social work curricula. As a result, social work education programs are now required, as part of an accreditation standard for both bachelor's and master's programs, to either teach about human biology or guarantee that students have adequate background in the subject from other sources such as their general education requirements in their bachelor's studies. This book is designed to help pursue the profession's historical and recently rediscovered emphasis on the biological aspects of the professional social worker's work.

NEW THINKING ABOUT BIOLOGY

But the traditional emphases on human biology may no longer be sufficient. In recent years, more and more scientists have discovered ways in which biology is a powerful determinant of human behavior and human potential—perhaps the most powerful determinant of all. For example, a venerable social psychology text (Baron & Byrne, 2000, p. 17) states, "We should note once again the growing influence of a biological or evolutionary perspective in modern social psychology. . . . Growing evidence suggests that biological and genetic factors play at least some role in many forms of social behavior—in everything from physical attraction and mate selection to aggression and helping behavior."

Science theory is going in so many different directions that it is important to keep up with it. A clear and extensive discussion of current thinking about genetics and inheritance in human behavior was written by Louis Menand for *The New*

Yorker in late 2002. He writes about two books, Steven Pinker's *The Blank Slate: The Modern Denial of Human Nature,* which was published in 2002, and Judith Rich Harris's 1998 book, *The Nurture Assumption.* Newcombe (2002) provides a critical analysis of the new works on the biological impact on human behavior.

Pinker and Harris both note that parenting and other environmental influences are not the sole determinant of variations in personality. In fact, Harris suggests that parenting doesn't account for personality variations. She suggests that half of personality comes from the genes and half from the environment. Of course, neither author suggests that parenting has no impact on children. However, "parents cannot make a fretful child into a serene adult" (Menand, 2002, p. 99). Identical twins raised in separate environments share many behavioral characteristics, for example. And even the best parenting, as prescribed by professionals such as social workers, teachers, and psychologists, does not always seem to prevent or overcome serious behavioral shortcomings in children. These biological and genetic approaches counter the theories of the "Blank Slate," which was the philosopher John Locke's assessment of the newborn—a blank slate on which experiences and socialization would replace the blank with knowledge, behavior, and personality.

Although even the most passionate advocates of the theory that heredity and genes influence behavior enormously, none suggest that the environment has no impact at all. However, it may be that advocates of the theory that the environment is the most important influence on behavior attribute only a minimum of influence to genetics. That is, more or less, Pinker's point of view.

This debate is important for social work because this profession has largely adopted the nurture or environment understanding of the ways in which people develop. The very name of the profession, social work, suggests the paramount importance of the social forces. However, new findings about the influence of heredity on behavior may be causing the whole social work profession to reexamine its largely environmental approach to assuring and attempting to deal with human behavior.

A theoretical physicist who received a MacArthur Foundation Genius grant has now written a book called a *New Kind of Science,* published by Wolfram Media. Steven Wolfram (2002) tries, in his new book, to redefine the basic foundations of every branch of science from physics to psychology and including biology. His attempt is to simulate the basic patterns of nature with computer programs. Should he be successful, he will have provided a new understanding of the nature of all science. Efforts such as his to synthesize science and show how it connects in every way and in every element are in the offing for those who want to understand science in the modern world.

One of the major theoreticians of evolution and heredity, Harvard professor Stephen Jay Gould (2002), who was widely regarded as Charles Darwin's successor, described his basic theories in a book over 1,400 pages long that was published shortly before he died in 2002.

Biology is now also much more complicated than it was when social work used it as a central part of its educational curriculum. And it is less exact, in some ways, than other sciences. Trillin (2001) cites experts who suggest that the biology of humans is too variable to be reduced to mathematics. Understanding the biology of illnesses, for example, requires judgment and knowledge that go beyond the technical and quantitative analyses that are to a greater extent sufficient for other sciences. Williams (2003) says that biology is now the most dynamic of the sciences, as it does not rest on fundamentals such as the laws of physics or chemistry's periodic table.

Part of recent discoveries about biology suggests that it is even more important than may have been imagined earlier. Tom Wolfe (2000), a popular novelist and essayist, focuses part of his attention in one of his newest books of essays, *Hooking Up,* on the works of Edward O. Wilson (2000), to whom the emerging field of "sociobiology" is attributed. Wilson first wrote *Sociobiology: The New Synthesis* in 1976. His original work was as a zoologist, a biologist who studies animal rather than plant life. His primary focus was entomology and within that field, ants. He later studied other animals, especially monkeys, and, eventually, human beings. His conclusion, after careful study, was that social phenomena were largely governed by biological forces, especially the genetic inheritances of human beings. Wolfe points out that Wilson believed that human brains were born not as blank slates but more like photographic negatives that were waiting to be placed in and finished with a developer. In other words, Wilson asserted that people were born with most of the genetic determinants of what they would do and how they would do it. Education, family nurturing, and other experiences could enhance the process, but much that is social about humans is fundamentally biological, he concluded. Sociobiology could explain much of what the world and its people were like—more, perhaps, than fields such as history, anthropology, or economics.

Although sociobiology itself is not a major emphasis in most social work programs or of this book, and although its tenets are controversial, the field points to the probably neglected degree of importance that should be given to the biological in understanding and dealing with human behavior. The concept is essentially that human behavior evolves just as the physical aspects of humans and other beings do. The idea is not popular with all observers of human behavior, and in some ways, it contradicts much of what social workers believe and toward which they work—that people can change and develop, especially with the help of social agencies and agents. The idea that social behavior is genetically built in suggests that less can be done than one would like about human behavior.

If behavior evolves, just as physical characteristics do, then the implications are enormous. Certain behaviors would have to be defined as more effective in the evolutionary process than others; certain elements of behavior would be based on biological imperatives rather than value choices and preferences. Marriage and reproduction could be a product of a male human's drive to perpetuate himself and his genes. War and other forms of violence could be understood as elements in the natural selection process, both physical in terms of who survives and in terms of the waging of violence as a means of working to dominate others.

Actually, there probably are behaviors—some more than others—that are biologically driven. Understanding why people choose to have children, why some behaviors lead to violent interactions, how and why people choose careers, and many other issues may require the recognition that such choices and actions may be biologically as well as emotionally and socially based. How much of behavior is defined biologically is a matter that is likely to be carefully studied over the years.

Another popular essayist and novelist Larry McMurtry (2000) also makes some significant points about the importance of the physical or biological in understanding the social and psychological. In 1991, McMurtry had heart bypass surgery in Baltimore at Johns Hopkins University Hospital. Such surgery is relatively common for heart patients and has saved lives that would have ended with heart disease only a few decades earlier. But McMurtry says that he had a nonfatal death from his surgery. As he writes (pp. 162–163), "My body lived on but my personality died, or at least imploded, disintegrated, shattered into fragments. For the past eight years I've been struggling to collect and reassemble these drifting fragments of personality and I believe I have now reassembled most of them. They fit together a little crookedly still, but that's only to be expected after one has been radically cut open."

McMurtry describes this phenomenon as fairly common (p. 163): "I'm far from being the only person to experience personality death while continuing physical life. Victims of stroke very often survive physically but lose all trace of personality—that which, in their view and the view of their loved ones, made them uniquely them."

The disorienting experience McMurtry suffered after heart bypass surgery is experienced by 30 percent of bypass patients in a condition they call pump head (Park, March 11, 2002). Surgeons blame the condition on the heart–lung machine, which takes over from the heart while it is being operated on. Some surgeons are now trying to operate on the heart while it is still beating, which seems to prevent the loss of memory, attention, and motor skills that appear to result when some patient hearts are stopped and substituted for by the heart–lung machine.

Barbara Kingsolver (2001), who writes novels and edited *The Best American Short Stories, 2001,* says she refuses to read fiction that fails to get its facts straight—an important concern for those who may have wanted their short stories to be selected for the volume she edited. She decries what she finds as occasional examples of "biological illiteracy" and notes one author who wrote that humans were separated from baboons and lemurs by the latters' lack of opposable thumbs. Kingsolver wrote that humans, baboons, and lemurs all have opposable thumbs, which makes them primates. Of course, written and spoken illiteracy can discredit a person's otherwise sound work, as can mathematical illiteracy, which John Alan Paulos (2001) calls "innumeracy." Now Kingsolver provides another literacy concern with her decrying of the biological variety.

It is often easy to forget the social and psychological elements of physical conditions. But clearly, personal and social behavior are often more affected by physical conditions than by the family and the environment. Inasmuch as so many social workers deal with patients with serious illnesses and their families, understanding the consequences of the physical is crucial.

SOME DEFINITIONS

What, exactly, is biology? It is the study of living things (Harkavy, 1998). That means it studies both animals, which is called zoology, and plants, which is called botany, the two broad classifications of living things. One of the earliest scientific developments in biology was the development of a taxonomy, a system of classifying that provides each living thing a unique name.

Biology has many subtopics: physiology, which is the study of organs and how they are affected by diseases; pathology, the study of diseases; as well as others. Biology is also connected to chemistry, through a field called biochemistry, and physics, through a field called biophysics. Molecular biology is also a subdivision that studies biological processes at the molecular level. Genetics is also a major element of the science of biology. This text deals with many of these subjects in addition to others, although the emphasis is on the biological effects on human behavior and development.

A fundamental focus of this book is on the centrality of the scientific method for understanding human beings and for defining and carrying out social programs. That is, of course, an emphasis in all human services educational programs. It simply means that decisions about who or what we deal with and the ways in which we serve them ought to be based on systematic observation. Ideally, we would use experimental methods to draw conclusions—experiments that, at minimum, compare randomly selected treatment groups with randomly selected control groups that do not receive the treatment. Conclusions about people and services based on sentiment, unproven theories, or political power are not sufficient for defining human problems or mounting services programs. An example of the opposite is the Drug Abuse Resistance Education program or DARE, which has been popular with both the federal and state governments as a means for keeping children away from illegal drugs. *Harper's* magazine (2000) reports that in 1999, $1.75 million in federal funds were allocated for the program, along with many more dollars in state and local financing. But, *Harper's* reports, evaluation research published in the *Journal of Consulting and Clinical Psychology* in 1999 showed that the program had no effect on drug use (Conn & Lapham, 2000).

Human biology is not one of the terms regularly used in defining the science of biology, which the *Webster's 21st Century Pocket Encyclopedia* (2000, p. 253) calls "the science of living things." It is a convenient term for social workers, though, because the profession's emphasis is on the biology of human beings as opposed to all animals, which are included under the rubric of the field of *zoology*. When the authors of this text write about human biology, however, they are including fields of study such as *physiology*, mentioned earlier, which the encyclopedia (p. 253) says deals with "the workings of organs and how they are affected by disease." The study of disease is called *pathology*. The same source goes on to discuss the connections between biology and psychology, biology and chemistry, genetics, and the study of the biology of molecules, the subdivisions of the field that are discussed above.

So this text deals with a broad range of biological phenomena as they apply to and affect human beings and their behavior. It deals with some of the traditional knowledge of the sort learned in introductory biology courses. However, it goes beyond all of that into emerging fields such as sociobiology, cloning, and the interactions of human biology with mental illnesses and drugs. Its emphasis is on the sorts of information human services practitioners, especially social workers, need to serve people competently. That is the subject matter covered in this volume.

One of the decisions that the authors had to confront was the extent of biological material that could be covered in a fairly brief and accessible text designed to be useful to social work students and practitioners. Introductory biology texts are enormous and cover a good bit about the science of biology—the structure and functions of cells, the molecular biology of genes, complete explanations of the Mendel principles of inheritance, and detailed discussions of evolution, for example. One biology text that the authors used in defining the material for this book is Campbell, Mitchell, and Reece's *Biology: Concepts and Connections* (2000). Its over 800 pages of text, including illustrations, has an extensive glossary of biological terms and covers much of what there is to teach about both animal and plant biology, which is, of course, related to the study of human biology. We also consulted Michael D. Johnson's *Human Biology: Concepts and Current Issues* (2001).

Not only is the classic material on biology extensive, daily reports on new developments in biology, new pharmaceuticals, and new discoveries about health conditions that are biologically related make much writing about human biology immediately out of date. It is a dynamic field, which is another justification for social workers to become better educated about it. There is probably no lesson more important than understanding how much and how frequently biological knowledge is modified or replaced by new knowledge.

Although during the writing of this book the authors attempted to stay current with new developments in biology, the realities of book production make it impossible to be completely up to date. So the authors chose to cover the kinds of basic information and phenomena that should be most useful to social workers in their professional studies and in their practice. Issues such as genetics, including the human genome, the basic physical systems, the biological elements of diseases, the biology of aging, and sexuality, are discussed in this text, among several other topics.

A full understanding of the science may require consulting comprehensive biology texts, many of which are available and some of which were consulted in the development of this text. Detailed descriptions of the various biological processes and the bases for them require much larger studies and volumes than are presented in this book.

Part of this book's purpose is to promote sophisticated knowledge among social workers about human biology. A social worker's knowledge about people has to be extensive. Obviously, it should include sound understanding of social functioning as well as some sophistication about mental processes and mental disabilities. But the social and mental functions of human beings are inherently related to their biology as well, as discussed earlier in this chapter. So this text is geared to helping social workers build that dimension of their understanding of people.

SCIENCE AND THE HUMAN SERVICES

In some ways, those of us in the human services professions sometimes seem as if we are refugees from mathematics and, by extension, from science. More often than not, social work students and others who are involved in planning or carrying out human services careers suggest they are less than enthusiastic about courses in research, statistics, and other work with similar scientific connotations. At the outset of their studies, graduate social work students, for example, are likely to suggest that courses in research are those they anticipate liking least. Many change that prediction and enjoy their work in the area of research, but some are nearly terrified of courses such as statistics and research methods. Although they may have been excellent students in literature, social science, and history, many had negative encounters with the sciences and with mathematics. It is sad to think that people with baccalaureate degrees and beyond may have significant gaps in their education. That is particularly true when so much that has changed the human services has resulted from scientific innovations and discoveries. It is likely that future improvements in those fields will also result from scientific achievements.

In some ways, human biology is a complex subject that requires at least a beginning comprehension of several other subjects, including some of the natural sciences. Students in the human services may focus more heavily on the social and behavioral sciences in their undergraduate careers, but it becomes increasingly clear that effective human services work is dependent on some understanding of the biological and natural sciences' impact on human growth and human behavior.

However, the connection between science and human services practice is often not made for students. Perhaps science information is taught without connecting it to real-life objectives or to matters that are of special interest to students whose inclinations are toward the humanities and social sciences. The primary purpose of this text is to help students understand the ways in which their biological and other science learnings have significance for their practice careers in the human services. Obviously, science educators, by and large, will not be able to make those connections for their human services–oriented students. Or it may be a lack of appropriate science texts that keep students from understanding the relevance for their careers of basic science information. But science cannot be left to the scientists alone. As the noted writer and editor Timothy Ferris (1991, p. xi) says, "The delights of science and mathematics . . . are too profound, and too important, to be left to scientists and mathematicians alone." He compares modern scientific discoveries to the epic poems of the Greeks and the landscape painting of the Sung Dynasty Chinese. However, he goes on (p. xi), "Technical matters customarily are announced in technical terms—in words and equations that make sense chiefly to initiates."

It is often surprising to human services program graduate admissions committees that applicants, with obvious interests in human beings, fulfill undergraduate science requirements by taking courses in fields such as geology, rather than more person-related fields such as biology or even chemistry. Often, such students explain that they were able to satisfactorily complete geology courses, something that may not have been true of courses in other sciences. Fortunately, accredited undergraduate social work programs currently require some study of human biology, either in the science programs of their colleges or universities or in special courses offered as part of the social work curriculum.

Much of what has been most significant for economic assistance as well as social services has been possible, for example, because of scientific innovations especially in information technology—computers. Keeping records and distributing assistance to the thousands who need food stamps, medical assistance, and financial aid would not be possible at reasonable costs were it not for computers. Would it be possible to effectively track and collect from absent parents who owe child support without effective computer services? Would we have known about the extent of the problems of child abuse and neglect without computer programs? And could child welfare agencies keep track of foster children without the aid of computers? Computers write the checks to pay for those services, maintain the rosters of clients, and ensure that service and care deadlines are met. Would Social Security for the massive number of people entitled to its benefits be possible without the giant computers that operate the program? And would the state and federal tax agencies be able to collect properly without computers? It is doubtful.

Health problems as well as many mental health issues are related to biology and other sciences. So working in hospitals and community health programs without some scientific knowledge can be a serious handicap. Dealing with the aging processes and understanding both the normal and pathological dimensions of advancing age, as well as the medications and medical procedures associated with them, require workers with older clients to master some scientific information. The transmission and course of diseases such as AIDS are understood only through biology and can be prevented only by educating people about the biological steps for preventing it.

Helping people adopt proper nutritional habits requires some capacity for understanding the science behind it. Understanding the fundamentals of genetics and heredity is also crucial in many human services roles. Essentially, all human services roles demand some sophisticated scientific knowledge if they are to be effectively discharged. Of course, a human services worker's knowledge is no substitute for the professional skills of physicians and geneticists. But being able to work effectively with those specialized professions, on behalf of clients, is enhanced when we know some of the fundamentals of the subjects with which we are dealing.

SCIENCE AND ITS ALTERNATIVES

Sometimes failing to expose oneself to scientific information not only means forgoing knowledge that can be helpful to clients but can also lead to embracing unproven or dangerous options. For example, one problem associated with the lack of scientific knowledge is the possibility of human services workers grasping for and lacking the ability to evaluate unproven and potentially harmful alternative approaches to service. Herbal solutions to health and behavioral problems when those problems demand expert care and proven medications can leave clients ineffectively served. Being unable to see the lack of help available from such "treatments" as homeopathic and naturopathic healing can keep professionals from providing the kinds of guidance their clients may need to maintain or restore their health. Even when the products and services do no harm, the major difficulty is the failure to obtain treatment that could make a life or death difference. And some unproven treatments may also do harm. One of the authors encountered a medicine package called "Nature's Way Cold and Flu Homeopathic Formula." It was offered under the auspices of a person with the title of M.P.H., who was identified as the founder of the Foundation for Homeopathic Education and Research. Several problems with the medicine were evident. First, M.P.H. means Master of Public Health, a human services field that provides some excellent services and research on health issues. (See Chapter 13.) However, developing medicines is not normally part of the curriculum of public health. Developing and testing pharmaceuticals is a function of pharmacists and pharmacologists, not public health workers. Second, the whole concept of homeopathy is suspect. According to Clayman (1989), homeopathy is a form of alternative medicine. Under the theory, minute quantities of medicine or substances that would induce symptoms of an illness in a healthy person are given to persons with that illness as a means of overcoming the illness. Although that is something like the process followed with some inoculations—mild forms of a disease are induced in a patient as a means of making the person immune from contracting the disease in the future—the use of the process is unproven for most treatment of illnesses. The analogy with scientifically based treatments has not been proven and, in fact, inoculations against diseases are only put into effect after careful and extensive research. Third, some of the homeopathic substances may be dangerous in themselves. The cold and flu remedy mentioned contained arsenic trioxide, which is primarily a poison, according to dictionaries and medical guides. It is used, apparently, in some heart disease cases as a blood thinner, but it is primarily used for killing, not for maintaining health. It is used in insecticides, for example. Most people may have traces of the substance in their systems, but high concentrations of arsenic trioxide may cause severe illness or death. Using a formula for supposed health improvement to those suffering from colds and flu that contains a noted poison seems unreasonable. However, *Men's Health* magazine (2002) reported that researchers in Seattle also believe that tiny amounts of what the magazine refers to as a deadly poison may be able to treat leukemia, too. Of course, homeopathic formulas are heavily diluted so that the small amounts of arsenic in the cold and flu formula would probably not directly harm a patient. Taking much more than the recommended amount could cause illness, it would seem. But what purpose can be served by diluting a supposed curative substance, even if it has a role in curing illnesses, to almost nothing? Would the patient be equally well off from just drinking water? Exactly what to believe about such alternative medical practices as homeopathy is a complicated issue.

A book on the emergency use of homeopathic medicine (Nauman, 2000) says that the approach was developed some 200 years ago by Samuel Hahnemann in Germany. The author says that the basic theory is that like cures like, so that a medicine that may induce vomiting might, in a small amount, prevent vomiting. So the arsenic, mentioned previously, which can kill, may be viewed as something that, in small amounts, promotes health. However, it is not clear whether any of these theories have been tested or proved with the use of accepted scientific methods.

Another form of alternative medicine, naturopathy, is based on the idea that disease results from waste products and toxins accumulating in the body. Disease symptoms are reflections of the body's efforts to get rid of the toxins and waste, naturopaths believe, according to the *American Medical Association Encyclopedia* (Clayman, 1989, p. 716): "Practitioners of naturopathy believe that health is maintained by avoiding anything artificial or unnatural in the diet or in the environment." It is not difficult to conclude that this form of health practice helped spawn the "natural" and "organic" food industries, which are major growth factors in the American economy. Those specialized foods generally cost more than the ordinary foods sold in supermarkets, some of which now carry both kinds of products. Naturopathic influence is also likely behind the amazing growth of sales and use of bottled water in the United States, which monitors and guarantees the quality of its public water supplies.

The problem with many alternative treatment medicines is that they are based on what their proponents call research. However, that research is not based on the controlled experiments that one would want in defining a health measure. Instead, the research is based on what scientific researchers would call *anecdotal* evidence—that some patients reported feeling cured or better after taking the substance. Without a control group that had similar health problems but did not receive the treatment, one cannot know, definitively, whether the "cure" was spontaneous or the result of the treatment.

That same problem may also be true with the popular practice called chiropractic medicine, which is based on theories of the involvement of the human spine in diseases. According to Clayman (1989), chiropractors believe that manipulation of the spine can help overcome a number of conditions. Clayman says that medical practitioners are not persuaded that chiropractic medicine provides cures or is based on accurate theories about the human body and diseases. The evidence sometimes used to justify it is often anecdotal—patients say the treatments helped. But pain, especially back pain, which is often what brings a patient to a chiropractor, is often susceptible to improvement with time and rest, regardless of whether or not specific treatments are used.

In late 2002, *Newsweek* published a series of articles on alternative medicine. In one, Cowley (pp. 49–53) describes alternative care as "integrative care." He reminds the reader that over one-third of Americans have used some form of alternative care such as acupuncture, massage, and the use of herbs for healing illness.

He also reports on the federal government's National Center for Complementary and Alternative Medicine. Some of the nation's major medical schools have centers for integrative medicine.

The rest of the series included materials on some of the potential strengths and problems of herbal cures and the contributions of Chinese herbal medicine. It also includes a chart showing that chiropractic medicine and acupuncture for some purposes may be safe and effective. The series also suggests that the injection of unproven substances and forgoing proven treatments are dangerous practices. But alternative (or integrative) medicine is becoming increasingly widespread and often acknowledged by some more traditional health care practitioners.

Other Sides

Perhaps a scientific approach to biological and health issues such as these has no other side. However, the authors regularly encounter well-prepared professionals in social work and other fields who believe that some alternative treatments have helped them greatly. Although that sounds like anecdotal evidence, it should be noted that many people are firm believers in some of what we have suggested is less than proven. Of course, it is possible that some things work that may not seem therapeutic. Worldwide, there is a heavy reliance on herbal preparations and alternative procedures to mainstream medicine. The best guidance we may be able to provide is to be sure that a trusted, professionally educated physician—M.D. or D.O.—or a similarly well-prepared pharmacist with a degree from an accredited school of pharmacy agrees that the procedure or preparation can help and that at least it would do no harm.

Part of the issue in alternative health care procedures and products are some relatively new government policies. One policy keeps a hands-off posture for the Food and Drug Administration where herbs and other "natural" substances are involved, which means that such substances do not have to be of proven benefit to be sold. A second is the establishment of a unit that deals with "alternative" medicine in the National Institutes of Health—perhaps providing a degree of legitimacy to these popular approaches—which may be a result of their acceptance by large segments of the public as well as the political influence of their proponents rather than an indication of their efficacy.

The National Organization for Rare Disorders, Inc. (2001/2002) reported that the Office of Inspector General of the Food and Drug Administration received only 2,547 adverse event reports about nutritional supplements between 1994 and 1999. However, according to the report, in 1999 alone there were 13,000 reports from poison control centers that treated people with adverse events arising from taking supplements.

These alternative treatments—perhaps they are alternatives to treatments of proven value—are not unlike the medicine shows which huckstered tonics and elixirs in earlier America. They also seem, at times, comparable to the examples one sees in Southeast Asia of pitchmen who push market attendees to eat prepared snakes—often cobras—as a means of rejuvenating their sexual performances or of the ingestion of aphrodisiac foods such as oysters and sea cucumbers for the same purposes. They are also unproven and usually products of folklore.

The difficulty with herbal and other nonprescription medicines for dealing with health is their lack of specificity. Although they can be sold without being regulated, unless they can be proven to be toxic, they also cannot be marketed as remedies. Therefore, although vitamins and such may state a recommended daily allowance, herbal formulas cannot suggest that they are effective in particular treatments for particular conditions. Obviously they cannot specify dosages. Since these remedies have not been proven in government-approved ways for specific conditions, they cannot be credited with curative powers.

Therefore, people use substances and quantities of those substances that are recommended to them by friends or by clerks in stores and therefore do not always get accurate information about the possible dangers of overdoses. Another complication is that such substances may interact in dangerous ways with other substances that the patient may be taking. For example, there are many prescription products used for depression. An herb, St. John's Wort, is also used for depression, particularly in Europe and more recently in the United States. There has been some research on its value in treating depression. However, standardized information on the amount of the substance that one should use, which depends on size, weight, the condition, and the recommended therapy for the condition, is not readily available and actually cannot legally be provided by those who make and sell the product. Some may substitute St. John's Wort for more proven products. They may take too much or too little. And, of course, depression is a dangerous condition that can lead to suicide. Some recent scientific research on the herb shows it has little effect on the body or mind.

Another danger is the example of the person who has been diagnosed with depression and told to take a prescription medicine for it. The patient may decide to try St. John's Wort. Combining the prescription with St. John's Wort, which the patient can purchase freely in all sorts of retail outlets, could cause a severe reaction.

The United States has not fully come to terms with nonprescription medicines and their use. The consequences of not regulating such preparations can lead to severe reactions.

Perhaps another side to this discussion is the ways in which other nations handle medicines that are prescription products in the United States. In much of Latin America, for example, patients can purchase what the United States treats as prescription medicines over the counter in whatever quantity they choose. So persons who feel ill in many Latin American nations may simply go to a pharmacy and purchase and use substances such as antibiotics, which make them, if used to excess, immune to their effects when they are really needed, or they may be toxic.

In many of those nations that do not use prescription procedures, severe restrictions are put on the importation and use of various medicines—and those medicines simply are not available. Medicines in those nations are prescribed by physicians who may simply jot them out on paper. The patient purchases and uses those that have been recommended but does not need a formal prescription to obtain them. Perhaps the dangers of unregulated prescription medicines are more dangerous than those of the herbal preparations.

The federal legislation that makes it difficult or nearly impossible for the Food and Drug Administration to evaluate and remove herbal and "natural" substances and supplements from the market is the Dietary Supplement and Health Education Act of 1994 (Solotaroff, 2002). The legislation exempts supplements from the usual drug approval processes used by the FDA by reclassifying supplements as foods. The logic used was that the supplements existed in the food and water that all people use and, therefore, were natural substances that were not drugs. The FDA wanted to regulate such substances after 38 people died in 1989 from taking an amino acid named L-tryptophan and 16 children died from iron supplement poisoning in 1991. The manufacturers lobbied Congress heavily, according to Solotaroff (2002), and contributed more than $100,000 to the campaign of Utah's Senator Orrin Hatch, who sponsored the legislation. Under the legislation, the FDA has to prove that substances are harmful or not found in normal food and drink to take them off the market. But congressional budgets have allocated few dollars for making such investigations or substantiating such charges.

Although consumers of herbal products may believe that government would prevent their being sold if they were either useless or dangerous, that is not the case. As suggested, legislation has made the FDA basically impotent in its abilities to deal with such substances. That increases the pressure on social workers, teachers, public health professionals, and others who have contact with potential users of such substances to be familiar with their characteristics and educate those they serve about them.

Body Building Substances

Mind altering substances are not the only kind that pose a danger to people. A variety of drugs used to enhance athletic performance and to build muscle have also caused serious health problems and some deaths (Solotaroff, 2002). Among them are androstenedione, a male hormone that is popularly called Andro. It was used by baseball player Mark McGwire when he set the now-broken record of 70 home runs in a season in 1998. During the same season, another baseball player, Sammy Sosa, who also broke the existing record but with 66 home runs, used an amino acid called creatine to help build his body. Another substance, ephedrine, which is a stimulant, may be used for treating asthma and joint pains. Some athletes believe it provides them with extra bursts of energy. According to Swanson (2002), the FDA reports that it has found 81 deaths since 1994 that are apparently linked to the use of the stimulant.

Young athletes are susceptible to using these kinds of "supplements" as a way of building the strength and appearance of their bodies or for improving their athletic performances. Swanson (2002) says the amino acid creatine is naturally produced by the kidneys, liver, and pancreas and can help in muscle regeneration. There are no documented side effects from the use of creatine, but some anecdotal evidence suggests that it can cause cramps, dehydration, and weight gain. Andro is structurally similar to steroids, and many believe that steroids may cause damage to the liver and heart and also lead to shrinking testicles, violent changes in moods, male breast development, and reduced sperm counts.

SEXUALITY AND REPRODUCTION KNOWLEDGE

Lack of knowledge of reproductive processes and sexuality can also render a human services worker ineffective with those he or she serves. The basic misinformation among the public one encounters in such important areas as reproduction, child development, and health can lead to undesired and sometimes tragic results. For one dramatic example, the media have frequently reported on the problem of rape in some African nations, especially South Africa. Somehow, the rumor spread that men could cure themselves of AIDS by having sexual relations with virgins. The problem of rape of young women and the concomitant spread of HIV/AIDS has been a tragic outcome in some environments. So a lack of scientific sophistication can inadvertently lead human services workers and their clients to commit sins of both commission and omission.

This book is not, of course, a resource that can compensate for all that human services practitioners and students may have failed to learn in their earlier educational careers. However, it is designed to help attain knowledge about critical biological facts that are essential for human services workers.

BASIC SCIENCE AND UNDERSTANDING THE WORLD

Although biology is a distinct scientific field, all the sciences are related and all depend on one another. This book makes reference to findings from chemistry and physics, which are essential contributors to biological theory. The late physicist Richard Feynman (1991), an expert in making scientific information accessible to nonscientists, says that of all the scientific knowledge that ought to be understood by contemporary people and passed on to future generations, the most important is the atomic hypothesis. That hypothesis is that all things are made of atoms, which Feynman (1991, p. 3) describes as "little particles that move around in perpetual motion, attracting each other when they are a little distance apart, but repelling upon being squeezed into one another." Feynman (1991, 1995) goes on to add that everything is made of atoms. "The most important hypothesis in all of biology, for example, is that everything animals do, atoms do" (Feynman, 1991, p. 17). He says that what all living things do can also be described from the point of view that atoms, acting according to the laws of physics, are doing it. And to help readers understand atoms, Feynman adds that if an apple is magnified to the size of the earth, each atom within it would appear to be the size of the original apple.

A similar explanation of the subject was written by Lewis Thomas, who first wrote his article "The Lives of the Cell" in 1971. It has since been collected and reprinted in numerous publications. Thomas, a great essayist of his time, was one of the first to emphasize the fact that human beings are very much a part of nature, composed of atoms and other smaller units that are constantly in motion. As he puts it, "We are shared, rented, occupied. At the interior of ourselves, driving them, providing the oxidative energy that sends us out for an improvement of each shining day, they are mitocondria, and in a strict sense they are not ours. They turn out to be separate creatures. . . . Without them we would not move a muscle, drum a finger, think a thought" (Thomas, 2000, pp. 358–360).

Thomas points out, as do other authors quoted in this text, that the body is made up of cells and that cells are made up of smaller systems. Human bodies are systems that are more complicated than cities or regions. And that is true not only of animals but also of plants, as he points out. The DNA in our cells is inherited and carries on genetically. That conception of the human body is, of course, crucial for understanding human beings in modern ways and especially for understanding them from a biological perspective.

Trefil (1991) says that the term *atom* comes from the Greek for something that is indivisible. Of course, since they were first defined, atoms have become divisible. Trefil also points out that the development of modern physics occurred at the same time as the development of knowledge about the genetic development of the universe.

Feynman (1991) explains that humans can rarely see atoms. Observation through powerful microscopes will show particles that are in motion—moving because the atoms are acting on them. But scientists created the concept of atoms long before they could see them by developing hypotheses and testing those hypotheses in laboratories. The hypotheses were proven true over and over through the results of scientific experiments.

It is unlikely that many human services workers—or many scientists for that matter—regularly view the world and all its components as massive collections of atoms, in constant motion, regularly bumping up against one another. But that is the reality of matter—and human beings are just an example of matter.

K. C. Cole (1997) cautions that learning about the functions of small things does not necessarily help with the understanding of larger things. She cites the example of knowing all about the atoms that make up a cat—which would not tell the owner whether or not the cat would scratch the furniture or sleep on the owner's head. She also writes that the arrangement of the electrons in atoms will determine color, smell, and other characteristics of the organ of which they are a part, but a single atom has no color, odor, or texture. Put another way, Andrea Barrett (2001) quotes the biologist Joseph Dalton Hooker as saying that the organic world consists of organisms. Cole carries the same subject to the social world and says that epidemics do not exist with one person alone—they require many. Nor can an individual alone suffer from mass hysteria. So the fact that all things consist of smaller things does not mean that perfect understanding can emerge from simply comprehending the tiniest components.

Biology has to be understood as a less exact science than its counterparts of physics and chemistry. Physicist Eugene Paul Wigner (1991) says that it would be difficult and confusing if someday a theory could be established of consciousness or biology, which is an animate science dealing with moving and changing organisms, that would be the equivalent in coherence and the convincingness of the theories of the inanimate sciences of chemistry and physics. He says that the Mendel laws of inheritance come closest. Freeman Dyson (1991), also a physicist, says that biology is full of miracles, and his prime example is the metamorphosis of the Monarch butterfly. Bertrand Russell (1950) quoted in Frank (2001, p. 756) would likely call Dyson's miracles matters of philosophy because, Russell wrote, science is what we know and philosophy is what we do not—a good corollary for miracles, that which we do not know or understand fully.

Although this book and its authors cannot cover all of science, the goal is to selectively cover some of the most important current issues in human biology—concepts and facts that are useful for understanding clients and working effectively. Knowing all of science is an unachievable goal as is knowing all of biology. However, knowing some of that science—defined by the chapters that follow—is both a possible and a helpful accompaniment to a professional career in the human services.

BIOLOGICAL MYTHS AND THEIR DEBUNKING

Part of the motives of the authors is to help readers better understand human biology and to become capable of debunking myths they might encounter. It is unlikely that social workers and other human services professionals will be able to communicate all that is true about human biology. But they ought to be able to refute that which patently is not true.

Americans are not free of susceptibility to witch doctors, native healers, and other primitive examples of biological mythology. In fact, everyday television and printed advertising promote health and wellness solutions that are neither proven nor necessarily safe. These are modern versions of the witch doctor or, in the Spanish, the curandero, native healer.

These are some myths about biology and humans and some information to counter them:

1. *Herbal formulas and other products purchased without prescriptions or health care professional guidance are proven to cure or improve health conditions.* Many such products are not of proven effectiveness—at least not with the standards of proof demanded by modern science. Some are based on anecdotes or theories that have little or no scientific basis. They are not always regulated by government agencies for quality or effectiveness. Using such products without proper guidance can cause illness or delay curative treatment. Physicians and pharmacists are reliable sources of information and direction on cures for health problems.

2. *Eating foods that are fat free can lead to weight loss.* In fact, many foods that advertise their freedom from fat use large quantities of sugar and flour, carbohydrates that are typically as capable of causing weight gain as fat—and sometimes more.

3. *Electric machines that vibrate against and therefore stimulate the tissue will build muscles.* It is not clear that vibrating body tissue has any effect on the muscles.

4. *"Alternative" health care such as chiropractic, homeopathy, and naturopathy are regularly safe and effective options for dealing with health problems.* In fact, these alternatives are generally not proven to be effective or even harmless through the kinds of rigorous research that conforms to the standards accepted by modern scientists. Relying on them may delay or counter adequate, competent treatment.

5. *Basically, human biology is well understood and fixed. Learning the fundamentals will serve the student of the subject for a lifetime.* Actually, biological discoveries are made almost daily and many contradict fixed truths from the past. Areas of nutrition, exercise, disease prevention, relationships between the mind and the body, and many other major human biology issues are constantly subject to reexamination and many of the expounded truths on the subjects are based on dogma rather than scientific inquiry.

6. *Scientific findings are absolute and unchanging.* One of the authors recalls from his limited study of and understanding of chemistry that many basic concepts seemed to change from his era of study to the chemistry knowledge base a few decades later. Scientists are constantly learning that their original ideas require change. Stomach ulcers, a disease, was thought to be a product of intense worry, poor diet, and other lifestyle patterns. Ulcer sufferers were required to consume bland diets and reduce their emotional tension. But it is now understood that stomach ulcers are a disease that can be treated and cured with antibiotic medicines. Famous scientist and science writer Isaac Asimov (1991) wrote that scientific truth is limited and not absolute and may need further refinement. Science is simply a product of the efforts of humans, and scientists, like other humans, have the ability to be absolutely wrong. A collapsed theory can be replaced by better theories, Asimov wrote. One of the most famous of all scientists, Werner Heisenberg (1991) is perhaps most famous for his theory of uncertainty. He asserted that observing or measuring an object of phenomenon changed that phenomenon. Pagels (1991) explained the Heisenberg theory with an illustration: if one located a tomato seed on a plate and thought its location was absolutely fixed, and if that measurer placed a finger or spoon on the seed in order to be exact about its location, the seed would move and the exactness would be disturbed.

CONCLUSION

This chapter introduces the balance of the text. The Table of Contents shows the various chapters that cover the elements of human biology the authors consider critical to the understanding of the subject for social workers and other human services professionals. The underlying subject of this chapter is the primacy of the scientific method, which is ideally used in all decisions about social work and other human services theory and practice. The focus is on the importance of scientific information about human biology in the practice of the human services. Better understanding of human biology will improve practice in all the human services. The balance of this text is about the elements of human biology that appear to be most crucial to building the effectiveness of the human services.

How to Learn More about Human Biology

The references in this text will lead the reader to books and journal articles that assist in better understanding the subject matter. In addition, however, many readers will want to access information through computers.

A variety of websites are available through the Internet or the World Wide Web. By the time this book is published, most readers will have good knowledge of use of the Internet for locating information. Those who do not may receive instructions from their college or university computer centers or at almost any public library in the United States.

The Internet and World Wide Web are well-developed sources for learning more about human biology. Generally, to locate information, one should connect to the Internet and look through information using a browser. The two more common browsers are Netscape and Microsoft Internet Explorer. However, America Online, Mindspring, Earthlink, and many other Internet service providers also provide their own browsers.

Once the Internet is accessed, one can use a "search engine" that will provide linkages to information that has been collected on the Internet. There are several search engines, such as Yahoo!, Google, and Alta Vista. Most will connect to a variety of sources of information.

In the box for the subject to be searched, just enter the term you are seeking, such as AIDS, cystic fibrosis, heart disease, or anything else. That will lead you to a number of websites and moving the mouse arrow to the site that is listed and clicking will bring you to that site. Some sites are better than others and one should always know the validity of the site before determining that its information is accurate and reliable.

For example, the Americans with Disabilities Act home page is sponsored by the U.S. Department of Justice and is highly reliable. Federal government agency sites are generally quite responsible. Nothing goes on them that has not been checked with experts in the appropriate government department such as the U.S. Department of Justice. The Learning Disabilities Association of America is a reliable organization that maintains a site. The ERIC clearinghouse on disabilities and gifted education is part of the National Library of Education and has a highly reliable site. The Children with Disabilities website is also helpful for learning about those issues. There is also a website associated with the American Association of People with Disabilities. There are particularly large numbers of Internet sites that deal with children's disabilities. There is a Child and Adolescent Bipolar Foundation site, which deals with children who have that mental illness. These sites can be accessed and used for research for term papers and other kinds of assignments as well as for augmenting the information provided in this text.

DISCUSSION QUESTIONS

1. Try to recall, as best you can, your education in biology from elementary and secondary schools as well as from your higher education experience. What are some of the basic concepts you remember? To what extent was the information you garnered applicable to your interest in human services work? Has the impact of biological knowledge affected your understanding of social work courses? Can you think of ways in which biological knowledge could help your understanding of specific social work content and the clients you encounter in your field practicum?

2. This chapter suggests that scientific knowledge, including the knowledge of biology, frequently changes. What is your reaction to that fact? Based on your knowledge of psychology, sociology, and political science, do you think that biological and natural sciences are more or less subject to change than the social sciences? Why might there be significant differences in their propensity to change between the social and the biological and natural sciences?

3. Visit a pharmacy and an alternative vitamin or remedy shop. Note the label descriptions and information on packages from the pharmacy and the alternative vitamin or remedy shop. What similarities and differences do you note? What seems to be included in one package label that is not included in the other? How would you compare the validity and reliability of the two products?

4. Interview your personal physician, on your next visit, about his or her reaction to herbal treatments and alternative medicine. (Some will be supportive and open to ideas of efficacy of such approaches, whereas others will be suspicious. See where your personal healer fits.)

5. Atomic and molecular theories are fundamental to understanding human biology. In what ways do these theories help or hinder your comprehension of human beings and human behavior? Do you believe that scientific theorists always look at the world and its inhabitants as collections of molecules and atoms or is that something that only occasionally occurs to them, when they are engaged in scientific speculation and research?

CHAPTER TWO

BASICS OF BIOLOGY, ANATOMY, AND PHYSIOLOGY

If anything is sacred, the human body is sacred.
—Walt Whitman (1855)

To delight in the human body without shame, to enjoy
it without adulteration, is no simple human prerogative:
it comes only at the summit of high culture.
—Lewis Mumford (1951)

This chapter deals with some of the fundamentals of human biology and its associated fields of anatomy and physiology. Part of the purpose of the chapter is to establish some common definitions as a backdrop for the chapters that follow. Chapter 4 provides a description of a human infant's first year of development as a means for showing the ways in which growth and human development initially and normally occur.

SOME DEFINITIONS

Some authors define biology as the study of living things. It is a vast and growing body of knowledge which ranges from everything from the smallest organisms, which are viruses, to complex systems. Social workers and social work students who are familiar with the concept of systems and systems analyses should have no difficulty understanding the complexity of biology, which ranges from small systems, which are impacted by environments, to larger systems, which are impacted by larger environments and which, in turn, impact smaller systems. Interestingly, biology may be easier to understand as a system than are social systems, which require application of the systems approach to nonphysical entities. The social systems approach is an adaptation of an understanding of physical systems.

LEVELS OF ORGANIZATION IN HUMAN BIOLOGY

The first chapter discussed some of the basics of biology and the importance of understanding it from the molecular level. The following, which is adapted from Johnson (2001), shows the systems under which human biology is organized, from the atomic and molecular levels to the biosphere.

The components of human biology consist of the following:

1. Atom and molecule—An atom is the smallest unit of matter whereas molecules are made up of associated atoms.
2. Cell—The smallest unit of life, which is composed of molecules.
3. Tissue—Cells associated with one another that have the same structure and function.
4. Organs—Several tissue types that are associated together and that carry out a specific function. The skin, the stomach, and the brain are examples of organs.
5. Organ system—Several organs that work together to carry out a more general function, such as the nervous system, the reproductive system, or the circulatory system.
6. Organism—One individual of a specific life form, such as a human or a fish.
7. Population—Several individuals of the same species who live and function together.
8. Community—Many different populations of different species that live in the same area and interact with one another.
9. Ecosystems—Collections of all the living organisms and the nonliving matter such as forests and lakes as well as energy in a place.
10. Biosphere—Brings together the ecosystems with the portion of the earth occupied by living organisms.

Specialized studies such as genetics, cell biology, evolution, microbiology, and human physiology are all included in the study of biology. Physics and chemistry underlie the basic understandings of the science of biology and are, of course, closely related to understanding biological systems, as discussed in Chapter 1. However, it is not necessary for social workers to understand all chemistry, physics, and other sciences that go into understanding human biology. It is enough to know that biological systems are complicated and that they interact with human behavior. Some biological phenomena are directly related to behavioral patterns as well as diseases of all kinds. Certainly physical diseases, and, in many cases, mental diseases are connected to human biology.

Basic biological theories suggest that mammals, of which human beings are a part, live in all the environments of the earth, from the oceans to the deserts. Mammals live underground, on the ground surface, in trees, and in the air. Mammals also have highly developed nervous systems and use memory in learning to guide their activities (Alcamo, 1995). Because mammals have been able to adapt to so many different environmental situations, they are considered to be the most successful animals on earth. Compared to fish, amphibians, reptiles, and birds, mammals have been much more successful, are much more diverse, and are more pervasive than any other kinds of animals. Humans are, of course, mammals, and most agree that humans are the most highly developed of all the mammals.

BIOLOGICAL SYSTEMS

As suggested earlier, biology is a systems-oriented science. The elements of human beings and all other living things are built from simple forms and structures to complex forms and structures. For example, all living things are composed of one or more cells. As Feynman (1991) noted, cells, genes, and all the components of all things are fundamentally composed of atoms and their sub-elements. Cells, in turn, are organized into tissues. Tissues are series of cells that accomplish a function. When tissues are organized into organs, they become part of large organisms. The organs of human beings include, for example, the heart, lungs, skin, glands, and other body parts. When organs work together, they become an organ system or an organism, and human beings are examples of one kind of organism.

DISSECTION

Understanding the ways in which human bodies function is partly a development of the use of dissection of corpses, both human and animal bodies. The use of dissection for understanding the human body and to learn medicine is very old but was also not used for a long time for ethical and religious reasons. According to Grice (2001), the first human dissections began in the third century B.C. in Egypt, but were performed by Greeks who invaded Egypt and who had fewer taboos about the human body than did the Egyptians. The earliest student of anatomy, Galen, who was a Greek physician living in the second century A.D., was one of the main students of human dissection, in Alexandria, Egypt. He also worked on other animals to better understand the functions of the body.

But for 1,000 years, under early Christian views, the body itself was not studied or examined as an object, but, instead, physicians used herbal medicines and other kinds of efforts that did not require great knowledge of human anatomy. Barbers carried out the medical procedures that were used, such as bleeding with leeches and even minor surgery. Medical schools taught anatomy only from theory and not by examining bodies, which is the practice today. Later, in the thirteenth century, professors would lecture about the human body while a student assistant would point to the parts and while barbers handled the bodies. In other parts of the world, according to Grice (2001), dissection of human beings was treated as a carnival attraction. People who had enough money could come look at the ways in which the body appeared after it was dissected.

In more recent times (the seventeenth century), dissection was again hidden. That was part of an effort to hide the uglier facts of life and this is why books such as Mary Shelley's *Frankenstein* became so popular, because they dealt with a subject that was taboo.

Today, of course, medical students and others involved in health care learn about the human body through the study of animal bodies, including human cadavers. Cadavers are shown on the Internet and "virtual dissections" are possible through computer use. A frozen and thinly sliced cadaver, which was the body of an executed murderer, has become a major source of study for large numbers of people who study human anatomy.

EVOLUTION

Most scientists agree that the human body, as well as those of all other organisms, has evolved over the millennia. The basic theory of evolution and natural selection—that the most viable organisms survive and pass on their characteristics genetically to their successors in the world—is essentially a given in the field of biology.

Most scientists believe that the theory of evolution, originally developed by Charles Darwin and enhanced by many scientists after his time, explains the ways in which people, animals, and plants have developed. Darwin began developing his theory in 1831 when he was only 22 (Campbell, Mitchell, & Reece, 2000). He basically discovered, after traveling to many parts of the world, that the earth and its inhabitants were very old but that they changed constantly.

Essentially, he believed that organisms evolved without supernatural intervention and that is, of course, the basic disagreement with the theory of evolution—that biblical sources say something much different about the origin of humans and animals. Biologists such as Campbell, Mitchell, and Reece (2000) believe that fossils make it quite clear that species have evolved. Comparative anatomy, comparative embryology, and molecular biology all point to the fact that species have evolved over the generations.

The fundamental idea was that the natural selection of the most fit examples, of, for example, offspring, are those that survive. As Darwin noted, many eggs might be laid, young might be born, and seeds might be spread, but only a small fraction completely develop and leave offspring of their own. As Campbell, Mitchell, and Reece (2000, p. 264) say, "the rest are starved, eaten, frozen, diseased, unmated, or unable to reproduce for other reasons." Darwin might be quoted as saying that the process of natural selection means that those that survive and pass on their characteristics are those that are most successful in life.

Darwin compared the natural selection process to artificial selection, such as breeding plants and animals. Humans, when they participate in artificial selection, are playing the same role as nature in the evolution of that which they are affecting.

Later works by theorists such as Mendel, who promulgated theories of inheritance and whose work is the basis for the science of genetics, were blended during the last century so that we now better understand evolution and the ways in which characteristics are inherited.

Most scientifically educated people are persuaded that evolution occurs as Darwin described, although Gould (2002) viewed the process a bit differently than Darwin. That does not negate, of course, the values of religion and faith. In some ways, religions develop to help people understand and explain phenomena that they otherwise would not understand. So the maintenance of faith should not be abandoned because new understandings make it possible for people to more effectively understand that which was considered a product only of faith. See Chapters 5 and 7 on evolution and genetics for more detailed discussions of these subjects.

INTERACTIONS BETWEEN ORGANISMS AND THEIR EXTERNAL ENVIRONMENTS

Living things also interact with their external environments. They receive information (in the case of humans through their eyes, ears, noses, taste buds, and touch) and they can change their environments by means such as moving into shady areas when it is hot or covering one's body when it is cold. Organisms also grow through taking in energy such as food and metabolizing that energy.

Living organisms can also reproduce themselves. Mammals do so through sexual reproduction. See Chapter 11 for a detailed discussion of sexuality and reproduction.

The study of the interaction between living things and their environments is called ecology, and social workers and other human service workers and human scientists are especially interested in human ecology.

Understanding these basics of biology and biological systems is a critical foundation for understanding the balance of this book and its discussions of the interactions between biology and human behavior, human social problems, and human functioning, in general.

The biology of human beings is to a great extent known—perhaps more completely known than is the psychology or sociology of human beings. Understanding the biology of human beings is a necessary precursor to understanding much of the rest the information one must have in working with people.

Human biology also includes the fields of anatomy and physiology. Fully understanding anatomy and physiology is a major undertaking because the subjects deal with complex processes and are significantly detailed. The fields of anatomy and physiology (anatomy studies the structure and relationship between body parts whereas physiology studies the function of body parts and the body as a whole) focus on the chemistry, cell structure, and tissues of human beings.

For convenience, human biology is divided into and focuses on a variety of body systems. Each body system is a complex collection of various elements. Each has its own chemistry, cell structure, and physical responses.

HUMAN BODY SYSTEMS

It is beyond the scope of this book to describe, in detail, human anatomy or physiology. However, it is instructive to note the diverse elements that go into human anatomy and physiology.

Pack (1997) describes the systems that make up the human body. Although most humans do not think very often about the complexity of their own bodies, the differentiation and varied factors are awesome, when they are examined.

The systems Pack describes are discussed in the following sections.

Integumentary System

The integumentary system consists of the skin, which is an organ (although many people do not ordinarily think of it as such), and several other organs that work within and as complementary organs to the skin; for example, hair, nails, sweat glands, and sebaceous glands are all organs that work within the skin.

The skin is, of course, an important organ because it protects the rest of the body; provides sensations for touch, pain, heat, and cold to nerve endings in the skin; helps in the storage of blood; and helps in the excretion of waste materials through sweat.

Skeletal System

The skeletal system is often what we think of when we talk about the human body. Understanding the skeletal system in detail requires knowledge of bones, bone structure, and joints, which connect bones to one another. There are many different kinds of bones, many different kinds of joints, and complex interactions among the bones and joints as well as within bone structures and joint structures.

Large numbers of illnesses and disabling conditions such as arthritis affect the skeletal system. Therefore, many who are defined as experiencing disabilities are affected by skeletal system disorders.

Muscular System

The muscular system includes muscles of the skeleton and the connective tissues. Although the heart and other muscles, which are defined as smooth muscles, are undeniably muscular, they are not usually discussed in connection with the muscular system. These smooth muscles are the heart, as mentioned, the digestive system, the urinary system, and various other components. Many of the smooth muscles are involuntary and, therefore, cannot be consciously manipulated by the human being. Therefore, although they are muscles, they are defined in other systems that are discussed next.

Understanding the muscular system also requires detailed understanding of the muscle tissue, which makes up the muscular system. Muscle tissue is subdivided into other categories, which are important in understanding human movement, growth, and development.

Nervous System

In some ways, the most complex of all body systems is the nervous system, which includes two major subsystems—the central nervous system, which is the brain and spinal cord, and the peripheral nervous system, which is the nerves that are outside the central nervous system. Some of those nerves originate at the brain and some at the spine.

Again, understanding the nervous system requires the understanding of the physiology of nervous tissue. There are two kinds of nerve cells: neurons and neurogia. Both these kinds of nerve cells are divided into subsystems, as were the muscular systems. Neurons are the basic nerve systems, those that transmit sensory impulses from the skin to the brain and spinal cord, motor neurons that transmit nerve impulses, as well as several others. Neurogia are the cells that support and protect neurons. These tissues maintain the balance of ions between neurons and control the exchange of materials between blood vessels and the neurons.

Complex processes connect the rest of the body, all of which contains nervous tissue, to the brain and the spinal cord. The nervous system interacts with all the other systems. For example, problems with the functioning of the heart may be related to ineffective regulations of the heart beat by the nervous system. The heart, itself, may be negatively affected but the treatment is of the nervous system, not the cardiovascular.

There appear to be fairly adequate understandings of the physical brain and its functioning. However, that does not mean that one can understand the human or human emotions, or the intelligence of individuals by understanding the brain as an organ only. Human functioning and behavior are less definitively understood than are the physical organs that comprise the individual.

Pope (2000) attributes the "triune" brain theory to a neuroanatomist, Paul McLean. McLean, Pope says, believes there are three levels to the brain. The first is the paleoreptile brain, which includes the brain stem and which lies between the spinal cord and other parts of the brain. It coordinates and controls motor functions such as breathing, reflexes, maintaining body temperature, and reacting to food. That is the kind of brain lower orders of organisms such as reptiles and amphibians have. But even they can learn with such a limited brain—as when a frog rejects poisonous foods.

In the triune theory, the level that transcends the three basic parts, Pope (2000) writes, is the neocerebellum. It processes concepts and language and has the most neurons of all the brain parts. It may have begun by being oriented only to physical movement but evolved into a brain part that carries on more complex functions such as dealing with language and symbolic thought.

The paleomammalian brain level carries attributes that nonhuman animal brains have. It deals with behaviors such as rage, hunger, thirst, sex drive, and fear. Pope indicates that animals have emotions such as those associated with the issues mentioned earlier. However, they probably lack, in terms of comparisons with human beings, the ability to plan and to have foresight. Of course, humans have this brain level. But they also have a third level, the neocortex.

The neocortex level in humans (all animal brains have a cortex) is large, thick, and covers the brain. The cortex, in animals and in humans, controls the higher functions of the species. Personality, language, the planning and foresight that animals lack, and other complex functions are centered in this highest level part of the brain. The cortex is also divided into lobes, each of which controls specific functions.

Pope (2000), as well as more popular sources, suggests that the hemispheres of the brain are significantly different. However, he says that both hemispheres discharge similar functions but each has more emphasis on one set than another. The left side of the brain is believed to be more oriented toward analytical and logical behavior—those who are right-handed have brains that are left-hemisphere-dominated. The right side of the brain, characteristic of left-handed people, is perceived as more emotional, creative, and holistic. Of course, all humans are influenced by and require the influences of both sides of the brain, as part of the need to be emotional, analytical, able to reason, and able to be creative.

According to Pope (2000), there are also some gender differences in brains. Males have larger brains, for example, but women have more neurons concentrated in the cortex. Women seem to use more of their brain in their usual functioning than do men.

It was believed until very recently that when brain cells and brain neurons died, the brain did not regenerate itself or its components. However, several researchers, particularly Ferando Nottebohm of Rockefeller University and Elizabeth Gould of the University of Pennsylvania (Specter, 2001), have led to discoveries of the ways in which the brain regenerates itself and creates new neurons.

Interestingly, Nottebohm discovered this new information about the brain by studying birds. He noticed that birds regularly learn new songs, have excellent memories about where they store food, and generally carry on activities associated with complex brain functions. Some scientists have learned about neurogenosis, which is the scientific name for the process of generating new neurons in the brain, by studying the actual physical brains of animals. They also use substances that study the development of new cells in cancer patients to determine how many, if any, new cells are generated by the brain. Although the substances were studied using injections of the chemical marker bromodeoxyuridine, it was essentially used to discover the extent of growth of cancer cells. The substance counts the development of all cells. It was clear that the brain generated additional neurons when the total number of cells was counted.

Some researchers have also found that exercise in animals, at least, also increases the numbers of neurons. Mice that have regular exercise (Specter, 2001) seem to increase their numbers of neurons.

Of course, these new findings about the brain have major implications for dealing with some of the significant diseases discussed earlier. Conditions such as Parkinson's disease, strokes, spinal cord injuries, multiple sclerosis, and the other brain-based conditions could eventually be addressed by these new understandings of the human brain.

Other health conditions that involve infections in the brain include encephalitis, an inflammation of the brain; meningitis, inflammation of the meninges, which are membranes of the connective tissue that help protect the brain and nervous system; rabies, an infectious viral disease of the brain usually contracted by direct contact with affected mammals; epilepsy, also discussed in Chapter 8; Parkinson's disease, a degenerative disorder that strikes primarily older people and results from a loss of dopamine-releasing neurons; Alzheimer's disease, a disease of mental impairment that results from a lack of acetylcholine, a neurotransmitter that affects the frontal brain lobe and the limbic system, which is discussed in a later chapter; and brain tumors, growths on the brain that may or may not be cancerous. Chapter 8 on health, illness, and treatment provides detailed discussion on some of these health problems as well as others that are associated with other body systems.

It is also true that stem cells, which are underdeveloped cells taken from fetal tissue, can be injected into the body and can be effective by becoming the same as other kinds of cells. That is especially true of brain cells—perhaps, some day, stem cells can be injected into the brain and enhance the process of brain regeneration.

Brain experts, using electroencephalograms to monitor the brain waves of people in an experiment, have monitored reactions to simple gambling games. According to Flam (2002), gamblers take more risks after they have lost. Their brains tell them that they have made a mistake and need to correct it. The same kind of phenomenon occurs when people make typographical errors, lose money in the stock market, and in other kinds of activities that communicate to the subject that he or she is losing. People who are down want to get back what they lost.

The brain activity may be the basis for the "gambler's fallacy," which makes people assume that if they have several losses in a row, they will very soon have a win. Of course, the statistical odds on winning or losing or, for that matter, drawing a head or tail, are equal for each event. The probabilities of change do not occur with a new event and the chances remain fifty-fifty. These brain tests indicate that there are organic reactions to loss which can lead to the basic gambler's fallacy.

The human brain is also a potential source of combinations with technological innovations that can make a difference in the ways in which physicians, social workers, and others deal with people who have disabilities. John Hockenberry, a network television news reporter who is confined to a wheelchair as a result of injury in an accident, describes the ways in which people with disabilities are in the advent of using assistive technology (Hockenberry, 2001). As he points out, for a long time people with disabilities have been using assistive technology by combining their bodies with technological machines.

Hockenberry describes physicians who drill holes in the skulls of people with disabilities and connect the electronic equipment directly to the brain. Brain cells connect with the electronics through wire and simply thinking seems to be communicated to machines. In other words, by producing brain patterns, people with disabilities have been able to move cursors on computers and even change facial movements, which they were not able to do directly through muscles because of their injuries, and were even able to move other body parts.

Other people with injured spinal cords have had electrical electrodes implanted in their hands to stimulate their nerves and thereby to exercise their arms and legs. In some ways, these combinations of the body with electronics are substitutes for any cures for spinal cord injuries, and they have significant amounts of public support and notoriety.

Currently some even better developed techniques are affecting the lives of many people with a variety of disabilities. Some time ago a technological device was developed that allowed blind people to place their hands over printed text and to feel that text directly. In other words, technological machines are now available to help people read printed materials with their fingers, bypassing Braille, which is difficult for people who have become blind in later life to learn.

For people who are hard of hearing, cochlear implants are inserted into the ears and direct signals are sent to the brain and the effect is comparable to that of hearing. Cochlear implants are controversial among some deaf and hard-of-hearing people because they are likely to replace some of the elements of "deaf culture," which includes sign language and other systems that deaf and hard-of-hearing people use to communicate with one another. For people who are not part of the deaf culture and lose their hearing later in life, the issues of technological solutions are not as significant. Famous author and radio commentator Rush Limbaugh lost much of his hearing but also restored much of it with the use of technology.

Another major development is the IBOT, which is increasingly available to people who use wheelchairs. The IBOT makes it possible for people who cannot walk or stand to stand in the wheelchair, climb stairs, and move on any kind of terrain. The IBOT makes many people with disabilities the equal of others who have no physical disability. The IBOT may also revolutionize the whole set of issues relating to access to and the use of facilities by people with disabilities. The inventor of the IBOT, Dean Kamen, is also the inventor of the Segway, a two-wheeled personal transportation device that may be used in urban areas by pedestrians, police, and service personnel, and that may also replace four-wheeled vehicles such as golf carts (Heilemann, 2002).

The connection of the human brain to technological solutions that enhance or extend the human functioning has grown dramatically in recent years, although the growth has not always been described as such. For example, the advent of the Sony Walkman and its counterparts has made it possible for humans to be continuously connected to recorded or radio sounds. Thus, being able to hear and use information as well as entertainment throughout the day and in every circumstance has changed the way people obtain and process information. If nothing else, that technology—connecting earphones to the brain through the ears—has revolutionized broadcasting, the music industry, newspapers, and magazines. It is almost impossible for printed publications to compete for immediacy with what people may hear (or even see through the advent of a small portable television) as it is happening.

Cerebral or brain aneurysms are a serious health problem that kill about half the people who have them. They involve a weak blood vessel in the brain that ruptures and that often causes death (Gupta, 2002). The typical treatment has been to drill a hole in the skull and put metal clips around the pouch to prevent bleeding into the brain. However, a new procedure has now been developed in which a surgeon inserts a catheter from the patient's groin into the blood vessel and then puts platinum coils into the aneurysms, which promotes clotting of the blood and prevents the need for a major operation. The coil procedure seems to work in about 85 percent of the cases in which it is used.

The Brain and Drugs.   One of the important physiological functions of the brain is the "blood-brain barrier" (Johnson, 2001). Johnson (2001, p. 273) states: "Most charged molecules and large objects . . . such as proteins, viruses, and bacteria, generally are prevented from entering the cerebrospinal fluid." Because of the barrier, infections of the brain by bacteria and viruses are rare. That is important because infections of the brain by these organisms are very serious. The protection against them is significant. However, some substances cross the barrier easily. These are the psychoactive substances such as alcohol, caffeine, nicotine, cocaine, and general anesthetics, according to Johnson. So the barrier does not prevent mind-changing drugs from entering the brain and causing the changes that are associated with them. As Johnson points out, psychoactive drugs were invented usually to deal with diseases. Some are called "recreational" drugs because of their use. All psychoactive drugs have as their common mode of action influencing the concentrations or actions of brain neurotransmitters. They only stay in the brain a short time and are short-lived. The physiology is such as to change "the normal patterns of electrical activity in the brain" (Johnson, 2001, p. 282). Chapter 10 provides a detailed discussion of the biological as well as the social significance of drugs and alcohol.

Intelligence.   An ongoing debate, often a highly emotional one, is over the influence of the physical being and inheritance on human intelligence. Is intelligence inherited or a product of the environment? Intelligence is generally regarded as a product of the brain. Alfred Binet (Pope, 2000) developed the first intelligence tests, which were later modified by Lewis Terman of Stanford University. The basic IQ tests became known by the name Stanford–Binet. Some of the same principles used in developing IQ tests were later applied to the development of the Scholastic Aptitude Test (SAT) and the Graduate Record Examination (GRE). Because all these tests are used for classifying people in education and employment and determining their admissibility for higher education programs, they have ongoing significance.

The tests are probably adequate predictors of potential academic success for many people but it is still far from certain whether or not the ability to score well on the tests is a product of inheritance. Most would agree that it is a combination of genetics and experience, but the argument is about the relative proportions of each.

Books such as *The Bell Curve* (Herrnstein & Murray, 1994), which seem to imply that there are major differences in intelligence between white people and minority groups of color, are a source of great controversy. Although there are consistent reports that the averages, comprising the scores of large numbers of people, of the scores of white and Asian American test-takers are higher than those of African American and Hispanic takers, the reasons for the differences and their implications are a source of extensive debate. Differential scores on standardized tests are likely to be a product of differential levels of opportunity, just as are many other characteristics of Americans. Chapter 6 of this book discusses human intelligence in more detail.

Sensory System

Sensory receptors, those that control the senses of smell, vision, hearing, touch, and taste, are specialized neurons that receive specific kinds of stimulants.

The ability to see is clearly a high sensory priority. Much of the rest of human functioning depends on vision. Blindness has been a serious problem of disability for all of human history. Technological measures are being used to help restore the sense of sight. One of the ways in which vision is being restored is through technology, a kind of marriage among electronics, medicine, and engineering. Experts are using digital cameras and computers, and are wiring devices into the brains of people who are blind (Cotler, 2002). Although not routine, in the future, it is likely that vision can be restored through technological devices and approaches such as these for many people.

The sensory system also deals with the sense of balance through the internal ear and has a major role in the maintenance of physical equilibrium.

The processes through which these senses are actualized are quite complex. Large books are available about each of the senses and the various disorders that may affect them.

According to popular Sunday supplement columnist, Marilyn Vos Savant (2001), the idea that there are five senses comes from the fourth-century Greek philosopher Aristotle. It is time to update the concept, she says, to include senses such as balance, pain, heat, hunger, and thirst. She seems correct and it is probably only an artifact of the remote past that still defines the senses as five rather than many more.

One of the practical issues associated with the sense of smell is halitosis or bad breath. According to M. Rosenberg (2002), the basic problem associated with bad breath is oral bacteria. He describes the concern about bad breath to be an American obsession and indicates that billions of dollars are spent every year on toothpaste, breath mints, mouthwash, and other items designed to prevent or cure bad breath.

The problem is with the microbes in the body. Tiny organisms that try to consume proteins and the chemical compounds that result from the digestion of these proteins are thought to be the cause of most bad breath. They cause distinctive bad smells that are comparable to the odors of rotting corpses, feces, sweaty feet, and other traditionally avoided odors.

The causes also include poor oral hygiene, some periodontal diseases, and other compounds that cause bad smells. There are even people who have obsessive concerns that their breath may be bad. They are among those who spend an aggregate fortune on remedies.

Bad breath odors originate, according to M. Rosenberg (2002), almost all of the time in the mouth—almost 85 percent of the odors originate in the mouth. Five to 10 percent originate in the nose, 2 percent in the tonsils, and 1 percent in other parts of the body. Basically, avoiding bad breath is primarily an issue of maintaining good oral hygiene. Rosenberg suggests that brushing and flossing the teeth, cleaning the mouth after eating foods with strong odors, occasionally using mouthwash by rinsing the mouth and gargling before sleep, chewing gum occasionally, and eating a good breakfast are sound remedies to the problem of halitosis. It is also useful to ask a family member to advise on the nature of one's breath, the author adds.

Endocrine System

The endocrine system deals with glands and hormones. Hormones in the blood have important effects on the other bodily systems and regulate, through their association with glands, functions such as growth, reproduction, and many other fundamental elements of human functioning. In many ways, the hormones produced in and secreted by the endocrine system impact every other bodily system.

Cardiovascular System

This system deals with blood, the heart, and blood vessels. As indicated earlier, the heart is a muscle. However, it is not one that associates clearly with the muscular system. The cardiovascular system has basic functions, one of which is the transportation of nutrients, oxygen, and hormones throughout the body as well as the removal of waste such as carbon dioxide and heat from the body. Also, blood protects the body against infections through white blood cells. The cardiovascular system also regulates body temperature and the water content of cells.

Blood Pressure.   A familiar measure of heart functioning is the blood pressure test. Two different kinds of pressure are tested. The higher number, systolic, is the pressure that is created when the heart muscle contracts and the large blood vessel, the aorta, recoils from the pressure when blood comes through it. The diastolic pressure is when the ventricles relax between beats and it measures the resistance of the small arteries and is an indicator of how hard the heart has to pump (Clayman, 1989). Most readers will be familiar with blood pressure tests. A young person who is healthy has a blood pressure reading of about 110 systolic and 75 diastolic, which may increase to about 130 and 90 for a person age 60 or older.

Pulse.   The pulse, which is counted by touching the wrist or neck and which should reflect the heart rate, is another measurement of the cardiovascular system.

According to Clayman (1989), most people have a heart rate between 60 and 100 beats per minute at rest. Exercise increases the heart rate. Some top athletes have resting heart rates under 60 beats per minute. Irregular heart beats as well as beats in most people below 60 or over 100 are considered signs of possible problems with the nervous system, which controls the rate, or the heart. The functions of the cardiovascular system and their implications for health and illness are also discussed in Chapter 8.

Artificial Hearts.   A long-time effort in health care is the search for an efficient mechanical heart to replace the failing hearts of patients. Transplanted human hearts have worked well for decades, but the use of mechanical hearts has not kept recipients alive for long periods. In July 2001, a 59-year-old man, Robert Tools, was given the AbioCor artificial heart, which made it possible for him to carry on with his life. He died in November 2001—not especially from a failure of the artificial heart but from multiple organ failure associated with bleeding in his abdomen, which was a complication of blood-thinning drugs. The artificial heart had worked well for the several months he lived with it implanted in his chest (Underwood, 2001).

Lymphatic System

The lymphatic system supplements the cardiovascular system. It collects excess fluids and plasma from tissues and puts them back into blood circulation. The material forms a fluid called lymph, which transports any material picked up in the body to the neck. From there, the material is emptied into the circulatory system, from which it is distributed. It also cleans the body. The spleen, lymph nodes, and the thymus are also part of the lymphatic system.

Immune System

The immune system is the defense system that combats bacteria, viruses, and other organisms. The immune system provides certain specific defenses against various possible invaders of the body, but the skin and mucous membranes provide the first line of defense against invasion of the body. The immune system is the system that first keeps human bodies well when viruses and bacteria invade beyond the skin and mucous membranes, often through their ingestion in the digestive and respiratory systems; that is, breathing a dangerous substance may not lead to negative consequences because of the defense provided by the immune system.

Respiratory System

The basic function of the respiratory system is to deliver air to the lungs. Oxygen in the air moves to the lungs from breathing and then to the blood through the lungs. Carbon dioxide is sent from the body as a waste material. The respiratory system includes the nose, the nasal cavity, the septum, the pharynx or throat, the larynx, and the lungs.

Digestive System

The digestive system provides digestion through the breakdown of food into smaller molecules which have been absorbed in the body. The gastrointestinal tract is a tube with openings to the mouth and anus. The digestive system connects the other systems and also makes use of accessory organs such as the teeth and the tongue, salivary glands, liver, the gallbladder, and pancreas. The digestive system is that through which humans absorb and distribute nutrients. Waste materials are excreted from the body through the digestive system.

Height and Weight.   Height and weight are related and persons who are too heavy for their height may be courting illness. Charts on height and weight are readily available; the general principle is that all but very tall women, over 6 feet, are considered overweight or obese if they exceed 180 pounds. Men who are shorter than 6 feet and 2 inches are considered overweight or obese if they weigh more than 200 pounds. Of course, persons of shorter stature are expected to weigh proportionately less than the maximums indicated here, if they want to avoid illnesses associated with overweight, which include diabetes, some orthopedic conditions, and, in come cases heart disease and cancer. Some suggest that obesity is a more serious cause of health problems than alcohol or tobacco use.

Urinary System

The urinary system regulates water balance and removes particle substances from the blood. Human blood is filtered by two kidneys, which produce urine. Urine carries away toxic substances and waste products. Urine is then expelled from the body through the urinary system.

Reproductive System

The reproductive system consists of the primary sex organs, such as the scrotum and penis in men and the uterus and vagina in women. Both male and female reproductive systems contain gonads, which for men are the testicles or testes and for women the ovaries, which produce eggs. Both male and female systems are much more complicated than is discussed here. A more complete discussion of sexuality and reproduction can be found in Chapter 11.

An important and artistic biological phenomenon of the early part of the century was the production of a play, performed on Broadway and in many other sites of the world, called the *Vagina Monologues*. The author, Eve Ensler (2001), produced the play and also wrote about her subject in a book. When the play is performed, famous movie and stage stars often perform in it. The essential theme of the play and the book is that women, especially U.S. women, do not know very much about their reproductive organs and often have a sense of shame about them. The play consists of the results of interviews with women of various ages who describe their experiences with their vaginas. Many have not seen the organ and found it repulsive when they looked at it in mirrors. Others relate their feelings about their vaginas to sexual abuse during their childhood as well as their adult years. The author's objective is to help women with their sexuality and with acceptance of an understanding of their most personal organ. The introduction to the book was written by Gloria Steinem, perhaps the best known American feminist of recent years, who remembers that for much of her life, the vagina was not described or defined in that way but was only discussed as "down there."

Of course, many of the issues that direct practice social workers encounter with clients are related to the ambivalent and less than perfectly understood relationship between female clients and their sexuality. Many prominent and leading women believe that Ensler has helped women come to terms with their sexuality and their reproductive organs.

Although there is no comparable play or book about the male sexual organs, there is a growing literature about the penis. There is even a play in which two men provide caricatures with their sex organs. The play is called *Puppetry of the Penis,* and the authors and performers are Simon Morley and David Friend (*Stuff,* November 2001). They manipulate their sex organs, on stage, into symbols such as the "Loch Ness Monster," "Beached Mollusk," and others. They have also produced a book based on their performance art: *Puppetry of the Penis: The Ancient Australian Art of Genital Origami* (Morley & Friend, 2000). There is also *The Penis Book* by Joseph Cohen (2000) and *The Book of the Penis* by Maggie Paley and illustrator Sergio Ruzzier (Paley & Ruzzier, 2000).

Another author, Jill Conner Browne (2001), writes humorous books. In one, she describes a visit to a sexual novelty shop that offered a "talking vagina." She imagined it to be something like a talking doll and wondered what it would say. She also found an ad for an "artificial vagina," called a vaginal substitute, that men could use without fear of the consequences of sexual activity with a real organ. She also jokes about the male sex organ. She suggests that the penis cannot always tell whether it is in the "home vagina," where it is supposed to be, or has wandered off into a neighbor's. She suggests getting rid of the male partner who cannot tell where his penis is but providing him a vaginal substitute as a farewell gift. Books and public performances such as these assist, perhaps, in normalizing human awareness of sexuality and sex organs.

Human Nutrition

One of the frequently changing areas of biological inquiry that is related to the digestive system is human nutrition—what is the proper diet. In the mid-twentieth century principles of nutrition were suggested, which have been largely discredited in the twenty-first century. The senior of the three authors remembers many of these—from elementary through graduate school and until recent times. For example, it was dogma that children should consume relatively large quantities of milk and milk products. Children in elementary schools were quizzed on a rigorous schedule about their daily consumption of at least a pint of milk daily. And that meant whole milk because the skim variety was practically unknown. We now know that many people's digestive systems cannot handle lactose and that whole milk is a source of cholesterol, which is associated in some cases with conditions such as heart disease. Generous donors to college football programs donated beef cattle so the players could consume quantities of meat and, in that way, improve their strength and endurance. Today's athletic teams are advised to concentrate on complex carbohydrates, which are the preferred current routes to energy and strength.

The ideal body, not very long ago, was a bit corpulent compared to today's weight and height chart recommendations. And one of the unchanging rules that seems to prove consistently true is that people are wise to keep their weight down, with less emphasis on what they consume and more on how much it does to their body weight.

Current nutrition concepts, which are promoted by the federal government as well as other organizations, are explicated in the *American Medical Association Encyclopedia* (Clayman, 1989). It says that the essential nutrients are protein, carbohydrates, fats, fiber, water, vitamins, and minerals. Information on the minimum daily requirements of each is available from many sources such as world almanacs or Internet. Most expert information suggests that the ingestion of mineral or vitamin supplements is unnecessary and sometimes ill-advised. Balanced diets should provide adequate nutrition, including adequate minerals and vitamins. However, the presumption that people have balanced diets is not valid in many cases and large numbers of health-conscious people take vitamins regularly. Vitamins and minerals with antioxidant properties, which are helpful in preventing coronary problems, seem especially important to some. Those with antioxidants include vitamins C and E and the mineral selenium. Also often used are multivitamins, which include the range of B vitamins along with some minerals and usually with A, C, and E included. Like almost any other ingested substance, excessive doses of vitamins may be harmful to one's health. That is particularly true of the "fat-soluble" vitamins such as A and E. But excessive doses of "water-soluble" vitamins such as the B's and C can also cause health problems. The mineral iron can be important for women who menstruate but can be dangerous for men and for children. Consulting reliable sources, including personal physicians, about vitamins is always a good idea prior to embarking on a program of vitamin use.

Food recommendations are divided into four groups. The milk group, which includes cheeses, milk, and yogurt, has a recommendation of two servings daily. Two servings from the meat group, which includes not only meat but also fish, peanut butter, and eggs, are supposed to be eaten daily. Four servings of fruit and vegetables and four servings from the bread and cereal group, which includes pasta and rice, are recommended. However, as suggested earlier, the key element may be avoiding over- or undereating and the problems that arise from obesity and malnutrition, including such conditions as anorexia nervosa, a major problem among young people in the United States.

COMPLEXITY OF THE HUMAN BODY

For social workers, it is instructive to note the complexity of the human body. It is also important to remember that diseases are typically related to one or more of the body systems. For example, many diseases such as heart disease and strokes are functions of the cardiovascular system. Cancer, which is also discussed in Chapter 8 on health, illness and treatment, of various kinds affects the functions of the respiratory system, the digestive system, and all others. Cancer specialists divide cancers into "sites," which are the various organs that are affected. HIV/AIDS is, as another chapter discusses, a disease of the immune system. Disabilities often result from problems in the vascular and skeletal systems or in the sensory system. Fully understanding a client or patient with a specific disease can best be accomplished by also understanding some of the biological realities of the condition.

The awesome complexity of the human body and the ways in which it functions help us understand why some familiarity with human biology is critical for effectiveness in the practice of social work.

Standard texts in biology, such as Starr and Taggart (1998), Johnson (2001), and others mentioned in this book detail these issues in greater depth. A good standard biology text will allow the reader to examine such basic issues as cell structure and behavior, genetic inheritance, chromosomes, DNA structure and function, evolution, and the many other issues that are included in any full understanding of human biology.

SUMMARY

This chapter outlines some of the basic definitions and understandings of the fields of biology and its associated fields of anatomy and physiology. The basic systems of the human body and some of the ways in which they interact are also outlined. In addition, it offers some introductory information on major biological subjects such as evolution. It is a backdrop for the other chapters that complete this text.

DISCUSSION QUESTIONS

1. Compare the functions of the nervous system with those of the circulatory system.

2. As a social worker or other human services worker, what do you believe are some of the reasons for better understanding the reproductive system?

3. What are some of the most important functions of the skeletal system? Describe some of the ways in which it supports other body systems.

4. Describe some ways in which the contents of this chapter might be made accessible to persons of more limited intellectual ability than that of the typical college student.

CHAPTER THREE

DETERMINISM, BIOLOGY, CULTURE, AND THE ECOLOGICAL PERSPECTIVE

The ecology of human development is the scientific study of the progressive, mutual accommodation, throughout the life course, between an active, growing human being, and the changing properties of the immediate settings in which the developing person lives, as this process is affected by the relations between these settings and by the larger contexts in which the settings are embedded.

—Bronfenbrenner, 1989, p. 188

Underlying the bioecological model is the cardinal theoretical principle emerging from research on theories of genetic transmission, namely, that genetic material does not produce finished traits but rather interacts with environment with environmental experience in determining developmental outcomes. Indeed, this interactive process is already operative in the earliest stages of embryological development.

—Bronfenbrenner & Ceci, 1994, p. 571

The societal ramifications of the nature versus nurture debate are widespread (Dennis, 1995). The profession of social work has not escaped the influences of this debate. Social work's knowledge base has been shaped by social scientists who have argued that environmental factors (i.e., nurture) play the most important role in determining human behavior. This has resulted in professional social workers minimizing the importance of the relationship of physiological and biological factors (i.e., nature) to human development and behavior.

The process of theory building has moved far beyond the initial debate of nurture versus nature. Research in medicine, genetics, chemistry, biology, psychology, and other scientific areas has expanded our understanding of human behavior and its antecedents. However, social welfare policies, clinical interventions used by social workers, and educational institutions that train professional social workers continue to use theories that are grounded almost solely in environmental explanations for human behavior. Practicing social workers often do not give much consideration to the deterministic epistemology of their knowledge base and the influence that the environmental versus biological debate has on that epistemology (Zimmerman, 1989).

The ecological model introduced by Urie Bronfenbrenner in a 1979 monograph represents both a longstanding lens through which social workers understand the people they work with and a way of understanding all of the factors that contribute to the development of human behavior. The ecological model integrates biological aspects with the many different environmental levels (meso, macro, micro, and exo systems) present in human society that appear to influence how humans develop. Despite Bronfenbrenner's extensive writing about the biological aspects of the ecological model, social work students are primarily exposed to the environmental aspects of the model, with little discussion of the biological aspects.

For the remainder of the chapter we will examine several concepts and theories. First, the concept of determinism and the division of determinism into environmental and biological determinism are examined. This leads to an examination of two popular theories of practice—the family systems theory and the cognitive theory—in an attempt to understand how this division influenced the theories that are typically used to underpin social work practice. Finally, the propositions, assumptions, and hypotheses associated with the ecological model are explored, with a focus on how the model integrates environmental and biological determinism using a weak biology approach. In the bioecological model, as the model is referred to by Bronfenbrenner, social work may find a theoretical framework for understanding human development and behavior that directs practice, research, and theory building.

DETERMINISM

Underlying both biological and environmental determinism is the concept of determinism, which is defined as the principle that life's events follow a set of natural laws or rules that cause the outcomes of all activities, even human development and behavior. These causes can be discovered and understood (Webster, 1989). The Greek philosopher Democritus first articulated the concept of determinism, and Aristotle built on his basic idea of cause and effect by adding the concepts of "formal cause (the idea to be realized in a causal process), material cause (the substance undergoing a change), efficient cause (external compulsion) and final cause (the goal to be reached)" (Zimmerman, 1989, p. 55). During the ensuing centuries many great scientists and philosophers, including David Hume, John Stuart Mill, and Karl Popper have debated about and refined the concept of determinism (Zimmerman, 1989). As Zimmerman (1989) points out, "causality continues today to be the cornerstone of theory building and empirical proof in all disciplines aspiring to scientific status," including social work (p. 55).

What is the importance of understanding determinism for social work students? Environmental and biological theories of human behavior have been used to explain the need for or the elimination of social welfare policy, immigration laws, and a variety of other cultural and legal structures that influence human behaviors. Even closer to home, the epistemological structures of theories have striking impact on the types of direct service interventions that they prescribe as being effective with individuals in need of social work services. The best way to show the effect that determinism, specifically its environmental/biological dichotomy, has on society is by citing some examples. Two recent examples of human behavior that have engaged both the popular press and serious social scientists in the nature versus nurture debate are domestic violence and homosexuality.

Domestic Violence

Social scientists from the Taylor Institute in Chicago believe that welfare benefit caps may increase the incidences of domestic violence nationwide. "Welfare reform that imposes limits on the length of time women can receive benefits may promote or exacerbate existing domestic violence according to research by the Taylor Institute in Chicago" (NASW News, October 6, 1996). This thinking highlights the belief that environmental factors play a primary role in affecting dysfunctional human behaviors. Implied in the statement from the Taylor Institute is that the amount of money offered by a governmental policy will influence the behavior of an individual by further destabilizing what may be an already unstable environment. This influence on the living environment of individuals receiving welfare may in basic terms make people violent toward their families. In contrast, Families in Society published an article entitled "Violence and Biology: A Review of the Literature" (Johnson, 1996). In the article Johnson reviews the available literature on violent behavior and finds that within the social work scholarly literature the contributions of biological factors associated with violent behavior are not discussed. Genetic and behavioral research have suggested that some violent behavior does have a biological basis (Johnson, 1996). An individual who has a biological problem that results in aggressive behaviors may not be the best candidate for treatment that solely focuses on environmental factors. In order to treat the problem of domestic violence, a more holistic view that includes cultural, economic, and biological explanations must be applied (Johnson, 1996).

Homosexuality

Homosexuality has also been at the center of recent nurture versus nature debates. An article by Herrn (1995, p. 32) in the Journal of Homosexuality examines the history of biological-based theories for homosexual behavior, stating that "biological theories of homosexuality fit into the discourse on reproduction and sexuality that began in the nineteenth century. They arose in the context of the early homosexual rights movement, with its claim for natural rights." In contrast, the religious right as well as the editors of the Diagnostic and Statistical Manual of Mental Disorders present arguments that homosexual behavior is the result of environmental factors (Kirkpatrick, 1993). These opposing beliefs about the underlying causes of homosexuality have helped to fuel debate on a number of policy and cultural issues, most notable of them being same-sex marriages. An in-depth understanding of homosexuality will never be reached without an awareness of how culture and biology interact (Looy, 1995). Research will most likely reveal that homosexuality is best described as a continuum where individuals have differing levels of biological factors that influence their behavior. Observations of single-sex institutions (e.g., prisons) indicate that there are times that individuals will engage in same-sex activities because of environmental factors (Aker, Hayner, & Gruninger, 1974; Eysenck, 1973). Other research has indicated there are differences in the brain structure of self-labeled homosexuals (Herrn, 1995). To ignore one of these findings in favor of another detracts from the scientific community's understanding of homosexuality (Looy, 1995).

DIVISION OF DETERMINISM INTO BIOLOGICAL AND ECOLOGICAL DETERMINISM

Theories with epistemological roots closely tied to biological explanations for human behavior have three typical features: (1) Heredity plays a significant role in biology, (2) biological factors play a significant role in determining human behavior, and (3) the biological factors at work in individuals shape society and culture. Environmentally based theories also have three typical features: (1) Environmental factors are the primary determinant of human behavior, (2) an individual's relationships and interactions with other people are the basis for human behavior, and (3) environmental factors (e.g., culture and society) shape the raw material provided by biology. These features associated with environmental and biological determinism will be used to provide a framework from which to evaluate family systems theory, cognitive theory, and the bioecological model. The two criteria used to evaluate theories in this chapter are (1) the theory's belief about the origins of (dysfunctional) human behavior and (2) interventions the theory prescribes to remedy problems created by dysfunctional human behavior.

Theories based in biological determinism often view dysfunctional human behavior as emanating from the individual and driven by a biological flaw. Interventions that are based on theories with epistemological roots tied to biological determinism will focus on controlling and maintaining the dysfunction or correcting the biological flaw using medically based procedures. In contrast, theories with culturally based epistemological roots view dysfunction in human behavior as arising from flaws in the environment (e.g., society or culture) or how an individual interacts with the environment. Interventions based on theories with epistemological roots tied to cultural determinism tend to focus on altering the environment individuals and groups live in or altering the behavior of an individual in a way that discontinues the dysfunctional behavior.

HISTORY OF DIVISION BETWEEN BIOLOGICAL
AND ENVIRONMENTAL DETERMINISM

Two important scientific discoveries in the mid-1800s set the stage for the modern nature versus nurture debate within the social sciences. Mendel, an Austrian botanist, was one of the first scientists to glimpse the power genetics had in determining the physical characteristics of living organisms. His basic pea plant experiment opened a new scientific frontier, which would later be called biogenetics. For the next century, social scientists would argue over the importance of genetics in determining a wide variety of animal and human characteristics and behaviors. Charles Darwin in the same era published *The Origin of Species* in which he put forth the theory of evolution. Unlike Mendel, Darwin's work had a significant and immediate impact on the epistemological roots of sociology, psychology, philosophy, economics, history, educational theory, and religion (Johnson, 1995). The societal and cultural ramifications of evolutionary theory are present even today, more than a 100 years after Darwin penned *The Origin of Species* (Asma, 1993; Dennis, 1995; Johnson, 1995; Smith, 1985).

Darwin's paradigm-setting theory of evolution and Mendel's manipulation of genetics through breeding were occurring simultaneously with the advent of the industrial revolution. Literature from the late nineteenth and early twentieth century reflect a sense of optimism about the human race's future tempered with a weariness about the modern technology that would make this future possible (Marcus, 1996). Examples of this fascination with modern technology can be found in Jules Verne's science fiction writings. Both *A Journey to the Center of the Earth* (Verne, 1966) and *Twenty Thousand Leagues Under the Sea: The Marvelous and Exciting Adventures of Pierre Arronax* (Verne, 1900) are excellent examples of the optimism and sense of purpose that the industrial and scientific revolutions brought to the western world. The advances of industry and science not only offered solutions to age-old problems, but also opened the door to new problems. This tension was well represented in Verne's novels. H. G. Wells, who penned *A Modern Utopia* in 1904 and *Anticipations of the Reaction of Mechanical and Scientific Progress Upon Human Life and Thought* in 1902 captured this feeling that modern society was moving toward perfection through the use of science and industry. Like Verne, Wells also wondered about the problems that modern science and technology would create.

"Nineteenth-century Britain was par excellence a technological nation: it invokes images of the Industrial Revolution and the workshop of the world; a world of heroic entrepreneurs, inventors and engineers" (Edgerton, 1994, p. 43). This sense of heroic inventors permeated the social sciences and helped to create an atmosphere conducive to the belief that science could solve many of the problems facing human kind (Smith, 1985). Intrinsic to this belief was a need to understand the irreducible underpinnings of human behavior. The reduction of the human condition to understandable parts in an attempt to seek the "ultimate truth" through scientific understanding is still hotly debated today as can be seen by the current popularity of the book *The End of Science* (Horgan, 1996) and Edward O. Wilson's two front-cover articles in the *Atlantic Monthly* (Wilson, 1998).

For the social sciences, this meant understanding how individuals were successful within the constructs of society and how to build on this success in a way that created a utopia. Evolution offered an accepted scientific paradigm in which to explore human behavior. The result of Darwin's theory of evolution being applied to social science was the creation of social Darwinism. David Smith (1985, p. 2) defined social Darwinism as a "philosophic and scientific movement during the late nineteenth century. The movement hinged on the idea that certain racial and ethnic groups are inherently inferior in intelligence and moral character and that, even within cultural or national groups, lower social classes are, by nature, inferior" (p. 2). From social Darwinism grew a fascination with testing procedures that reflected the scientific methods of the natural sciences (Dennis, 1995). The creation of intelligence testing lent support to the belief that human behavior could be fully understood and controlled in a way which led to a utopian society (Dennis, 1995).

Francis Galton, a half-cousin of Darwin, fellow of the Royal Society, and educated at Trinity College, became intrigued with Darwin's theory soon after it was published (Freeman, 1983). By the mid-1860s Galton had coined the term *eugenics* in several papers that took an extreme view of heredity's effect on human behavior (Freeman, 1983). The concept of biological determinism arose out of this movement and helped to shape much of the scientific debate, theory building, research, and social policy concerned with the human condition for the next century (Dennis, 1995; Smith, 1985). Galton and Goddard argued that all human traits, including physical appearance, moral character, and personality, were directly derived from a person's genetic make-up (Asma, 1993; Dennis, 1995; Freeman, 1983; Smith, 1985). For eugenicists, culture, upbringing, and family life played an insignificant role in shaping human beings lives. An example of this extremist view is that eugenics researchers believed that naval officers had a sex-linked recessive gene that gave them an inborn love of the sea (Smith, 1985). Galton, Goddard, and other followers of the eugenics movement were dogmatic about their belief in the power of genetics. "So convinced was he [Galton] of the efficiency of Eugenics, or controlled and selective breeding, as a tool to racially regenerate his native England that he urged the adoption of the idea as a new religion" (Dennis, 1995, p. 245). This rhetoric, coupled with the same optimism about science and the new industrial age that drove the eugenics movement, spawned the equally extreme view of human behavior, cultural determinism.

Franz Boas, considered by some scholars of academic history to be the father of American anthropology, was the driving force behind the theory of cultural determinism (Freeman, 1983). Boas was from a middle-class German family that was strongly invested in the enlightenment movement (Freeman, 1983). By the late nineteenth century Boas was teaching at Columbia University, where he would have Margaret Mead as a student (Freeman, 1983). His theory of cultural determinism was in direct response to the zealous eugenics movement (Freeman, 1983). Boas proposed that culture was a creation separate from biological influences and that human behavior was shaped by culture and not biological factors (Freeman, 1983). However, Boas did allow for biology to play a role in human development. His students, most notably Mead, took Boas' theories further by concluding that human behavior was almost entirely determined by culture (Freeman, 1983). This extremist view limited the importance of biology to the point of being insignificant.

Family Systems Theory

The family systems theory has its roots in the cybernetics movement of the 1940s (Hoffman, 1988). This movement focused on the feedback mechanisms, information processing, and patterns of communication among human beings (Becvar, 1995; Hoffman, 1988; Merkel & Searight, 1992). Early focus of family systems on interaction and process helped to move it away from traditional intraperson explanations of human behavior (Becvar, 1995). External forces (i.e., relationships with other human beings) and context (i.e., environment) were used by early family systems theorists to explain human behavior (Becvar, 1995). Human behavior, from a family systems perceptive, originated from the interactions and relationships between family members. Ultimately, these relationships shape the biological material known as a human being. An example of this is by Bateson, Jackson, Haley, and Weakland (1956), whose early experiments with schizophrenia tried to link the disorder's origins to the afflicted individual's family functioning.

By the 1960s, the family systems approach was applied to a variety of problems in an attempt to understand their origins and in turn offer possible solutions. Don Jackson, Virginia Satir, and Salvador Minuchin put forth subtheories of family systems that focused on the family as creating much of an individual's behavior (Lappin, 1988). Very little—if any—attention was paid to biological explanations for human behavior. For Jackson, Satir, and Minuchin, an understanding of individual human behavior could best be derived from an in-depth understanding of the individual's family (Lappin, 1988). Some of family systems' basic concepts include a focus on processes, and context, which gives meaning to events in individuals' lives (Merkel & Searight, 1992). Reality is created by persons, and individuals exist in the context of relationships in which each individual influences the other and both are equally the cause and effect of each other's behaviors. The origins of dysfunctional human behavior for the family systems theory are the faulty social constructions created by family interactions and relationships. This belief about the origins of human behavior links the family systems theory to its epistemological roots of cultural determinism.

The types of interventions prescribed by the family systems theory also indicated epistemological roots in cultural explanations for human behavior. How a social worker using the family systems theory would intervene with a depressed client would be based on the following three assumptions: (1) The depression experienced by the client makes sense, as it is behavior embedded in the social context of which the client is part; (2) the depression is symptomatic of a family disturbance (depression is a logical reaction to family dysfunction); and (3) the depression is a communication about the family (Shields, 1996, p. 12). All three assumptions lead professionals to believe that depression has an environmental basis with no physiological explanations.

In contrast, numerous medical research articles have presented findings that indicate strongly that there are biological factors associated with the occurrence of depression (Maranto, 1987; Steingard et al., 1996). That is why some patients experiencing depressive episodes respond well to medication interventions (Schiffer &

Wineman, 1990). Medication is an attempt to maintain and control the sympto-mology of depression, two characteristics of interventions derived from theories using biological explanations for behavioral dysfunctions.

Clearly, family systems theory is closely tied to cultural determinism. Its post–World War II roots might explain family systems' attempts to explain human behavior as being caused by culture rather than biology factors. The birth of family systems came on the tails of the eugenics movement and Nazism. This under-standable reaction to the devastating misuse of biological explanations for human behavior has outlived its usefulness. The limitations of the family systems theory can be linked back to the fact that it does not acknowledge the power of biological determinants of human behavior.

Cognitive Theory

The cognitive theory focuses on the individual and their cognitive processes (Beck, 1976; Payn, 1991; Thyer & Myers, 1997). In contrast to the family systems theory, cognitive theory purports that problems arise when individuals have irra-tional beliefs about the environment. "Individuals respond to cognitive represen-tations of environmental events rather than the event *per se*" (Thyer & Myers, 1997, p. 29). The origins of dysfunctional human behavior arise out of the indi-vidual; a belief more closely tied to theories with biological determinants as epis-temological roots.

However, the connection between the environment and the individual is an intrinsic part of cognitive theory's epistemological roots (Beck, 1976; Thyer et al., 1997). An individual's perception of the world "links their thoughts and feel-ings with the external social world" (Payn, 1991, p. 188). If an individual is to have a positive perception of life, the harmonious interaction of self-conception (being), perceiving self (knowing), and intentional self (becoming) needs to be present (Payn, 1991). This belief neither necessitates that the environment be conducive to empowerment or self-determination or any of the other social con-structs traditionally thought to effect positive self-image nor does it require that the individual be functioning at an optimum level biologically. In a sense, the cognitive theory accepts the environment and biological factors as they are and requires the individual to shape his/her perception of the world in a way that helps him/her to adapt to it, no matter what the underlying causes of a dys-functional behavior.

The cognitive theory states that individual change is brought about by working on one's internal functioning or thought processes (Beck, 1976; Payn, 1991; Thyer & Myers, 1997). Thyer and Myers (1997) state: "At least some forms of cognition can be altered" (p. 29). The point of intervention for social workers who use the cognitive theory is the internal functioning of the client. An unstated aspect of this belief is that therapists cannot realistically impact the environments that most clients live in or the individual's biology, but therapists can help clients formulate functional perceptions of the world. This intervention point implies that dysfunction in human behavior is socially constructed and therefore much more malleable than what is typically attributed to biological factors.

Despite this apparent bent on internal functioning, the cognitive theory does not address biological determinants of human behavior as seen by the interventions most cognitive practitioners use. Thyer & Myers (1997) cite four major types of interventions used in cognitive therapy. These interventions are (1) changing mis-conceptions, unrealistic expectations, and other faulty ideas; (2) modifying irrational statements to oneself; (3) enhancing problem-solving and decision-making abilities; and (4) enhancing self-control and self-management. Once an individual's irrational assumptions are modified, the individual should be taught how to be more strategic, tactical, and adaptive in his or her learning style no matter what the underlying causes of the problem (Payn, 1991). Payn (1991) defines strategic learning as "acquiring information and skills towards some set objective" (p. 189). Tactical learning is defined as being able to adapt to the pressures of "daily living," and adaptive learning is defined as being able to "alter the self and its construc-tions of the world as part of a process of dealing with life in a different way" (Payn, 1991, p. 189). The interventions used by cognitive therapists help to further clarify the theory's epistemological connection to the beliefs held by early environmental determinists. However, the cognitive theory does seem to provide a more balanced perspective of the relationship among individuals, their biology, and the environ-ment. This more balanced perspective does not offer an integration of the two determinisms.

Bioecological Model

Most social work students in the United States are exposed to some version of the bioecological model during their studies. Often the focus of this exposure is the environmental aspects of the model (exo, meso, macro, micro environments). However, Urie Bronfenbrenner, the Cornell University scholar who developed the model, clearly envisioned it as one based on interaction between an individual as defined by their biological composition and the environment. Beyond just inter-acting, Bronfenbrenner identified the process of interaction, resulting in a melding of the two and creating a reciprocal relationship that is ever-changing.

> Development involves interaction between the organism and environment: The external becomes internal and becomes transformed in the process. However, because from the very beginning the organism begins to change its environment, the internal becomes external and becomes transformed in the process. The bidirec-tional nature of these transformations is rooted in the fact that genetic potentials for development are not merely passive possibilities but active dispositions expressed in selective patterns of attention, action, and response. The process of transforming genotypes into phenotypes is neither so simple nor so quick. The realization of human potentials requires intervening mechanisms that connect the inner with the outer in a two-way process that occurs not instantly, but over time. (Bronfenbrenner & Ceci, 1994, p. 572)

The underlying implication of this interaction is that a person's genetic make-up does not translate easily or directly into finished traits (phenotypes), a version of weak biology that is discussed in a number of other chapters. Using a fairly classical approach to knowledge building, Bronfenbrenner identifies three propositions that, in turn, underpin six assumptions about the bioecological model. How biological and environmental determinants are integrated in a living and complex relationship is seen in examining these parts of the model.

The propositions represent the logical underpinning for the model. For the model to be of any value, the propositions should be accepted as valid explanations of how humans develop. Bronfenbrenner and his colleague Stephen Ceci, also from Cornell University, use a number of pieces of research to support the bioecological model's propositions. There are three propositions.

As identified in the introduction, central to the bioecological model is the interactive relationship between the individual and the environment. In particular, Bronfenbrenner believes that for the interaction between the individual and the environment to be effective, it must occur on a regular basis consistently throughout life. The identified interaction is referred to as proximal processes, and Bronfenbrenner cites a number of examples of enduring proximal processes in parent–child and child–child activities, group or solitary play, reading, learning new skills, problem solving, performing complex tasks, and acquiring new knowledge and know-how (Bronfenbrenner & Ceci, 1994, p. 572). This is the first proposition.

The second proposition of the bioecological model states that the "form, power, content and direction of the proximal processes effecting development vary systematically as a joint function of the characteristics of the developing person, of the environment—both immediate and more remote" (p. 572). This highlights how the proximal processes are reciprocal interactions between the individual and the environment, leading to changes in each.

Finally, the third proposition that provides the logical underpinning of the bioecological model is that proximal processes are the mechanism by which genetic material within the individual is actualized in terms of psychological development. The power of proximal processes on the realization of genetic material in an individual varies in relationship to the three factors identified in proposition 2.

Based on these three propositions, Bronfenbrenner makes six assumptions about human development. These assumptions are as follows (Bronfenbrenner & Ceci):

1. Proximal processes not only actualize genetic potentials but also give genetic potentials substance and content by the very interaction with the environment.

2. "Not all of the genotypic possibilities that a given child possesses find realization in phenotypic form. The nature of the emergent phenotypes will depend on the activities that take place in the principal proximal settings in which the child is growing up. These activities, in turn, depend for their content on the characteristics

of the persons, objects, and symbols present in the immediate environment. In sum, only those genetic predispositions of the individual can find realization for which the necessary opportunity structures exist, or are provided, in the particular immediate settings in which that person lives. Thus proclivities for acquiring a foreign language, mastering a musical instrument, or debugging a computer program require for their realization the presence of opportunity structures (e.g., teachers, computer manuals)" (p. 575).

3. "Some aspects of the immediate setting become partially transformed through the child's capacity to shape his or her own environment. However, early in life, such capacities are still limited in scope; they produce appreciable effects only in a restricted segment of the environment; namely, they influence the reactions of parents and other caregivers to behaviors of the infant that reflects its own emotional state and dispositional tendencies. By contrast, the range of possibilities for changing the immediate environment by parents is much greater. Not only by responding to the infant's cues and initiatives but they can also engage the child in new kinds of activities involving interaction not only with themselves and others but also with objects, toys, symbols, and other stimuli" (p. 576).

4. "For parents to further their children's learning and skill typically requires knowledge, know-how, and materials that, at some point, originated in the external world and, in effect, had to be imported into the family from the outside." This takes into account the environmental differences that surround families, such as socio-economic status, historical period, cultural norms, etc. "For example, parents with limited education may not have the knowledge or skill to help the child with his homework in math" (p. 576).

5. "Resources are not the only features of the environment that are required for proximal processes to operate successfully. A second essential is some degree of stability. . . . A growing body of evidence documents the disruptive developmental effect of unstable environments, characterized by inconsistent and unpredictable patterns of activities and relationships in the immediate settings in which the developing person lives, particularly within the family" (p. 576). Bronfenbrenner cites research that examined the effect of environmental stability on the development of children between the ages of 8 and 20. Findings suggest that changes in family structure, daycare and school arrangements, or parental employment; the number of family moves, and the frequency of parental absence "was associated with greater insecurity later in life, as well as a higher incidence of problem behaviors such as submissiveness, aggression, early sexual activity, excessive smoking, drinking, and delinquency" (p. 576). "In short, environmental contexts influence proximal processes and developmental outcomes not only in terms of the resources that they make available, but also in terms of the degree to which they provide the stability and consistency over time that proximal processes require for their effective functioning" (p. 576).

6. "Proximal processes not only require environmental stability for their effective functioning but they also engender psychological stability in others, particularly in children and youth" (p. 576).

The propositions and assumptions underpinning the ecological model taken together indicate in a general sense that the relationship between the individual and the environment is flexible and ever-changing. In the ecological model both the environment and the biology are viewed in more complex terms than the family systems theory or the cognitive theory, with interactions such as those between mother and child understood as having a number of environmental contexts such as family, culture, and historical period that play roles in influencing the various biological aspects associated with individuals. Like the environment, biology is viewed in terms of different levels or components, including individuals' genetic make-up, their brain development, and their physical health, all of which are different yet inseparably intertwined like the different levels of society.

Bronfenbrenner examines the example of low birth weight as a way of understanding the interrelationship between biology and the environment. Citing a number of studies that researched the impact of low birth weight, Bronfenbrenner states that children born with a birth weight under 5½ pounds experience the following: problems in physical growth, susceptibility to illness, impaired intellectual development, and poorer classroom performance. In examining the results of the research cited, Bronfenbrenner found that mother–child relationships, management of the home, and family health practices influenced the level of negative impact on life outcomes caused by low birth weight. The data indicated that the more effective maternal care was, the better the developmental outcomes for low-birth-weight children. "In other words, where the mother is willing and able to make the effort, she can do much to reduce the developmental risk that this handicap entails" (Bronfenbrenner, 1989, p. 198).

Bronfenbrenner goes on to point out that maternal care does not accomplish the task of improved developmental outcomes for low-birth-weight babies independent of the babies themselves. "Living organisms have the capacity, and indeed the active disposition, to heal themselves over time" (p. 198). Citing findings that the somewhat retarded intellectual development that is present initially in low-birth-weight babies decreases over time with the most marked recovery occurring before age two, Bronfenbrenner (1989) concludes that "in sum, significant resources for counteracting effects of prenatal handicaps exist both on the side of the environment and of the organism itself" (p. 198). Bronfenbrenner calls this interaction between biology and environment the "person-process-context model."

Bioecological Model and Genetics. The bioecological model recognizes the importance of understanding the genetic component of human development and behavior. Bronfenbrenner believed that understanding the extent of variation in individuals' innate capacities for "realizing individual talents and buffering against dysfunction" provides insight into the mechanisms involved in determining the outcomes of human development (Bronfenbrenner & Ceci, 1994, p. 570). Although the bioecological model does rely on a weak biology approach to understanding the importance of genetics in human development, it does integrate the concept of heredity as a central feature of understanding human development.

Bronfenbrenner points out that human genetics and heritability have limitations in understanding several important issues associated with human development. First,

> heritability . . . describes only the extent to which genetic endowment contributes to observed differences in developmental outcome between individuals growing up in the same environments. It provides no information whatsoever about another domain in which genetics can exert an important effect—observed differences in developmental outcomes between groups of persons growing up in different environments. (p. 569)

Second, there is no understanding of how environmental factors create variability in developmental outcomes for individuals and what is the genetic limitations of that variability. Third, heritability "only deals with individual differences and hence can tell us nothing about the absolute level of competence around which the individual variation is occurring" (Bronfenbrenner & Ceci, 1994, p. 569).

Summary of Bioecological Model.   Bronfenbrenner (1989) in an examination of other theories of biology (in particular regarding the brain) found that they are based on the assumption that genetic and other biological aspects intrinsic to the individual are invariant across place and time.

> This assumption characterizes a wide range of measures, including objective tests of intelligence, academic achievement, or personality; assessments of Piagetian or neo-Piagetian stages of cognitive or moral development; analyses of cognitive and personality styles; characterizations of persons based on their patterns of response in laboratory experiments; and modes of cognitive functioning based on information theory and theories of artificial intelligence. (Bronfenbrenner, 1989, p. 203)

The bioecological model differs from these theories in that the individuals' biology is both changing and flexible in relationship to the environment, including the social structure they live in, their relationships with other human beings, their culture, and the historical era. The weak biology approach used in the bioecological model states that "proximal processes can produce appreciable differences in developmental outcomes that cannot be attributed to genetic selection. The findings also imply that any effects of proximal processes on heritability cannot be interpreted solely as the products of a genetic component in proximal processes" (Bronfenbrenner, 1989, p. 195). The power of this approach for Bronfenbrenner was how to understand the environmental niches that encouraged the best possible development of an individual's biology. To be able to identify the best niches, the influence of biology must also be understood.

CONCLUSION: SOCIAL WORK
KNOWLEDGE BUILDING

By understanding the long-term effects of the scientific debate between the proponents of environmental determinism and biological determinism, social work researchers, educators, and practitioners will be better prepared to shed some of the remaining taboos created by the debate. In turn, the social work profession may then move toward the creation of theories of practice that more readily integrate both biological and environmental explanations of human behavior. To date, most theories used in social work practice can be directly linked to cultural explanations, with only a cursory consideration of biological factor (Zimmerman, 1989). Although the social work profession has rightfully embraced the notion that culture plays an important part in the lives of people, there can be no denying that biology is also a strong determining factor of human behavior (Johnson, 1996). What is problematic for the social work knowledge base is not the existence of two opposing views of human behavior determinants but the lack of integration of the two. The dichotomy between environmental and biological determinism restricts the possibilities for both theory building by social work researchers and implementation of theoretical knowledge by social work practitioners.

Both biological and cultural factors have played important roles in the theories social scientists use to explain human behavior. The particularly negative history and connotations attached to biological explanations of human behavior have wrongly led to their elimination from mainstream social work theory. The problem now facing social work is twofold: (1) The integration of biological explanations for human behavior into social work theory and (2) the presentation of biological factors as being one of many factors influencing human behavior. The bioecological model, which has been long used in social work does represent one of the few theories that addresses these problems and effectively integrates the biological and environmental aspects of human development.

Unlike recent attempts to illuminate biological determinants of human behavior (e.g., Murray and Hernnstein's *The Bell Curve* (1994), social workers should not attempt to resurrect the problems created by simplistic models of intelligence. Instead, social workers should attempt to alter the three features typically associated with biologically based theories of human behavior: (1) Heredity plays a significant role in biology, (2) biological factors play a significant role in determining human behavior, and (3) biological factors at work in individuals shape society and culture. The most controversial of these features is the influence of heredity. Medical and biological research have not borne out the theories of early eugenicists and followers of social Darwinism. New theories about biology's influence on human behavior need to place heredity in its proper place, based on the vast amount of genetics research conducted by the scientific community. Also included in any new theories about the role of biology is the inclusion of the individual's physiological functioning. Social science's focus on heredity has detracted from medical research, which has found chemical reactions (both intrapersonal and between the environment and individuals), hormonal fluctuations, brain wave patterns, diseases, and many other physiological conditions that affect human behavior. These biologically based influences should be integrated into social work theory and practice.

DISCUSSION QUESTIONS

1. Discuss how the nature versus nurture debate has influenced theories of human behavior.

2. Identify three features typical to biological and environmental theories for human behavior.

3. What are the three propositions and six assumptions underpinning the bioecological model?

4. What role does genetics play in human development as identified by the bioecological model?

CHAPTER FOUR

BIOLOGICAL DEVELOPMENT AND THE HUMAN LIFESPAN

There is no cure for birth and death save to enjoy the interval.
—George Santayana

Our existence is but a brief crack of light between two eternities of darkness.
—Vladimir Nabokov

Man is born to live, not to prepare for life.
—Boris Pasternak

This chapter is about human development throughout the lifespan, from birth through the end of life. Social work literature, especially when it discusses human behavior, focuses on the ages and stages of human beings, often from social and psychological perspectives. The focus here is on physical development.

The most dramatic developments of the physical human being are in the early and later years. For a variety of reasons, less is said about the years between the beginnings of adulthood and the onset of the senior or aging years.

In order to best explain the information that is most reliably known about the developmental stages, this chapter includes an excerpt from the literature. It deals with the first year of life in an article written by a nurse, Susan Biasella, published in *Lamaze Baby*, and reprinted here with the permission of that publication.

YOUR BABY'S FIRST YEAR

Please note: Each step listed represents an average of a 6-to-sometimes-12-week time span that is considered within normal range for that behavior. Don't be concerned if your baby is not doing something exactly the month on this chart. And each baby develops at his or her individual pace—don't compare.

Although the time of skill development may vary, the sequence of developmental tasks progresses the same. Babies usually focus on developing one major task at a time. For example, when your baby is learning to babble new sounds, she will slow down in developing her body movements or rolling over. Then, when her verbal development has achieved a new proficiency level, she'll change her focus to exploring new body movement again. Be aware, by the way, of how these changes affect your need to make your baby's environment safe and secure.

A PREMATURE ANALYSIS
Premature babies, too, should develop in the same sequence as full-term babies, but the timing will probably differ. The rule of thumb for accounting for the variance in timing is easy: To use this chart for a premature baby, subtract the length of a prematurity from his age. For example, if your two-month-old baby was born one month early, his development should probably be compared to a one-month-old's.

For more specific guidance, discuss your baby's expected rate of development with a pediatrician, pediatric nurse practitioner or developmental specialist.

1 MONTH
Body Movement
Arms and legs are usually flexed and movements are jerky.

Startle reflex: When baby's position is quickly changed or he hears a sudden loud noise, he extends both arms with open hands, then brings his arms to his chest with an embracing movement. He may also cry out at the time.

Step reflex: When baby is held upright with his feet touching a firm surface, he will make little stepping movements forward.

Lifts head for a few moments and turns head to side when lying on his tummy.

Eye–Hand Coordination
Eyes may cross due to lack of good muscle control.

Blinking reflex: Blinks in response to bright light.

Turns head from side to center to follow a slowly moving object with her eyes.

Stares at objects held 8–12 inches from her face.

Prefers to look at the human face, focusing on the eyes or mouth. Stares at simple black-and-white contrasting patterns, such as stripes, bull's eye or checkerboard. Looks more at the outside edge than the internal pattern.

Grasp reflex: Grasps anything placed in her hand, clenches it briefly, then just lets go.

Biasella, S. (1999, Fall/Winter). Your baby's first year. *Lamaze Baby,* 53–62.

Thinking Skills

Makes eye-to-eye contact for five to ten seconds; quiets to stare at a face. Will look at his mother's face longer than a stranger's face.

Focuses his attention on one quiet activity; shuts out the rest.

Listens to voices and responds to a higher-pitched female voice with throaty sounds and movement of his arms and legs.

Distinguishes his mother's voice from a stranger's. Quiets to hear soft music, singing or talking.

Soothes when swaddled in blanket; being rocked and patted; sucking; hearing monotonous, swooshing noise.

Emotional Development

Reflexive smile during drowsiness or sleeping, accompanied by the rapid eye movements of dreaming.

Adjusts body posture to cuddle into person holding her.

Sucking reflex: Sucks on anything placed in her mouth in hopes of food or to soothe herself.

Rooting reflex: In search of food, opens mouth and turns head toward the side where her cheek is stroked.

Responds positively to comforting action and cries loudly during painful activity. Often fusses through bath time.

Feeds every two to three hours and may sleep three to four hours between nighttime feedings. May spit up after feeding because cardiac sphincter valve at top of stomach does not close tightly until baby is walking.

When two to three weeks old, may develop **fussy crying** for a few hours every evening. Eats seven to ten times and has about eight naps over 24 hours. There's usually no regular pattern of eating and sleeping yet.

2 MONTHS

Body Movement

Arm and leg movements become smoother, more rhythmical.

Reflexes gradually fade to be replaced by voluntary movement.

Lifts head a few moments when lying on tummy and extends legs.

Makes creeping motions on tummy and may scoot forward in crib until head is securely lodged against bumper pad.

Makes bicycle movements with legs when lying on back.

Tries to hold head erect when sitting upright.

May begin to roll from back to side. May surprise himself by accidentally pushing over from tummy to back.

Eye–Hand Coordination

Focuses clearly eight to ten feet away. Her eyes will follow you as you move from her. Likes bright colors better than pastels.

(continued)

YOUR BABY'S FIRST YEAR (CONTINUED)

Prefers to watch moving objects, like a black-and-white mobile.

Prefers patterns of increasing complexity with curved lines and shapes. Studies the interior pattern plus the outside edges.

Relaxes fist to open hands and fingers. Sometimes begins sucking and mouthing fingers and hands.

Quiets and stops sucking to study each person's face.

Attempts to push at a dangling toy. Holds a toy placed in her hand for a little longer than she did earlier.

Thinking Skills

Turns head and eyes together toward an interesting sound.

Quiets and stops sucking to listen intently to a variety of sounds. Prefers the human voice to other sounds.

Coos and gurgles with vowel sounds "ah, eh, oh" in response to what he sees, hears and feels inside his body.

Begins to suck at sight of breast or bottle, anticipating feeding.

Becomes excited in anticipation or a regular activity like bath time. Begins to enjoy bath time.

Soothes and relaxes himself by sucking on hands or pacifier.

Startles and looks surprised at a sudden loud noise.

More visually alert when sitting upright. Beginning to associate lying down with sleeping.

Imitates your exaggerated facial expressions.

Stares at himself in mirror.

May become distracted during feeding by watching other people and activity in room or even just by hearing mother talk.

Emotional Development

Responsive smile in reaction to parent smiling at her. Smiles for pleasure and delight.

Turns away from eye-to-eye contact when tired of interacting.

Begins sucking, wrinkles up face, stares vacantly, yawns, begins to squirm or cry when tired of playing.

Expresses the emotions of delight, excitement, distress and protest with total body movements.

For colicky baby, crying may peak at six weeks and continue to 10 weeks; gradually fades by 12 to 16 weeks.

Demonstrates individuality in temperament and personality.

Settles into feeding and sleep pattern with more alert responsive time in the day. May sleep five to seven hours at night.

3 MONTHS

Body Movement

Lifts head when lying on tummy. When head on adult's chest, will push away and look over your shoulder. Turns head from side to side while on stomach and propped up on forearms.

When on stomach, with weight on elbows and forearms, arms can lift chest. Legs remain fixed when lying on stomach.

Sits erect when supported at the hips.

Arm movements are more purposeful. Enjoys moving arms and legs vigorously when lying on back, sometimes symmetrically or in bicycle motion.

Eye–Hand Coordination

Eyes can follow a moving object held about six inches above her face vertically and in a circular pattern. She can see objects 15 to 20 feet away.

Hands open most of the time. Voluntarily shakes and holds a rattle. Grabs onto your clothing and hair.

Looks at her hand held in front of her face. Enjoys watching her fingers move. Grabs one hand with other one. Sucks on fist.

Swings and reaches for dangling objects. Likes to feel different textures of objects. Explores her own face, eyes and mouth with her hand.

Loses interest in mobiles if they're beyond her reach.

Thinking Skills

Semi-upright sitting position best for learning and play.

More sparkle, recognition in his eyes. Smiles spontaneously.

Still prefers to look at the contrast of light and dark.

Pays more attention to detail. Likes shapes and colors.

Responds to his name more consistently.

Smacks lips and tongue together.

4 MONTHS

Body Movement

Arm and leg movements are better controlled.

Rolls over from tummy to back with ease.

When lying on tummy, his legs straighten, and he will make swimming movements with both arms and legs.

Makes single vowel sounds. **Coos and gurgles** while eating. Babbles in response to someone talking to him. Can screech, squeal, holler, growl.

Emotional Development

Different cries for different needs; pauses for your response.

Face expresses emotions—frowns, smiles, and grimaces.

(continued)

YOUR BABY'S FIRST YEAR (CONTINUED)

Face lights up when he recognizes parent. Flaps arms as a nonverbal signal indicating, "pick me up."

Stops nursing to smile at mother, then resumes sucking.

May sleep 15 hours, divided into 10 hours at night with remaining 5 hours divided into three naps during the day.

Holds head erect when sitting.

Kicks legs a lot. Splashes hands and feet in bathtub.

Eye–Hand Coordination

Head and eyes move in coordinated motion.

Both hands grasp at approximate size of object to manipulate it, and then baby puts objects in her mouth.

Easily tracks objects with her eyes.

Watches moving people and gazes across a room.

Explores own body with hands.

Looks for complexity and novelty in surroundings.

Thinking Skills

Mouths everything to explore objects.

Prefers bright colors of red and yellow to black and white.

Begins to realize he is distinct from objects "out there" and to realize his actions cause something to happen.

Enjoys listening to speech and music. Babbles for his own pleasure with chuckles, giggles, shrieks, and laughs.

Listens to himself talk. Says "da, ba, ma, pa, ga" consonant sounds. Notices how his speech influences adult actions—"m-m-m" brings Mom to feed him.

Looks around to find source of a sound. Is quieted by music.

Emotional Development

Responsive to play for one hour at a time.

Show signs of being tired—will yawn, rub eyes, refuse to play, suck thumb or become restless and irritable.

May drool and be fussy if teething.

Is developing her unique personality within a predictable daily routine—how active she is, how intensely she responds to things, what her patience and tolerance for frustration are.

Senses if her behavior is unacceptable to parent during daily interactions. Reacts to your tone of voice and expression.

Expresses joy, unhappiness, contentment, tiredness. Crying decreases as she expresses feelings with new sounds, gestures.

Recognizes family members she lives with. Loves to laugh and play with people. Vocalizes more to real person than picture.

Demands social attention by fussing. Cries if play is disrupted.

Attempts to soothe self when cries. Yells, fusses if frustrated.

5 MONTHS

Body Movement

Can lift chest higher off floor by pushing up on hands.

May creep or "commando"-crawl a few feet when on tummy.

Enjoys changing body position and moving.

Leans head forward to grab his toes when lying on his back.

Can hold his entire weight on his legs when supported in a standing position.

Helps pull himself to a sitting position by lifting head and flexing elbows. Enjoys sitting propped with pillows. (Note: It's not safe to leave baby alone in this position.)

Is too active to stay in infant seat. Don't delay. Babyproof the house now!

Eye–Hand Coordination

Reaches with her eyes first, then her vision guides her hands to precisely grasp an object. Turns and shakes the object.

Begins one-handed reaching for toys; may transfer objects hand to hand, then puts in mouth.

Hand begins to adjust to shape of object when reaching.

Enjoys grabbing another person's hair, glasses or necklace and enjoys grabbing her own feet to suck on her toes.

Thinking Skills

Compares part of self to an object to differentiate himself from objects outside in the world—for example, sucking on his thumb, then sucking on toy to feel the difference.

Learns to anticipate result of his action—hitting a dangling toy will make it swing.

Adds new elements to speech, such as yell, purr, blow "raspberries" and smack lips. He mimics adult expressions and gestures as he babbles. Listens very intently to the human voice.

Develops rhythmic dialogue to take turns in "conversation."

May vocalize to draw his mother's attention when she is conversing with someone else.

Vision is improved to adjust focus to near and far. Developing depth perception. Sees in full color; likes orange, blue, green.

Watches and follows a familiar person leaving the room. Looks where you look.

Emotional Development

Indicates discomfort by pulling, poking or scratching at self.

Shows dislike by pushing things away from her.

Enjoys genitals by poking and pulling.

(continued)

YOUR BABY'S FIRST YEAR (CONTINUED)

Enjoys loving exchange with caregiver during feeding time. May increase sucking time at breast or bottle.

Wakes quickly in the morning. May comfort herself by playing with a toy before you get her from the crib.

Hesitates and studies people outside her immediate family.

Has attention span of 10 to 15 minutes to play with toys alone.

Gives easily read behavioral cues. Extends hands, legs and body to you for "pick me up"; looks down to floor, squirms and fusses, meaning "put me down"; expressionless stare means "I'm bored"; cranky and nothing soothes means "I'm tired."

Likes to play peek-a-boo.

Learns to cough at will in order to attract attention.

6 MONTHS
Body Movement

Lifts chest and most of tummy off floor by pushing up on extended arms.

Rolls from back to tummy easily.

Rocks and kicks a lot. Rolls around in delight.

Sits erect briefly, using hands on floor for balance and support.

Bounces when held erect. Likes seeing world when standing.

Eye–Hand Coordination

Uses one-handed purposeful grasp to shake, bang, put object in mouth, then finally drop it. Enjoys dropping objects repeatedly to learn the noises they make.

Uses whole hand to rake in and pick up object.

Regularly reaches for objects out of her reach.

Grabs and sucks on her own and your body parts to differentiate herself from you as two separate individuals.

Thinking Skills

Follows your direction of pointing. May point at new things.

Babbles and "talks" to toys and to himself in mirror. Intently listens to his own voice.

Understands your speech by the tone of your voice.

Recognizes names, basic words, familiar household sounds.

Enjoys manipulating other people's faces by poking, pulling and studying them to understand his separateness from them.

Emotional Development

Very sociable—smiles, laughs hilariously and enjoys being with people. May be more selective about whom she socializes with.

When she can't do something, **may become frustrated,** whine or explode in rage.

Smiles at herself in the mirror (but does not recognize it is her reflection until she is more than one year old).

Is very curious to explore the world around her.

Plays by herself longer because she can sit better now.

Appears to make decisions when choosing to play with toys.

7 MONTHS

Body Movement

Can now sit unsupported, leaving hands free for another activity. Lunges forward onto floor from the sitting position.

Begins creeping backward or forward by pulling himself along with his stronger arms while his tummy and kicking legs drag behind.

Eye–Hand Coordination

Reaches and grasps a toy using her fingers rather than the palm of her hand. Will shake, bang, poke, push, squeeze, roll everything. Transfers a toy from one hand to the other.

Holds two objects simultaneously, one in each hand. Uses both hands for one task.

Learns voluntary "controlled release" of an object and puts it down in a specific place.

Distinguishes near and far objects in space with accurate depth perception.

Enjoys splashing toys in the bathtub.

Thinking Skills

As he explores an object, he **matches the feel** of the object with the appearance of the object. His attention is more concentrated and focused.

Recognizes a familiar toy if all but a small part is covered up. Does not realize a completely covered-up toy is still under there—beginning the concept of "object permanence." Searches the floor to find a dropped object.

Plays rigorously with noise-making toys, such as bell, music box or rattle, to explore what happens.

Tries to imitate more sounds and series of sounds. Vocalizes several sounds in one breath.

Knows he will attract attention if he cries or babbles.

Is learning the meaning of "no!" by the tone of your voice and your immediate actions.

Emotional Development

Wiggles with excitement in anticipation of playing.

Begins to show a **sense of humor.**

Reaches out to pat and smile at her mirror image.

Resists pressure to do something she doesn't want to do.

Experiences frustration as she begins the determined effort to stand and walk.

(continued)

YOUR BABY'S FIRST YEAR (CONTINUED)

Curiosity motivates her to leave a parent's side to explore but she comes back for frequent reassurance. She may be devastated if you are gone.

Separation anxiety: Begins to be shy with strangers—unfamiliar people outside her immediate family.

Cuddles before bedtime to help her relax after a busy day of exploration. Usually sleeps through the night.

8 MONTHS

Body Movement

Becomes more coordinated as muscles in neck, back, hips grow stronger.

While creeping, **holds his weight on one hand** to reach for toy.

Crawls up on hands and knees with chest and abdomen parallel to floor.

May stand up by leaning against something with hands free.

Sits without support when legs are out flat in front.

Likes playing with his toes; reaches for his feet with both hands.

Eye–Hand Coordination

Grasps larger object with thumb and first and second fingers.

Still **reaches** for an object with fingers overextended.

Enjoys banging objects to hear sound and see the effects on the object. Is able to bang two objects together. Sill mouths, chews and shakes objects.

Uses either hand indiscriminately. When you hand her an object, she will sometimes use her right hand to grasp it and other times she'll use her left hand.

Develops throwing as a controlled motion from hand to arm. Will throw an object repeatedly to see what happens.

Thinking Skills

Explores the idea that an object always remains the same. Repeatedly explores the size, texture, firmness, shape, taste, sound, smell and weight of an object.

Explores the concept of cause and effect—that when he performs an action, it causes the same effect repeatedly. When he manipulates a busy-box toy, each hand movement causes an effect, such as a noise of reflection of his face in a mirror.

Notices objects with his eyes and points to things he wants.

Pays greater attention to the details in his world.

Has the mental model of a human face in his mind and studies everyone's faces for comparison and contrast.

Continues babbling dialogue, expecting verbal answers from other people. May imitate noises for toys, like "brrr" for a car.

Enjoys listening to simple books being read to him. Enjoys singing and simple hand games like Pat-a-cake, This Little Piggy or How Big is Baby?

Develops favorite music among the regular songs he hears.

Can identify household and outdoor sounds.

Imitates rhythmic banging sounds.

Emotional Development

Expresses separation anxiety by becoming nervous, bashful, turning away, whining and crying around unfamiliar people.

Likes to be near her parents.

Smiles at and tries to kiss her image in the mirror.

Expresses emotions of anger and frustration. Changes emotions easily—from laughing to crying, for example.

Has no awareness of danger to herself or her surroundings as she constantly explores the world around her.

May have trouble sleeping at night as she awakes to practice crawling and standing in crib. Offer reassurance: "It's time to sleep now." (Remove all toys except a baby mirror to make crib place for sleep, not play.)

9 MONTHS

Body Movement

Sits steadily without support for 10 to 15 minutes. Pushes up to a sitting position when lying down.

Leans forward when sitting to pick up a toy without losing balance.

Crawls while holding something in one hand.

May pull up to stand; holds on to support with both hands.

Shifts weight from one leg to the other. Balances on tiptoe with feet turned in.

May not know how to get down from a standing position. (Help him to bend from waist and to bend knees from waist and to bend knees to squat.)

Begins climbing on anything. Can get up, but often cannot get himself down!

Eye–Hand Coordination

Grasps with thumb against the side of her index finger in developing pincer grasp to pick up small items.

Pokes with finger at small things. Points at distant objects.

May show a preference for using right or left hand now, but this can change over the next three to five years.

Can bang two objects together symmetrically or can hold an object in one hand while banging with one another.

Enjoys pulling things apart.

Fits small object through the hole of a larger one, like placing rings on a spindle.

Thinking Skills

Recognizes/responds to his name, names of familiar objects.

Deliberately imitates sounds by a parent.

(continued)

YOUR BABY'S FIRST YEAR (CONTINUED)

Understands simple one-word instructions, such as "no!"

Enjoys games with cue words that trigger a predictable response such as "kitchey, kitchey, coo" that leads to tickling and laughter.

May find object hidden under cup if he sees you hide it. Further understands the concept of object permanence.

Emotional Development

Enjoys dancing to music.

Expects a predictable response when she expresses emotion. Example: When she smiles, she expects a parent to smile back.

Is driven by curiosity. Nothing in her surroundings is sacred or off-limits to her inquisitive mind and busy hands!

Has difficulty coping with "don't" or "no." May express disappointment with a new limit by a hurt expression or anger. Note: This is not done to manipulate you, and you cannot control her reaction to the reasonable limits you set.

Slows down in new major accomplishments as she concentrates on perfecting her newly acquired skills.

Loves simple games with family members, like Chase the Baby. Will initiate peek-a-boo by placing a cloth over her face.

Develops fear of the vacuum cleaner . . . it's a big loud monster.

Deliberately chooses a toy to play with and may fight to keep the toy from other people.

Begins to understand that she is a separate person from her image in the mirror.

May take two naps, sleep about ten and a half hours at night.

10 MONTHS

Body Movements

Pulls up to stand; holds on with one or two hands.

May cruise around furniture with a high and deliberate sidestep motion.

Can sit from a standing position. Can move from a sitting position onto stomach.

Fascinated with climbing up stairs, but doesn't know how to crawl down yet! Climbs up and down from a chair.

Crawls into corners or narrow spaces, then doesn't know how to get back out.

Does not like lying on back except when sleeping. Tries to escape from diaper changes.

Eye–Hand Coordination

Opens drawers to explore the content.

Is interested in fitting things together.

Continues to refine ability to pick up small items.

Pokes finger into objects to explore depth.

Thinking Skills

Tries to figure out how big his body is by crawling into small spaces to see how (if) he fits in there.

May have a few words, such as "hi," "bye-bye," animal sounds.

Begins requesting objects to pointing to them.

Imitates "shh" with finger over mouth to signal quiet.

Imitates phone conversations on toy telephone.

Searches for a hidden object if he sees you hide it.

Follows a one-step instruction, such as "Go to Daddy."

Emotional Development

Seeks companionship and attention. Has very strong attachment to caregivers. May stop exploratory behavior when approached by a stranger. Turns around to check your presence as she crawls away.

Expresses the emotions of hurt, sadness and happiness. Is learning emotions by directly experiencing a situation and by watching how others react when things happen to them.

Begins to cooperate with getting dressed and drying herself with a towel at bath time.

Loves to swish toys in water, wade in water and drops things into water, including the toilet. (Note: Put lid lock on toilet!)

11 MONTHS

Body Movement

Holds on loosely as he cruises along the furniture. May forget to hold on.

May be able to push up from floor with hands to stand momentarily.

May stand alone briefly and be able to turn.

Bends halfway over to look through legs to see an upside-down view of the world.

Climbs down backward without falling down.

Eye–Hand Coordination

Has a firmer grasp; can hold two objects in one hand.

Watches intently what her hands are doing.

Pats, pokes, pinches and rolls various objects.

Places objects down deliberately.

Enjoys putting small objects into a large container.

May carry a spoonful of food to her mouth, but spills most of it because her wrist action is still developing.

Thinking Skills

Classifies objects by shape and size. Explores the weight of objects; likes watching how fast they fall.

(continued)

YOUR BABY'S FIRST YEAR (CONTINUED)

Finds an object hidden under another object. May understand that a toy moved from one hiding place to a second place is no longer under the first place. He may follow the movement and now look under the second place for the toy.

Follows a verbal direction after a demonstration, such as "Squeeze the toy."

May use a few meaningful words or offer sound substitutes for words—for example, "ta" may mean, "cat."

Recognizes words as symbols for objects. May start learning names for his body parts and common objects in his world.

Emotional Development

Learns attitudes and respect by watching her parents.

Imitates household tasks and self-care tasks. Pulls off socks and unties shoelaces. Cooperates with dressing.

Becomes bored with toys. Enjoys playing games with people. Can be encouraged to play independently near you.

Develops preference for certain books. Can turn pages in book.

Struggles to learn a new task. (Encourage her to persevere and solve the problem on her own. She will master skills only with much repetition over time.)

Begins to discern between "good" and "naughty" behavior.

Calls attention to good behavior, seeks approval and repeats action for additional praise. Tries to avoid disapproval.

May be quiet for a long period of time. This may mean she is into something, such as playing in the toilet. (Warning: She needs to be watched constantly!)

12 MONTHS

Body Movement

Loves to stand and resists sitting down.

Is very mobile; uses a combination of crawling, cruising along furniture and walls or walking. Can walk holding your hand.

May take first independent steps. Independent walking may start from 11 to 14 months. Will fall often while learning to walk.

May push up from squatting stance to stand independently.

Can sit down on a small child-size chair easily.

Likes to climb inside or under things to see how he fits.

Eye–Hand Coordination

Explores objects by rolling, spinning, and pushing them. Is fascinated by motion and prefers toys that move.

Uses another object to obtain a toy out of reach.

Reaches for an object while looking away from it.

Likes to pound pegs with a hammer and play with blocks.

Can hold two objects, one in each hand, then place one in her mouth or under her arm to allow her to hold a third object with her free hand.

Thinking Skills

Figures out different ways to make the same thing happen.

Enjoys water play to test sinking or floating of toys.

Imitates use of objects as he observes other people use them.

Expresses interest in what adults are doing.

Enjoys supplying a word for a singing game.

Loves to open and close cabinet doors, then empties out cabinet to play with contents, such as plastic food containers.

Says one to three words, such as "mama" and "dada."

Waves bye-bye.

Emotional Development

Gives affection to people and favorite toys.

Undresses herself frequently.

May resist naps because she is busy exploring, playing, and learning.

Play next to—not with—another child in parallel play.

Experiences stranger anxiety—the fear of people outside her immediate family—again, especially outside the home.

Distinguishes herself as separate from other people.

May begin temper tantrums to express frustration or anger when she can't have or choose between two things.

Repeats action that makes people laugh. Loves an audience.

CHILDHOOD STAGES

Understanding the development of children in their first year is critical because there is an amazing amount of growth and change during those first 12 months, as the foregoing description makes clear. The biological issues associated with old age, which are described in detail in Chapter 12 in another reprinted magazine article, are also relatively well defined as an era of major change and development for human beings.

Not so clearly delineated, however, are the stages of development between infancy and adulthood and between the beginnings of adulthood and the older years.

Social work has long been interested in and has taught about the developmental processes in which humans are engaged. For many years, large numbers of schools of social work taught the stages of development propounded by Sigmund

Freud, who was a physician in Vienna and who developed a major theory of personality and the process of psychoanalysis. Much of what was believed about human psychological development and psychological behavior for a long time came from Freud's work (Rathus, Nevid, & Fichner-Rathus, 2002). Freud's theories included major suppositions about the ways in which the personality develops, about the unconscious mind, defense mechanisms, and repression of instinctive behavior. A good bit of psychoanalytical theory also deals with human sexuality and psychosexual development at various ages. These ages or stages of development deal with both emotional and biological needs and drives. The five Freudian childhood stages are (Rathus et al., 2002): the oral, anal, phallic, latency, and genital.

The oral stage, of course, deals with the need of the infant to bring the world to himself or herself through the mouth by sucking and eating. The anal stage has to do with sphincter control functions dealing with excretion of waste. The phallic deals with early sexual development and the awareness of one's sexual identity. The latency period is one in which there is not great change, in the Freudian frame of reference, but the following stage, the genital, deals with the maturing physical sexual development of the individual and the capacity to engage in sex and to reproduce.

More contemporary theorists such as Erickson (Schriver, 2001) developed different approaches to stages of development, which are widely taught and studied in fields such as social work and psychology.

BIOLOGICAL DEVELOPMENTS
AT VARIOUS STAGES

In childhood, a variety of conditions develop that can make the difference between the adequate functioning of the child in school and as a peer. In many ways, future success in education, careers, and life, in general, is affected by some of the biological developments of childhood.

Circumcision

One of the early biological issues facing parents of boys is whether or not to have circumcisions performed on their children. Circumcision involves cutting away of the foreskin of the male penis or part or all of the female genitalia, which is uncommon in the United States (Cheers, 2001). For Americans, circumcision is an issue primarily for parents of boys. The use of circumcision for health purposes is not universally accepted, although it is a common procedure for males in the United States. It is primarily an important religious ritual for Jews and Muslims. Some advocates of male circumcision say that it can help prevent penal cancer as well as urinary tract infections and can help prevent sexually transmitted diseases. Opponents of the practice say that it is easy to keep the foreskin clean and therefore is an unnecessary and probably disadvantageous form of surgery for males.

There are conflicting findings about the effects of circumcision on sexual satisfaction. Female circumcision is almost universally opposed except among those who practice it in Africa, the Middle East, and Southeast Asia. When it is used, it is a religious ritual and is also believed by its proponents to improve hygiene, preserve virginity, and promote marital fidelity. In some cases, the procedure is used to remove the clitoris, which is the center of female sexual arousal and pleasure. In other cases, much of the genitalia such as the labia are removed and the vaginal opening is sutured as a way of promoting sexual abstinence.

Learning Disabilities

It is during childhood, especially during the school years, that learning disabilities may become apparent. These may include, although they may not be diagnosed, such disabilities as visual and hearing problems as well as the inability to properly read letters, called dyslexia; the inability to write, called dysgraphia; and agnosia, the inability to put ideas on paper. Another basic learning problem, dyscalculia, deals with the inability of the child to effectively perform mathematical functions. School age is also the time of the development of conditions that interfere with school functioning and general functioning, such as attention deficit disorder and attention deficit hyperactive disorder, widespread problems among children that are often treated by medical practitioners, sometimes with stimulant drugs.

This is also a time when children become differentiated in athletic ability, a primary focus of interest and concern among young children through at least the adolescent years. Children who are athletically talented, which is often a result, at least in part, of biological development, become leaders of other children whereas those who are lacking in athletic ability may become outcasts and isolates among their peers. This is primarily true for boys but it is sometimes also the case with girls.

Biological Benchmarks of Adolescence

The biological benchmarks associated with adolescence have to do with many hormonal changes and developments in the reproductive and sexual systems. Adolescence begins with puberty, which is a biological phenomenon that deals with the initial appearance of secondary sex characteristics such as pubic hair, development of breasts in women, and development of deeper voices in males. The reproductive organs also change, grow larger, and become capable of reproduction. Puberty is also the time of the menarche or the onset of menstruation (Rathus et al., 2002). Humans become capable of physical reproduction at puberty but, in industrialized societies, education and economics usually require the postponement of reproduction and marriage.

According to Rathus et al. (2002), a variety of other physical changes occur in human males and females. Note that the ages at which these phenomena occur overlap. That is, some early age developments in some children occur at later ages in others. In girls, between the ages of 8 and 11, the hormones stimulate the ovaries to increase the production of estrogen and the internal reproductive organs begin to grow.

Between ages 9 and 15, girls develop areola, which are the darker areas around the nipples. The breasts grow and become rounded. The pubic hair darkens and becomes coarser. The body grows taller. Girls develop vaginal discharges and the reproductive organs, both internal and external, grow. Between the ages of 10 and 16, underarm hair begins to grow. When menstruation begins, the ovaries begin to release eggs that are capable of being fertilized. They also begin regular menstrual cycles. Between ages 12 and 19, female breasts may have the same shape and size as adult breasts. Pubic hair covers the mons and spreads to the top of the thighs. Girls may also develop deeper voices. The body may change during their early twenties, too.

Among males, between ages 9 and 15, the testicles begin to grow, pubic hair appears, and the skin of the scrotum becomes redder and coarser. The areola also grow larger and darker. Boys grow taller and develop more muscle mass. Between ages 11 and 15, the testicles and scrotum continue growing and the penis becomes longer. Pubic hair becomes more coarse and spreads to the area between the legs. Male shoulders broaden, the hips narrow, the larynx enlarges to make for a deeper voice, and facial as well as underarm hair begins to grow.

Between the ages of 11 and 17, the penis grows in length and in circumference and the testicles continue to increase in size. Adult pubic hair texture develops. In half of all boys, breast enlargement occurs, which decreases in a year or two. Between the ages 14 and 18, the adult height is nearly reached and the genitals have adult shape and size. In many cases, chest hair appears. Shaving is very frequent because facial hair is growing. There are also significant physical changes in some males in their early twenties.

Erections become rather frequent for boys 13 to 14 years old, and Rathus et al. (2002) relate the common concern of early adolescent boys of being found with erections in school or in restrooms. The first ejaculation occurs between the ages of 11 and 17. Some boys ejaculate as early as age 8 and some as late as their early twenties. There are also common events of nocturnal emissions or wet dreams in which seminal fluid is ejaculated while the boy is asleep.

Masturbation becomes a major sexual practice for adolescents—both boys and girls—although masturbation seems to be more common among males than females. Chapter 11 on reproduction provides more specific information on the implications of the stages of development for the continuation of the species.

Pregnancy and Childbearing

Many of the most important biological implications of the adult stage of life has to do with reproduction and childbearing among women. It is instructive that the *Merck Manual* (Beers & Berkow, 1999) devotes some twenty pages to the abnormalities of pregnancy. This manual, which summarizes much of what is known about medicine, notes dozen of conditions that interfere with normal childbirth.

One condition that is often of special interest to social workers is preeclampsia and eclampsia. These are related conditions that affect, in the case of preeclampsia, 5 percent of pregnant women and, in the case of eclampsia, about 2.5 percent, who usually are those who have preeclampsia, too. The eclampsia condition if untreated usually leads to death and the basic treatment for the condition is, before eclampsia develops, bed rest and careful monitoring, often within a hospital. But the only full resolution of the problem is in delivery of the child. The condition seems to develop largely in persons who have other kinds of health conditions such as hypertension and other serious functional health problems.

These conditions are of special interest to social workers because they often develop among low-income women who had not had treatment for the conditions that are associated with the illness. There are also many other health conditions that cause the miscarriage of a child.

Of course, a highly controversial issue in the area of childbirth is abortion. However, it is more an issue of social policy than of biology. Abortion is a well-understood medical procedure. The issues of whether a fetus is a human being or not is at the foundation of the debate over abortion—a debate that is not part of the content or design of this book.

Hormone Replacement Therapy

A major health issue emerged in 2002 about hormone replacement therapy, which is a significant matter for middle-aged women who are dealing with menopause. Over the years, large numbers of American women of ages around 50 and above were prescribed estrogen or a combination including estrogen (often with progesterin), a hormone that declines during menopause. In 2001, pharmacies filled 67 million prescriptions for the hormone.

Hormone replacement therapy, which has been used by 6 million American women, was studied by the National Institutes of Health and the results announced by the National Heart, Lung, and Blood Institute (Rousseau, 2002). Dr. Jacques E. Rousseau (2002), who is a coronary expert and acting director of the Women's Health Initiative, a national study of which the hormonal studies were a part, further explained some of the implications of the study. He points out that although there had been studies of hormone replacement therapy—which involves taking Prempro, the most commonly prescribed estrogen-progesterone replacement formula or a similar treatment—observing the conditions of women who used it compared with those who did not, the studies were not as valid as they could be because those who took the therapy were more health conscious than those who did not.

The Women's Health Initiative study was the first large, "double blind" study of the therapy, an accepted way of evaluating health care treatments. That means that the experimenters and the patients did not either know who was and was not using the real hormone therapy rather than a placebo.

In describing the implications of the results, Rousseau (2002) explains that if 10,000 women take the hormones for one year, those 10,000 will have eight more cases of breast cancer than 10,000 women who do not take the therapy. A particular woman who uses the therapy will have less than one-tenth of 1 percent greater risk of breast cancer than a woman who does not. But when translated to the 6 million who use hormone replacement therapy, it means an additional 25,000 cases of breast cancer in the United States over a 5-year period. The study was suspended when the experimenters saw a 26 percent increase in invasive breast cancer—cancer that spreads to surrounding body tissue. They also found significant increases in the rates of strokes, heart attacks, and blood clots in the legs and lungs.

Rousseau (2002) also says that birth control pills, on which there are more data, involve the same hormones. He hopes to combine studies of birth control pills with these new findings to evaluate the long-term effects of long-term hormone therapy.

According to Rousseau (2002), women who do not have high risk factors, such as breast cancer, in their immediate families may find it advantageous to use the therapy for two or three years. That can help them control hot flashes, vaginal dryness, and mood swings. Nothing is better for such conditions. But longer-term therapy may not be advisable.

Rousseau (2002) also suggests alternative treatments such as antidepressants for mood swings; diet, exercise, bone-building drugs for osteoporosis; and cholesterol-lowering drugs as well as proper diet and exercise to prevent heart attacks. For hot flashes, vaginal dryness, and mood swings, nothing works better than estrogen-progesterone. Over long periods, however, there is little benefit and real potential for harm (Rousseau, 2002).

Cowley and Springen (2002) further explain the study results by indicating that 10,000 users of the therapeutic drugs were compared with a control group of 10,000 who received a placebo. The study found that those who used estrogen had greater numbers of heart attacks, strokes, breast cancers, and blood clots. However, they had fewer colon cancers and hip fractures. The results were considered significant enough to immediately end the experiment and inform those who were receiving the therapy that their health was in danger because of it (Cowley & Springen, 2002). The overall differences between those who took the estrogen and those who did not were statistically significant but not numerically as great as they may have seemed. That is, the stroke rate for women who took the estrogen rose from 21 to 29 per 10,000 cases. The breast cancer rate increased from 30 to 38 cases. The heart attack risk went up from 30 heart attacks in those who did not use the replacement therapy to 37 among those who did. As indicated, the numbers are not incredibly high for either group but the differences reached statistical significance—enough differences so that the researchers ended the study and warned those who used the hormone about the possible dangers associated with it.

Critics of the use of hormone replacement therapy said that no full and reliable studies had ever been conducted on the basic uses and dangers of the therapy, as Rousseau (2002) also found. Women who took hormone replacements indicated that they were able to reduce their incidence of osteoporosis and that they also were able to reduce problems such as insomnia, hot flashes and night sweats, mood swings, and forgetfulness.

According to other studies (Kalb, 2002), there are alternative and less dangerous ways of dealing with some of the conditions treated by the hormones, as Rousseau (2002) also believes. A glass of warm milk, an over-the-counter sleep aid, exercise, and weight loss, all seem to have some value in dealing with the problems of insomnia, mood swings, and forgetfulness. Hot flashes can be prevented or reduced with diets that are low in spicy foods, alcohol, and caffeine. Calcium helps deal with osteoporosis. Vaginal dryness, another symptom of the loss of estrogen, can be addressed with lubricants and moisturizers. Also, estrogen ointments and devices are available that deal with the problem but that prevent the release of the hormone into the bloodstream.

By 2003, there was great controversy in the medical community and among women patients who use hormone replacement therapy about the future directions in such treatments. "Women were told for decades that hormone-replacement therapy would protect their hearts and preserve their youth. Now the evidence is in, and an era is over" (Cowley & Springen, 2002).

Hormone replacement is also an issue in the care of older men (Groopman, 2002b). Both consumer magazines and publications aimed at physicians have focused on the virtue of providing hormone replacement therapy for men who have "andropause." Andropause is defined as a condition that results from androgen deficiency, a loss of testosterone, which can be treated, according to some, with the administration of testosterone, a male hormone. The symptoms of the condition are fatigue and loss of sexual capacity. According to Groopman (2002b), early efforts to replace testosterone with pills led to liver damage. Injections resulted in mood swings and fluctuations in libido and energy. A patch appeared to be more effective than pills and a gel applied to the skin appeared to be most effective of all. However, many question the validity of testosterone replacement therapy. The tests for testosterone levels are not as accurate as would be desirable. Therefore, diagnosis of the condition is problematic. Groopman (2002b) suggests that the value of the treatment as well as its safety are in serious question, despite active campaigns from pharmaceutical companies to promote hormone replacement therapy for men as well as women. The safety issues, which are not as well publicized because male hormone treatment is relatively new compared to the use of such treatment for women, are not yet as well known as those that have been identified for women. However, they may be equally severe. "An accurate assessment of its [male-hormone replacement therapy] effects on the heart, blood vessels, and prostate would require many years of observing many thousands of men—a male counterpart to the Women's Health Initiative" (Groopman, 2002b, p. 38).

AGING

The social work literature on aging is extensive. The primary emphasis is on social and economic issues facing older adults, some of which are serious impediments to satisfactory lives for the elderly. It is especially true that adults who had low incomes when they worked are likely to have even lower incomes and assets when they are elderly because the basic governmental program for retired people is Social Security and it is pegged to one's earnings while working.

Medicare, which is available to all Americans 65 and older, provides health coverage in many circumstances but not for all health needs. However, Medicaid provides the difference for very-low-income people, including older adults, and also provides nursing home care and other long-term care for those who are eligible and who need it. Supplemental Security Income provides a minimum monthly cash stipend for low-income older people as well. Details on all these issues, programs, and services are available in the many texts and many other books written on aging with an emphasis on social work with older people.

The growing proportion of aged in the United States is a significant fact. In 2000, there were nine workers worldwide for every recipient of Social Security. That number is expected to shrink to four workers per Social Security recipient by 2050.

Biological Issues in Aging

However, aging is also a biological phenomenon. As people approach the end of life, it is obvious that there are physical changes from their earlier years. But there is probably no age group with a broader range of biological differences than older adults. Normally developing children, adolescents, and young adults, and, to a large extent, those of middle age, have a great deal in common. However, some people in their senior years are biologically very old and some others are relatively young. A good bit of the difference depends on the health care, lifestyles, and diet in the younger years, but there are also genetic and little understood biological differences that differentiate older people from one another. In fact, older adults in their sixties are often caretakers for their elderly parents who are in their eighties and nineties.

Many older adults through their seventies work full-time, maintain households, are active in sports, and are generally fully functioning adults. The public health service maintains a measure of the number of days of healthy living. These vary significantly among older people. Some have almost all active, healthy days every year whereas others may be invalids and bedridden.

Normal Biological Changes in Old Age

There are some biological changes in the senior years that are common among most older people and that are the products of changes in the human body as it ages. For example, exercise physiologists established a measure for target healthy heart rates for all people. The rate is based on the formula of 220 minus the person's age. So the target heart rate for an older person who wants to exercise to his or her maximum is much lower than the heart rate expected for a younger person. A 65-

year-old, for example, will have a target heart rate of 155 whereas a 30-year-old will have a target heart rate of 190. The formula simply recognizes that as people age, the rapidity of their heart rate decreases.

There is widespread belief that older adults are often subject to the disease osteoarthritis. While it may be true that older adults are the most likely to feel the effects of the disease, new medical knowledge shows that the condition often begins in the much younger years—-even the twenties (Gorman & Park, 2002). The condition now affects more than 20 million Americans but by 2020, it could reach 40 million. Part of the reason for the growth is the large number of people who were born after World War II and who constitute the "baby-boom generation." Many of that generation have reached or will soon reach their fifties, which is a prime time for suffering from osteoarthritis. Although the condition may not be a product of old age, its major effects are primarily felt in the senior years. More information on osteoarthritis can be found in Chapter 8.

Older people are more susceptible to falls than younger people. Falls in older people often lead to permanent disabilities or even death. Broken hips are a common consequence of an older person's fall—an accident that may be only a minor inconvenience for a young person—because of deterioration in the skeletal system that is often associated with aging. Depending on the amount of weight-bearing exercise one engages in during the younger years and the amount of calcium taken in, older people may be subject to osteoporosis, or brittleness of bones. But even for those who do not have osteoporosis, bones still become more brittle in the senior years and what might have been a bruise for a younger person may well be a broken bone for an older adult. Of course, these physical conditions may often make some forms of work difficult for older people. Those who are accustomed to and have less physically active jobs may be able to work longer and into the later years than older adults of the same age whose work patterns are based on physical strength and agility. There is usually some decline in sexual functioning and sexual activity among most older people.

There are other normal processes associated with aging. For example, presbyopia is a nearly universal phenomenon in which the eyes fail to accommodate to close-up viewing such as is required for reading. Therefore, it is almost universal for persons in their forties and above to require reading glasses, even if they have no farsightedness, nearsightedness, or astigmatism because of the simple changes in their eyes' ability to accommodate. Diseases of the eyes such as cataracts and glaucoma are also common developments in later years.

Other senses may also deteriorate, especially hearing. Although it is not universal, older adults, especially those who have been exposed to hearing trauma in their earlier years, may find it difficult to hear and may find themselves needing hearing aids in order to participate in normal conversations and to hear television, radio, and social conversations.

And, of course, there are cosmetic differences associated with age. Dark spots called liver spots often appear on the hands of older people. These spots are not associated with illness but with aging. The hair becomes gray and, in some cases, sparse; teeth deteriorate from age and other dental problems such as gum disease become more common, especially among those who have not had adequate oral health care in their younger years.

However, most of these health changes and conditions are more annoying than they are debilitating. Older adults may well live full and active lives.

Diseases of Aging

Alzheimer's disease is a name now given to some forms of dementia and senility and is a specific disease. The disease can strike people in their middle years as well as in their elderly years, but there is definitely an association between aging and the onset of Alzheimer's. The disease is not curable although there are some treatments for it. There is also some evidence that its onset can be prevented through maintenance of extensive mental activity, through proper diet, and exercise. At this point, however, the disease is not well understood, except that it affects many older people and that as one grows even older Alzheimer's is increasingly likely to strike. Additional material on Alzheimer's can be found in Chapter 12.

Heart disease and stroke, conditions that can occur at any time, are more likely to occur among older people. The public health service even age adjusts death rates from these conditions because of the expectation that as people age, they are increasingly likely to have heart attacks or strokes and are increasingly likely to die from them. As mentioned, osteoporosis and arthritis are mobility diseases that are associated with aging.

Organic Mental Health Issues and Aging

Hales and Hales (1996) say that people retain key information, vocabulary, and verbal intelligence at about the same level as when they were younger when they grow older. They explain why grandfathers lose computer games with teenage grandchildren. Clearly, there are some losses associated with the aging brain, which actually shrinks in size when people become older. Hales and Hales (1996, p. 630) say that humans lose "reaction time, intellectual speed and efficiency, nonverbal intelligence, and the maximal speed in which we can work for short periods . . . by the age of seventy-five."

Memory falters in the older years and that can be addressed by older adults by keeping lists, taking notes, and documenting what they do and what they are working on. About 5 to 15 percent of people over the age of 70 develop more serious mental symptoms such as errors in judgment and impaired thinking, some of which result from illnesses. They also may forget the names of people, things, and events.

According to Hales and Hales (1996), the American Psychiatric Association thinks that 15 to 25 percent of the elderly have significant symptoms of mental illness. Many of these are the result of physiological changes and others result from medicine they have taken. Hales and Hales (1996) suggest that older people are most likely to suffer from loss and grief, depression, anxiety disorders, and sleep disorders. About 15 percent of men and women over 65, who are not in nursing homes or other facilities, are depressed. Anxiety disorders increase with age, and about 20 percent of older people report some physical and psychological signs of anxiety. Sleep is much less efficient in older people than in younger. Confusion, delirium, and the effects of alcohol and medications are also a factor in the mental functioning of older adults.

More detailed information on the biological aspects of aging can be found in Chapter 12, devoted to the subject of older adults.

SUMMARY

The human lifespan has been a subject of consuming interest to all the health and human sciences professions for most of their histories. As suggested by this chapter, the greatest amount of study and therefore the greatest amount of knowledge, especially in terms of biological development, are at the extremes—child development and the aging process. Some knowledge is available about young childhood and adolescence but there is a significant dropoff in understanding about adults, both young and middle-aged.

However, most of the problems that occur in human lifespans and most of the programs designed to assist people in their functioning are centered on children and older people. For most individuals, the adult years are relatively placid. People are able to care for themselves, serious illnesses have either been left behind in childhood or are in the offing for the later years. So the critical periods of human life are at those extremes—youth and aging. It is no accident that most of the financing of human services programs and most of the preoccupations of social workers in their professional work is with younger and older people.

This chapter summarizes significant portions of the knowledge biological scientists of various kinds have been able to develop about human life, from its beginnings to its end. The information provides a background for understanding some of the rest of this text and the ways in which biology affects human functioning.

DISCUSSION QUESTIONS

1. Understanding the body systems is central to understanding human biology, as a totality. What are some of the ways in which the circulatory system interacts with the larger environment? Although the circulatory system may appear to be a closed system, it can develop disabling conditions when it interacts with other systems and with the larger environment in which the person lives. Describe some of those ways in which the circulatory system connects to the rest of the world.

2. Summarize the ways in which disturbances to the brain can lead to social problems and require the intervention of social workers. Be as inclusive and specific as possible.

3. Using an Internet search, what can you find out about attention deficit disorder? Specify the sites you find and some of the information they provide.

4. In what ways do 5-month-old children differ from 11-month-old children?

PART II

EVOLUTION, GENETICS, AND INHERITANCE

Among the many areas of biology that are important to understand in order to comprehend modern biological theory is evolution. This section of the book describes some of the ways in which personal characteristics are passed from one generation to the next.

The whole issue of evolution, which is a critical concept in understanding biological development, is discussed in Chapter 5. Also discussed is genetics, which is the transmission process for evolution. The chapter culminates in an application of genetic and evolution theory to understandings of human behavior.

Subjects such as genetics and evolution have not always been central to the kinds of knowledge provided to social workers as they prepare for their professional practice. However, it is clear that many health conditions or propensities for health conditions are inherited. It is also clear that genes determine some parts of human behavior or some of the elements of human physiology that can affect human behavior. Some of the theories about these matters are discussed in this part of the text.

Chapter 6 deals exclusively with human biology and intellect. The argument over the role of genes in human intelligence is long-standing, and this chapter deals with much of what is known about the impact of genetics and inheritance on the intellect.

During the past few years, one of the largest issues in the area of biology discussions has been the Human Genome Project. Chapter 7 describes the Human Genome Project. A history of the project and its various points of development is reprinted from *Science* and included in the chapter.

The concepts covered in Part II are fundamental to understanding the science of human evolution and the process of genetic inheritance. They are important concepts for comprehending health, illness, and other more practical matters that are major parts of the rest of this text.

CHAPTER FIVE

EVOLUTION, HEREDITY, AND HUMAN BEHAVIOR

*I have called this principle, by which each slight variation,
if useful, is preserved, by the term of Natural Selection.*

—Charles Darwin

Charles Darwin's controversial perspective that humans and primates share a common ancestry, and that, in fact, all organisms descended from a common ancestry, created the first serious challenge to the previously held belief that God created humans and all living organisms. The debate between what has become known as creation science and evolution continues today, although there are few serious scientists who consider creation science a legitimate scientific theory. Fossil records, studies of comparative anatomy, embryology and biochemistry, coupled with recent findings from comparing the genomes of humans to a number of other organisms, support evolution. The occurrence of evolution is considered a scientific fact and is strongly supported by 150 years of research that has produced an overwhelming amount of evidence. The debates within science concerning evolution cited by creation science as demonstrating that evolution is an unfounded theory are about how evolution occurs and not whether or not it occurs.

The application of the evolutionary theory to the understanding of human behavior is not a new concept. William James, considered the father of American psychology, in his seminal book *Principles of Psychology* (1890), discussed the existence of human instincts and how these instincts are "hardwired" into humans much like in other organisms.

Less appealing theories concerning the influence of evolution and heredity on human behavior, including social Darwinism and eugenics, also arose between the end of the nineteenth century and the beginning of the twentieth century. As a result of these theories, for many years there was a conscious effort by modern scientists interested in human behavior to move away from strong biological explanations for human behavior and to focus solely on environmental explanations. Starting in the late 1970s and early 1980s, after many years of focusing on the cultural aspects of human behavior, some psychologists and anthropologists have begun applying evolutionary principles to understanding human behavior.

As discussed in the introductory chapter, history shows that significant shifts have occurred in how much heredity and the environment are believed to influence human behavior. These shifts in belief about the extent of heredity and evolution determining human behavior have had a direct impact on the theoretical underpinnings of many social and natural sciences, including social work. Beyond impacts on science, history also shows that these shifts often influenced social welfare policy as well as the practice methods used by social workers and other helping professionals. The remainder of this chapter is devoted to defining the basic concepts and terms of evolution and understanding the role of evolution and heredity in human behavior. The goal is to provide social workers with a foundation from which recent applications of evolution can be discussed.

BASIC CONCEPTS AND TERMS

Before examining the relationship between evolution and human behavior, we should discuss generally what evolution is and how it has been researched through the examination of other organisms. Evolution is the unpredictable changing of the genetic make-up of a population over time. These changes result in physical traits and behaviors that are adaptive to the environment. The environment does not create changes, but instead helps shape the changes that do survive. There are two types of evolution: microevolution and macroevolution. Microevolution is the slow process of changes from generation to generation of individuals, resulting in the creation of new behaviors and physical traits that may lead to the development of a new species. Macroevolution refers to large-scale changes that effect groups of species and are typically caused by catastrophic events. The most commonly known example of macroevolution is the extinction of the dinosaurs and the ensuing rise of mammals approximately 65 million years ago, at the end of the Paleocene age. Darwin based evolution on three basic observations that hold true today. The first observation was that living organisms generally increase their population size at a rate greater than simply replacing the number of organisms that die. Thomas Malthus (1993 [1789]) originally made note of this phenomenon in *An Essay on the Principle of Population*. Second, no single animal or plant dominates all of the earth's environment. The third observation was that individual variation exists within a group of similar organisms (DeMoss, 1999).

The central feature of evolution is the concept of heredity. Darwin did not identify genes as the biological underpinning of how heredity works. One of Darwin's contemporaries, Gregor Mendel, first studied genes and heredity in 1866 using pea plants. For a variety of reasons, Darwin and Mendel did not know each other's work. During their lifetimes, the two pieces of research were never connected and it was not until the 1930s that scientists combined Darwin's and Mendel's findings in a meaningful way (DeMoss, 1999; Gribbin & Gribbin, 1998).

Since then, genes have generally been considered the biological basis for evolution and the mechanism by which heredity works.

Offspring receive half of their genes from each parent; genes have different forms called alleles that produce various possible versions of phenotypes. For example, in the pea plants studied by Gregor Mendel, one gene was associated with pea pod color (the phenotype) and there were two forms, or alleles, of that gene. One allele produced green pea pods and the other produced yellow pea pods. Gene alleles are considered either recessive or dominant. Recessive alleles do not produce a phenotype unless matched to the same type of allele, which is referred to as homozygous combination of alleles. In the case of pea pods, the color yellow is produced by the recessive allele and the color green by the dominant allele. This means that plants producing yellow pea pods receive two gene alleles for the color yellow, one from each parent. If one of the genes from the parents is the allele for the color green then the pea pods are green because recessive alleles do not produce a phenotype when matched with a dominant allele, a situation referred to as a heterozygous combination of alleles. Dominant alleles produce a phenotypic effect whether paired with an identical or a dissimilar allele. In the case of pea pods this means that green pea pods occur when both parents contribute an allele responsible for the color green as well as when one parent contributes an allele for yellow pea pods and one contributes an allele for green pea pods.

Phenotypes are the physical manifestations of genes, which are typically pro- duced by an interplay between environmental and genetic factors. For pea plants there is not an environmental factor that produces pea pod color, but for more com- plex phenotypes such as homosexual behavior in human beings, there is clearly a mix of genetic and environmental factors that contribute to the final manifestation of the phenotype. In essence, complex phenotypes such as most human behaviors are the end results of genetic predisposition that is shaped by the environment. However, there are human physical traits that are like pea pod color. Common rec- ognizable physical phenotypes for humans that have minimal environmental influence and are therefore dominated by genetic influence include earlobe shape, hairline, freckles, and eye color.

The third observation made by Darwin, that individual variation exists within a group of similar organisms, is central to understanding the process of evolution and its relationship to genes. Individuals within a species or population do not evolve during the course of their lifetime; their genetic make-up remains the same. Changes in populations occur typically over long periods of time and are directed by a number of different mechanisms. Because there is variation within populations, particular individuals, based on their genetic make-up, are either likely to survive to produce offspring that carry their genetic composition or are not likely to survive and therefore do not produce offspring that carry their genetic composition. The genetic variations within populations are random and the environment has nothing to do with the creation of these variations, but instead the environment is either detrimental or conducive to survival of a particular variation.

In *The Origin of Species* (1979 [1859]), Darwin suggested that the process of natural selection is the agent by which evolution works. As our knowledge of genetics and evolution has expanded over time, so has our understanding of the mechanisms that influence changes in the gene pool of a population to include additional mechanisms. Three of the mechanisms add new alleles to the gene pool: recombination, mutation, and genetic flow. Two of the processes remove genes from the gene pool: genetic drift and natural selection.

Because natural selection is the most widely known, we will address it first and in the most detail. Natural selection is the environment selecting individuals for survival, which ultimately leads to successful procreation. Natural selection merely favors beneficial genetic changes when they occur and, over time, as the environment changes, what was once a genetic composition that was favorable may become less favorable for survival and procreation. One of the most commonly cited examples of natural selection involves the moth species, *Biston betularia*, which resides in England (Kettlewell, 1955, 1956). The moth has two primary color schemes, one light and another dark, which are determined by one gene (two alleles). Although some have disputed the scientific rigor of the methodology used to examine this interesting case, it still provides a clear and easy way to understand natural selection in action.

Dark-colored moths comprised less than 2 percent of the total population of *Biston betularia* in England prior to 1848. This distribution of dark- and light-colored moths within the population predates the industrial revolution in England. Between 1848 and 1898, the dark-colored moths came to comprise 95 percent of the total population of *Biston betularia* in Manchester and other highly industrialized cities in England. The change in the rate of the color scheme from 2 percent to 95 percent represented an actual change in the gene pool of the *Biston betularia*.

Why did this shift in the distribution of light- and dark-colored moths occur? Between 1848 and 1898, the Industrial Revolution caused a significant expansion of factories in English cities such as Manchester. These factories discharged large quantities of black carbon ash that darkened the environment of the moths. Against the dark background the moths' primary predator, birds, could see the lighter-colored moths better, resulting in light-colored moths being less likely to survive to reproductive age and therefore less likely to procreate descendants. The greater number of descendants left by dark-colored moths because they had a higher rate of survival to reproductive age resulted in their increased frequency in the population. This is an example of natural selection at work within a population (Kettlewell, 1955, 1956).

Natural selection did not create the two color schemes within *Biston betularia*, but instead favored one color scheme over another during a specific period of time. Obviously, based on the distribution of light- and dark-colored moths prior to 1848, the process of natural selection favored light-colored moths. With the significant change in the environment caused by the Industrial Revolution, the environment no longer favored the light-colored moths. Without the genetic variation that created two different-colored moths, this process would not be possible.

The other mechanism for removing gene alleles from the gene pool is genetic drift, which is the simple change in allele frequencies created by chance. The occurrence of particular gene alleles within a population is random. Scientists are in debate about how significant the role of gene drift is in creating shifts in the frequency of particular alleles. Some believe that in smaller populations, gene drift can play a significant role whereas in larger populations it has less of an impact.

Of the mechanisms that add variation to the gene pool of populations, gene flow, much like gene drift, plays a small role in creating variation. New organisms entering a population and mating with organisms already in the population cause gene flow. This rarely occurs between closely related species and is almost unheard of between species that are more distantly related.

The process of recombination is the most common form of creating new alleles within a population. Recombination happens in humans at the time of conception. The male and female each contribute half of the chromosomes necessary for the offspring. The numerous combinations of possible gene pairings mean that genes in the offspring are a mix of alleles from the parents. This makes the offspring both genetically unique as well as genetically similar to the two parents.

The more dramatic mechanism that creates new alleles within a population is mutation. Occasionally, a gene is copied imperfectly through the process of recombination and a new allele is created. If the new allele confers some advantage on the phenotype produced, the allele will spread. However, most mutations are not beneficial and often result in the immediate death of the organism or bestow a negative phenotype that lessens the likelihood of procreation.

Other important terms worth considering when discussing evolution include adaptation, co-opted, and genotype. Adaptation is a term that has two possible and applicable meanings. One is a reference to a positive trait or phenotype present in an animal or human. The second meaning is a reference to the process of gene mutation and the passing of beneficial traits on to future generations (DeMoss, 1999). Co-opted refers to when a trait has evolved for one purpose over time and later is taken over by another purpose (DeMoss, 1999). A genotype is defined as the genetic constitution of an organism as distinguished from its physical appearance, or a group or class of organisms having the same genetic constitution.

Stephen Jay Gould and Niles Eldredge theorized that evolution was not a linear process but a dynamic one that contained long periods of aimless change followed by brief periods of radical change. Before his death in 2002, Dr. Gould completed a rewrite of evolution that incorporated punctuated equilibrium into Darwin's work.

SCIENTIFIC PURSUIT OF UNDERSTANDING EVOLUTION AND HUMAN BEHAVIOR

Evolutionary biologists focusing on animal behavior have dominated the study of the relationship among heredity, the environment, and behavior (Daly & Wilson, 1997). Much of the reason for the focus on animal behavior rather than human behavior is linked to the controversial ideas of eugenics, which was a theory of the biological perfectibility of human beings. The idea was also one of the basic underpinnings of Nazism. This has recently begun to change with the growing number of scientists working on and interested in the Human Genome Project, gene therapy for curing inherited diseases, DNA matching, and brain research.

Between 1945 and 1990, there were three areas of scientific research that provided the basic findings that are used in applying evolution to human behavior. First, biologists studying animal and insect behavior have focused on the relationship between genetics and the environment. Most of the terms and basic structures underpinning theoretical discussions of evolutionary psychologists come from the study of animal behavior. Over the years, some behavioral biologists have ventured into applying their knowledge to human behavior. An example of a prominent evolutionary biologist who studies animal behavior (specifically bird behavior) who has also examined human behavior from an evolutionary perspective is Stephen T. Emlen from Cornell University. For the American Association for the Advancement of Science (AAAS), Dr. Emlen presented a paper titled "The Evolutionary Study of Human Family Systems," in which he identifies correlations between family structure and the well-being of children with a specific focus on stepfamilies. His findings included:

1. "Stepchildren suffer much higher rates of physical abuse and even death than children in intact families."
2. "Stepparents invest less time and effort in the offspring from their partner's previous marriage than they do with their own children."
3. "Stepchildren are at greater risk for sexual abuse than children in intact families, and stepparents are overwhelmingly the abusers. The incidence of sexual abuse of stepdaughters in one study was eight times that of biological daughters."
4. "Children in stepfamilies leave home significantly earlier than children in intact families."
5. "Stepfamilies are less stable than intact families. The incidence of subsequent divorce is higher in second marriages and increases with the number of stepchildren present." (Emlen, 1995)

The second area of scientific research with data supporting evolution as influencing human behavior is brain research. Starting in the 1970s, there were a number of techniques developed, including brain imaging, which allowed for the examination of how thoughts and words alter metabolic processes in the brain. These technical advances significantly improved research methods for studying live brain functioning (DeMoss, 1999). The primary contribution of brain research has been to strengthen the evidence supporting a biological link between human behavior and emotion. Researchers, in general, believe that the brain has developed through a long evolutionary process.

The third area of fruitful scientific research has been genetics. During the mid-1990s, scientists began to develop a number of techniques for identifying particular genes likely to be linked to the existence of diseases long believed to have an inherited component. Recently, there has been a growing movement within psychology to reexamine the importance of evolution through the identification and study of universal behaviors. This growing subfield of psychology is known as evolutionary psychology.

MODERN DISCUSSION CONCERNING THE RELATIONSHIP BETWEEN EVOLUTION AND HUMAN BEHAVIOR

There are varying views within several different scientific groups about the influence of evolution on modern human behavior. Because the work of evolutionary psychologists is directed at understanding human behavior, in particular, the arguments used by scholars in that field provide much of the basis for the following discussion. The presence and identification of universal behaviors within the human population is the strongest evidence of genetic influence on human behaviors. For example, Rozin (2000, p. 971) states that there "are a surprising number of common, perhaps universal themes: meals, marriage, cuisine, designation of family relationships, facial expressions of emotion, religion, the existence of languages and syntactic language universals." Beyond universal social behaviors, there are also physical behaviors that are common to all human beings.

Detractors of evolutionary psychology have pointed to the impossibility of separating environmental conditions from the influence of genes. "Complex human behaviors of the kind that have interested psychologists—beliefs, intentions, emotions, personalities—do not have localized biological or genetic causes in the sense that stroke lesions cause aphasia or a single gene cause phenylketonuria" (Turkheimer, 1998, p. 789). Because of direct links between behavior and genetics, researchers often accept a "weak" biological explanation for human behavior. In this scenario all human behavior has a biological base, but that base does not represent a very good explanation of why the behavior occurs. The acceptance of a weak biological interpretation of behavior can result in a discounting of genetic influences.

A refinement of weak biological explanations relies on the concept of canalization, which attempts to identify the level of genetic influence over a phenotype by examining the degree of universal presence across a number of normal environmental variations (Cummins & Cummins, 1999). By taking this approach, the level of genetic contributions to behaviors can be seen as varying depending on the relationship that the behavior has to the environment (MacDonald, 1998). The question when examining universal behaviors then becomes to what degree is a behavior robust across normal environmental variations? For example, breathing remains a constant behavior across all environments. In contrast, the social behavior of participating in organized religion is seen to have wider variability across a number of environments.

Another way of studying the relationship between evolution and human behavior is to research behaviors that seem to violate the norms of evolution. For example, altruism researcher Hoffman (1981) described empathy in a way that attempted to incorporate an evolutionary underpinning to empathy. "Empathy may be uniquely suited for bridging the gap between egoism and altruism, since it has the property of transforming another person's misfortune into one's own feeling of distress . . . an aversive state that may often best be alleviated by helping the victim" (p. 133).

The largest problem confronting researchers interested in understanding the relationship between behavior and genetics is isolating the influence of environmental factors. The classic solution to this problem when studying human beings has been the use of twins, or "twin studies," which allow the researcher to assume that the two subjects are genetically the same and that the only factors that created variation were environmental in nature.

DRAWING CONCLUSIONS FOR SOCIAL WORKERS

Eric Turkheimer (1998) in his paper "Heritability and Biological Explanation" asks a tongue-in-cheek question that captures the fears of social workers and other helping professionals whenever issues of genetics are discussed. He asks: What would you say to a computer programmer assigned to correct a problem with your computer's software that started out with a pile of computer chips and a soldering iron? Attempts during the early twentieth century by social Darwinists and the Nazis to affect human behavior at such a base level were inhumane, unethical, and reflected the worst tendencies in human society. When applying the computer analogy, attempting to fix a software problem with radical changes to the hardware seems ridiculous and mistaken.

Furthermore, within the various theoretical arguments that surround the modern discussion of evolution and human behavior when talking about genetics, heredity, and evolution, often the assumption is that the concept of innate means that the biological underpinnings for particular behaviors are present at birth. This theory is not congruent with growing brain research findings, which show that the physical manifestations of language and emotion are not necessarily present at birth, but may develop over time as a result of environmental stimuli.

Findings from behavioral biology, genetics, and brain research during the past 30 years have expanded the complexity in which the relationship between evolution, heredity, genes, and human behavior are discussed. Despite the leaps in understanding about this relationship, the basic question of what influence heredity has on direct service interventions provided by social workers remains. Perhaps, for direct practice social workers, evolution in and of itself has very little importance in the provision of direct services. Evolutionary concepts, however, can help social workers better understand possible hereditary factors in family background and client behaviors.

In conclusion, evolution is one of the most complex theories in human biology. For some it remains controversial, but almost all serious scientists believe that it is an accurate portrayal of the way in which species develop. Social workers must be aware of the basic concepts of evolution and heredity, which as this text discusses in several other sections, are important for understanding many health problems and, as scientists increasingly believe, many of the manifestations of human behavior.

DISCUSSION QUESTIONS

1. What are the two types of evolution in the chapter?

2. On what three observations did Darwin base his theories of evolution?

3. Discuss the importance of universal behaviors in understanding the relationship between human behavior and evolution. Cite examples.

4. What are some of the conclusions social workers may draw about human behavior being related to evolutionary forces?

CHAPTER SIX

HUMAN BIOLOGY AND INTELLECT

You don't realize that you're intelligent until it gets you into trouble.
—James Baldwin

Intelligence is quickness in seeing things as they are.
—George Santayana

Intelligence alone, without wisdom and empathy for suffering, is hollow.
—John G. Stoessinger

Social work practitioners and social work students, BSW, MSW, or PhD, should be eager to leap into any discussion regarding human biology and intellect (used interchangeably in this chapter with the term intelligence), or the lack thereof. Nor should it matter what arena the discussion emanates from or resonates within. Social work practitioners and social work students undoubtedly already realize that a meaningful attempt to understand the connection between human biology and intellect has conceptual, scholarly, political, and societal implications. Of course, a basic understanding of the issues inherent in the human biology and intellect discussion is central to meaningful social work practice and the afore-mentioned discussions. This is true for generalist social work practice and becomes even more pronounced in nearly every area of specialized practice, examples of which include social work practice with persons with developmental disabilities or chronic mental illness. Also, social workers in particular practice settings, such as schools, hospitals, long-term care facilities, and/or hospices face a nearly con-stant need to assess the impact on intellect of biological improvements or reduc-tions in functioning.

Social work practitioners and social work students should also feel a sense of confidence when they enter any human biology and intellect discussion. Although the reasons for this presumed confidence are many, the chief one is that the field of intelligence research and the body of knowledge regarding intelligence is dominated by uncertainty (Ceci, 1996). In fact, in the intelligence research community there is more agreement regarding answers than there is regarding what questions these answers answer. For example, it is well accepted that on conventional tests of intelligence, members of certain racial and ethnic groups score differently. However, what does such a difference show? What questions does it answer? Does it answer the question of whether there are differences across groups in intelligence, whether the tests are differentially biased for members of different groups, whether different groups have had different educational opportunities, or whether different groups differ on a narrow subset of skills that constitutes only a small part of intelligence, or some other questions still (Sternberg & Kaufman, 2001)?

As well, social work practitioners and social work students have a keen interest in helping persons gain a greater sense of self-awareness. An increased sense of self-awareness is believed to enhance the functioning of people. Also, increased self-awareness is thought to be helpful when people are facing problems in their lives. Self-awareness can also be helpful when social workers are assisting people to restore previous levels of functioning (Axinn & Stern, 2001). Social work practitioners and social work students realize how important the dynamic of self-understanding and self-knowledge is to the helping process, for both the practitioner and the person being helped. Self-understanding and self-knowledge are believed by a number of theorists to be central to the intelligence of people (Hamachek, 1991). Most important to remember though is that theories abound as to what is intelligence, what are its central features, what influences intellect in general, and what specifically are biological influences on intellect. Although impressive advances have been made in the understanding of human biology and intellect as separate entities over the past decades, and even as joined entities in the last two decades, the fact remains that mythology, societal and individual assumptions, interpersonal intuition, and unspoken conclusions have contributed as much as have the social sciences.

This chapter includes a historical and scientific understanding of the concept of intellect, including the practice of IQ testing and measurement of intellect. Readers are exposed to the progression of language and the process by which ideas about human biology and intellect have been socially constructed. Additionally, the chapter includes recommendations for critical thinking skills for assisting social workers to make informed judgements about the use of intellect as a predictive or diagnostic tool in practice.

BIOLOGICAL THEORY OF INTELLECT

Theories of intelligence have a long history, predating such prominent historical intelligence researchers as Galton, Spencer, and Binet by at least 2,000 years. From the time that Plato (427–347 B. C. E.) first described the characteristics of intelligence in terms of the soul's entrapment of ideas to the modern day idea that intelligence is information processing there have been hundreds of theories of intelligence (Ceci, 1996).

The understanding social work practitioners and students have of intelligence is credited most often to their study of the work of psychologists (MacLullich, Seckl, Starr, & Deary, 1998). Galton and Spearman, two pioneering researchers of intellect, put forth the idea that to understand human intelligence, and differences in human intelligence, one first had to discover the biological mechanisms of thought. The biological approach to understanding intelligence evolves from a tendency to reduce the relationship between the results of intelligence tests with the ability of the brain to help people make sense of what is happening around them. Recent attempts, with potentially an even more reductionistic tendency, reflect the intent of scientists to discover genes that are associated with psychometric intelligence and the biological pathways from genes to the ability of people to think. Scientists are still a long way from truly understanding what are the mechanisms of human intelligence, particularly as related to biological theory (MacLullich et al., 1998).

To understand the biological theory of intelligence it is necessary to understand three terms: (1) psychometric intelligence, (2) biological intelligence, (3) social or practical intelligence—and one major concept, the g factor of intelligence. Spearman's g essentially defines something called psychometric intelligence, as measured by IQ tests. Nevertheless, the term *intelligence* has additional meanings. Biological intelligence refers to the basic anatomical, physiological, and hormonal properties and functions of the brain that underlie all forms of thinking. In addition, they act as a go-between and help explain individual differences in cognitive ability. Social, or practical, intelligence refers to the successful application of IQ to the events of a person's life.

The distinction between biological and psychometric intelligence is important to the gaining of a basic idea about any theory of intelligence. The importance of the distinction between biological and psychometric intelligence harks back to the two protagonists, Galton and Binet. Essentially, Galton believed in a unitary, or singular, concept of intelligence, and Binet believed in a multiplicity of functions or faculties, such as memory, imagery, imagination, attention, comprehension, suggestibility, and persistence. Galton is regarded as the originator of the g factor concept, and Binet of the "primary abilities" movement. Galton laid stress on genetic factors in producing individual differences in intelligence. Binet, as an educational psychologist, was more interested in environmental manipulation as a means of determining how intelligent a person might be. Binet, however, did not deny the possibile role of genes in determining a person's intelligence (Eysenck in Detterman, 1994).

Noted researcher and scholar Stephen J. Ceci (1996) claims there are five basic facts that are known to all members of the intelligence research community and embraced wholly by biological theorists of intelligence. In the following discussion of those five basic facts, it is important to keep in mind that Ceci places a great deal of emphasis on the context and the "bio-ecology" that a person lives within.

The first fact is that there is a "positive manifold" of correlations among test scores. Simply put, if a group of persons is administered a battery of cognitive tests or tasks, the performances of the persons tend to be consistent across the tests or tasks.

The second fact is that if the correlations among a battery of test scores are analyzed by factor analysis, an entity known as the "first principal component" can be extracted. The size of the first-principal component reflects the average correlations among the test scores. The greater the intercorrelatedness found among the test scores, the greater will be the size of the first principal component, .30, for example. In other words, how well the test scores are associated with one another helps the researcher identify what is the most important, or principal, component in judging how intelligent a person might be.

A third fact is that the first-principal component is viewed by many researchers as a replacement for general intelligence, or *g* factor. General intelligence or *g* is thought of as a singular intellectual resource that underpins all intelligent behaviors. Note that this view does not deny that specific intellectual skills exist in addition to *g*, only that most intellectual tasks require some degree of this general resource for their successful performance. In other words, that one identified component, the principal component, is the most important thing in whether an individual is intelligent or not.

The fourth fact is that a number of associations, correlations, exist between *g* and academic and social accomplishments. For example, *g* is strongly correlated with IQ, anywhere from .4 to .9. Moreover, *g* is somewhat predictive of school grades, work efficiency, everyday problem solving, social attainment, and criminality, and other important life outcomes. In other words, if one has a lot of *g* factor, one will do better in school. But on the other hand, one may also be a better criminal. Both things, doing well in school and being a good criminal, seem to be better accomplished if one is intelligent—makes sense.

The *g* factor of intelligence is positively associated with such outcomes as mental health, marital dissolution rates, years of school completed, and managerial level attainment. The important thing to keep in mind about the *g* factor and such correlations is that they validate the *g* factor as a measure of the biological capacity of the individual person to adapt in order to shape their environment. This is a central belief of the biological theory of intelligence. The ability to adapt means that theoretically persons with high *g* can retrain themselves to do many different tasks in one lifetime and often at a highly creative level.

The fifth fact is that a number of studies have reported that *g* can be inherited. Quite understandably, heritability of intelligence is another central belief of the biological theory of intelligence (Ceci, 1996). Arthur Jensen, a major figure in the community of intelligence researchers, and his colleagues studied the biological basis of *g*. Their studies led to present-day studies of behavioral genetics and the impact of genetics on intelligence, reaction time, and speed processing of information. An additional outgrowth of Jensen's work with small-scale reaction time studies and his interest in a biological foundation of intelligence is the study and identification of a number of biological/physiological correlates of *g*. Jensen showed that the speed with which research participants could execute a number of more specific cognitive processes, such as encoding information, scanning information in short term memory, or retrieving information from long-term memory was indicative of their "g" factor. His studies of the biological basis of g also yielded significant correlations between the g factor and IQ scores (Eysenck, 1993).

No discussion of the biological theory of intelligence is complete without consideration of the relationship between the physical size of the brain and intelligence. Although head size has been dismissed as having a positive correlation with intelligence, it appears that brain size is somewhat correlated with intelligence (Eysenck, 1993). The assumption is that the larger the brain the more information it can process. This is what Jerison has called the "principle of proper mass." However, humans with large amounts of brain mass should be conservative in their celebration. We know that some large biological organisms with large convoluted cortices, such as cows, are not much brighter than some of the insects (e.g., bees) with no cortices at all. Mass can be just bulk.

There is little controversy that the biological theory of intelligence includes the notion that intelligence belongs to the brain. And biological theorists believe that a number of brain regions exist and have evolved for the function of problem solving. There is great specialization in the older parts of the brain. These older parts can be viewed as a massive set of modular, parallel processing systems all working on different aspects of physiological and behavioral coordination. As humans evolved it is speculated that there were a number of ways to solve problems the biological human faced in nature. Human brains evolved to recognize problems, to invoke solutions, to test hypotheses using a background of knowledge, and to act quickly. If the hypothesis does not work and if the brain is sufficiently evolved, it will come up with other possible solutions by invoking other hypotheses to test. Problem solving is selective trial and error. The brain is thus a massive computing device. It is constantly thinking. Nature exploits a number of resources to attain the same function, in this case, planning. From the amoebae to little children, intelligent systems in nature adapt and generate hypotheses to resolve dilemmas, or solve local problems. It is important to keep in mind, however, that the potential effectiveness of any thinking process is in part biologically limited and in part limited by the nature of one's knowledge (Sternberg & Kaufman, 1998).

The important questions remain, however. What is intellect? What is the relationship between human biology and intellect? What is the connection between intellect and human behavior?

COGNITIVE SKILLS ASSOCIATED WITH INTELLECT: THE INFLUENCE OF CULTURE AND SOCIAL CONSTRUCTION

As noted earlier, the majority of psychologists who study intelligence believe that there exists some undivided mental entity—g—which flows into virtually all cognitive activities. This would also be true of intelligence researchers who are housed in other disciplines (e.g., biology, neurobiology) and believe in a biological theory of intelligence. Those who would argue against the biological theory of intelligence tend to argue that (1) there exists not one underlying intelligence g, but multiple forms of intelligence, and (2) it is logically impossible to separate these intelligences from acquired knowledge (Ceci, 1996).

Sternberg and Kaufman (2001) strike for some sort of middle ground among the biologists, the culturalists, and the cognitionists when they state that different approaches to understanding or researching intellect raise somewhat different questions, and hence produce somewhat different answers. They have in common, however, the attempt to understand what kinds of mechanisms lead some people to adapt to, select, and shape environments in ways that match particularly well the demands of those environments. They are trying to answer how it is that some people are better at adapting to, selecting, and/or influencing the environments within which they live. Does intelligence help people do these things?

Although the new phrase for learning and adaptive abilities, metacognition, or the ability to understand and control oneself, introduces a complex set of ideas, the idea is actually not new. The Greeks, particularly Aristotle, emphasized long ago the importance of intelligence for knowing oneself (Sternberg & Kaufman, 2001; Hamachek, 1991). The Greeks are most often cited as speaking early to the elements of intellect, but other cultures have done the same. Although the timing of their claims about intelligence are seemingly overvalued, it is actually the cultural differences in perceived valuations of skills of intellect that are most meaningful for understanding a biological theory of intelligence.

For example, the Western cultural emphasis on speed of mental processing is not shared by many cultures. In fact, other cultures may even be suspicious of the quality of work done very quickly and may emphasize depth rather than speed of processing. The Chinese Confucian perspective emphasizes the characteristic of benevolence and of doing what is right. In this Eastern perspective, the intelligent person spends much effort in learning, enjoys learning, and persists in lifelong learning with enthusiasm. The Taoist tradition emphasizes the importance of humility, freedom from conventional standards of judgement, and full knowledge of oneself and external conditions. The difference between Eastern and Western conceptions of intelligence persist even in modern times. Taiwanese conceptions of intelligence include five underlying factors: (1) a general cognitive factor, much like the g factor in conventional Western tests, (2) interpersonal intelligence, (3) intrapersonal intelligence, (4) intellectual self-assertion, and (5) intellectual self-effacement. Three factors underlying Chinese conceptualizations of intelligence are (1) nonverbal reasoning ability, (2) verbal reasoning ability, and (3) rote or repetitive memory. These factors differ substantially from those identified in people's conceptions of intelligence in the United States: (1) practical problem solving, (2) verbal ability, and (3) social competence (Sternberg & Kaufman, 2001).

In all cases, people's understood theories of intelligence seem to go quite far beyond what conventional psychometric intelligence tests measure. The importance of culture in the social construction of a theory of intelligence cannot be overestimated. Reasoning skills, both verbal and nonverbal, the ability to relate to other persons (i.e., social skills), oratory ability, numerical skills, and memory are just examples of the exhaustive list of cognitive skills that can go on any list of what it takes to be intelligent in any particular culture.

Western cultures and their schools of thought tend to emphasize "technological intelligence." Western schooling also emphasizes as indicators of intelligence (1) the ability to generalize, or going beyond the information given, (2) speed, (3) minimal moves to a solution, and (4) creative thinking. Silence in Western culture, and particularly in the United States, is interpreted as a lack of knowledge. In contrast, people may be viewed in another culture as more intelligent if they speak less. A number of cultures on the African continent have conceptions of intelligence that revolve largely around skills that help facilitate and maintain harmonious and stable intergroup relations. The social aspects of intelligence are emphasized.

The reader is cautioned, however, to keep in mind that no one description of culture can capture the complexity of culture for places as diverse as China, Africa, and the United States. Nor is the difference between "Western" and "Eastern" culture as distinctive as the terms appear to indicate. For example, any claim of the culture of the United States and the view of the relationship between human biology and intelligence misses the diversity of views from within European, Latin, Asian, and indigenous groups. As well, each of these groups has a differing perspective on the valuation of a variety of cognitive skills.

Whatever intelligence is, or is not, cognitive skills and adaptive behaviors connected to it are numerous. The list might include such skills as adaptive behavior, learning, problem solving, knowledge acquisition, goal achievement, planning, information coding and processing, attention, symbol manipulation, judgement, attribution, a hodgepodge of cognitive capacities, understanding, purposive thinking, apprehension of experience, mental self-governance, and many more (Eysenck in Detterman, 1994).Cultures (or groups of people) tend to designate as intelligent the cognitive, social, and behavioral attributes they value as adaptive to the requirements of living in those cultures (groups). Although conceptions of intelligence may vary across cultures, the underlying cognitive attributes seemingly do not (Sternberg & Kaufman, 2001).

HISTORY AND BIOLOGICAL APPROACHES TO INTELLIGENCE

Early biological approaches, all pre-1990, included Halstead's suggestion that there were four biologically based abilities: (1) the integrative field factor, (2) the abstraction factor, (3) the power factor, and (4) the directional factor. Halstead attributed all four of these abilities to the functioning of the brain's cortex of the frontal lobes. More influential than Halstead's ideas of biological intelligence were those of Hebb. Hebb distinguished between two basic types of intelligence: Intelligence A, which equated with innate biological potential, and Intelligence B, which equated with the functioning of the brain as a result of the actual development that has occurred. Both Intelligence A and Intelligence B had a biological foundation and Hebb distinguished them from Intelligence C, or intelligence as measured by conventional psychometric tests of intelligence. Hebb's early theory also suggested that learning, an important basis of intelligence, is built up through cell assemblies, by which successfully more and more complex connections among neurons are constructed as learning takes place. Luria's early theory included the idea that the brain consisted of three main units with respect to intelligence: (1) a unit of arousal in the brain stem and midbrain structures; (2) a sensory-input unit in the temporal, parietal, and occipital lobes; and (3) an organization and planning unit in the frontal cortex. Modern biological approaches to intelligence, research, and recent theories have dealt with more specific aspects of brain and neural functioning. Brain nerve conduction velocities, glucose metabolism, and behavior genetics are but a few of the very complex studies recently and presently being pursued (Sternberg & Kaufman, 2001).

Application of the new complexity in brain research can be seen in intelligence research focused on children with disorders such as attention deficit disorder. Neuropsychological processes of alertness, orienting, and executive control and concepts from the neurosciences, and consideration of neural networks with anatomical foci in right prefrontal, posterior parietal, and anterior cingulate brain regions are all being used to help understand the concept of attention deficit (Swanson et al., 1998).

PSYCHOMETRIC APPROACH TO INTELLIGENCE

The psychometric approach to intelligence is among the oldest. In its purest sense it is the operationalization of the biological theory of intelligence. Psychometric tests can be divided into two categories: static and dynamic testing. Static tests are the conventional kind in which people are given problems to solve, and are expected to solve them without feedback. Their final score is typically the number of items answered correctly, sometimes with a penalty for guessing. Psychometric instruments are designed to test basic intelligence and related abilities. A variety of factors can be included in the tests. For example, the third edition of the Wechsler Intelligence Scales for Children offers scores for four factors—verbal comprehension, perceptual organization, processing speed, and freedom from distractibility— but the main scores remain the verbal, performance, and total score. The fourth edition of the Stanford-Binet Intelligence Scale drifts away from the past sole orientation toward general ability that characterized earlier versions and now yields scores for crystallized intelligence, abstract visual reasoning, quantitative reasoning, and short-term memory (Sternberg & Kaufman, 2001).

In dynamic assessment, individuals learn at the time they are completing the psychometric test. If they answer an item incorrectly, they are given guided feedback to help them solve the item. The notion of dynamic testing is generally based on the notion that cognitive abilities are modifiable, and that there is some kind of zone of proximal development, which represents the difference between actually developed intellectual ability and latent capacity (Sternberg & Kaufman, 1998).

Traditionally, psychometric tests of intelligence have focused on the use of maximum performance procedures. Although the modern trend has been for intelligence researchers to move away from the singular focused psychometric instrument and toward multifaceted views of intelligence, not all have agreed.

BELL CURVE CONTROVERSY

The ongoing debate on the singular or multifaceted feature of intelligence has been fueled by the recent publication of books by biological determinants, most notably *The Bell Curve: Intelligence and Class Structure in American Life* (Herrnstein and Murray, 1994). Although this work, and others, are notably focused on the interrelationship among race, socioeconomic status, and social problems, they are based on two central premises: that one's ultimate social position is, to a large extent, the consequence of the inherited characteristic of intelligence (biological); and that the major racial groups differ significantly on this largely predetermined characteristic. Biologically inherited differences in intelligence and other inherited differences among racial groups are then put forth as explanations for black–white differences on such personal and social problems as criminality, parental investment, illegitimacy, and welfare dependency. Moreover, one of the unstated assumptions of this biologically deterministic position is the assumption that race is predominantly a biological rather than a social construction (Gorey & Cryns, 1999).

BROAD THEORIES OF INTELLIGENCE AND OF KINDS OF INTELLIGENCE

The theory of multiple intelligences challenges the notion that intelligence can be considered a general ability, the *g* factor, which cuts across all areas of competence. Rather, Gardner, the developer of the theory of multiple intelligences argues for the existence of seven relatively autonomous intellectual competences: linguistic, musical, logical-mathematical, spatial, bodily-kinesthetic, interpersonal, and intrapersonal. Gardner defines each of the intelligences as the capacity to solve problems or fashion products that are valued in one or more cultural settings. The idea is that intelligence cannot be considered apart from the uses to which it is put or the values of the surrounding community. Intellect cannot be conceptualized or assessed in the abstract. A theory of context is needed to complement a theory of individual competence in order to describe fully and accurately the range of human intelligences (Krechevsky & Gardner in Detterman, 1994).

The trend toward broad theories of intelligence continues with consideration of successful intelligence, emotional intelligence, and others. Successful intelligence is hypothesized as the ability to adapt to, shape, and select environments to accomplish one's goals and those of one's society and culture. A successfully intelligent person theoretically balances adaptation, shaping, and selection, doing each as necessary. Three broad abilities are important to successful intelligence: analytical, creative, and practical (Sternberg & Kaufman, 2001).

Emotional intelligence is an idea introduced by Salovey and Mayer and is the ability to perceive accurately, appraise, and express emotion; the ability to access and/or generate feelings when they facilitate thought; the ability to understand emotion and emotional knowledge; and the ability to regulate emotions to promote emotional and intellectual growth (Sternberg & Kaufman, 2001). Research studies continue in the area of emotional intelligence. For example, Mehrabian (2000) recently defined emotional success as general happiness and satisfaction with life and attempted to look beyond IQ as a measure of intelligence. He speculated as to the use of emotional intelligence as a broad-based measurement of individual success potential.

IMPLICATIONS FOR SOCIAL WORK PRACTICE

The implications of a social work practitioner and/or a social work student understanding the relationship between what we know about human biology and intellect are many and profound. Social work practitioners and students, aware of the complexity of biological theories of intelligence, both historical and present day, can resist the inclination to rely on simplistic models of intelligence. Understanding the uncertainty that pervades the community of intelligence researchers and our limited ability to operationalize the concept of intelligence allows social work practitioners and students to (1) feel more confident, (2) understand the impact of intelligence testing or assessment on the lives of their clients, (3) challenge the notions of limited intelligence unfairly or unknowingly placed on their clients, (4) utilize biologically based assessments of intelligence, primarily a measure of g via the implementation of psychometric testing, in adaptive case planning, and (5) understand the potential for cultural bias. Social workers with a basic knowledge of the theoretical foundations of intelligence can play a more meaningful role in systemic assessment of people and their environments. The different theories of intelligence can help social workers understand how people and their environments influence one another. This will help social workers to acknowledge, at least in theory, the importance of multiple factors (not just heritable intelligence) in the development of both personal (e.g., bipolar disorder) and social difficulties (e.g., race relations) (Gorey & Cryns, 1999).

Well-informed social work practitioners will be able to explain the uncertainty of any determination of a client's "intelligence." If so, social workers can more easily recognize and possibly soften the negative effects of intelligence testing and intelligence research on clients who are members of oppressed groups. Well-informed social work practitioners and social work students will be able to explain at least the basics of the g factor, the biological theory of intelligence, and the difference in merits of singular factor (g) or multifaceted factor (schooling, family income, social versus emotional versus general intelligence) considerations of intelligence.

Social work practitioners and students aware of the concept of "contextualism" in any theory of intelligence, but particularly as it relates to the biological theory of intelligence, will understand that the nature of context is quite broad. Contextualism, the recognition of the impact of environment, includes consideration of the physical, historical, and social contexts within which a person's thought process unfolds. As well, contextualism includes consideration of relevant background knowledge that individuals bring with them to the intelligence testing situation and the attainment value that people attach to successful performance on intelligence tests.

DISCUSSION QUESTIONS

1. What are the differences between the concepts of biological intelligence and psychometric intelligence?

2. If researchers have been studying the concept of intellect for so long, what are some of the reasons why it is so hard to specify exactly what it is?

3. What are the merits of psychometric testing for social work practice?

4. How can intellect be positively associated with both a positive outcome, such as years of school completed, and a negative outcome, such as participation in criminal behavior?

5. What does the emphasis in Western culture on speed of thinking as a sign of intellect mean for social work clients who are members of oppressed groups?

CHAPTER SEVEN

THE HUMAN GENOME PROJECT

Humans are much more than simply the product of a genome, but in a sense we are both collectively and individually, defined within the genome. The mapping, sequencing and analysis of the human genome is therefore a fundamental advance in self-knowledge; it will strike a personal chord with many people. And application of this knowledge will, in time, materially benefit almost everyone in the world.

—Dennis, Richard, and Campbell (2001)

Humanity has been given a great gift. With the completion of the human genome sequence, we have received a powerful tool for unlocking the secrets of our genetic heritage and for finding our place among the other participants in the adventure of life.

—Jasny and Kennedy (2001)

The human genome underlies the fundamental unity of all members of the human family, as well as the recognition of their inherent dignity and diversity. In a symbolic sense, it is the heritage of humanity.

—Universal Declaration on the Human Genome and Human Rights

The history of genetics research that predates and underpins the widely publicized Human Genome Project (HGP) started in the late nineteenth century. Amazing leaps in understanding the relationship among genetics, human biology, human behavior, and the general quality of human life have been made during the past 140 years of genetics research. As with past genetic research, the HGP is both singularly important and also one more piece of knowledge in the larger puzzle of human biology. Unlike much of the past genetic research, which has either been obscure or maligned for misguided intentions, the HGP has been viewed positively by the public. Numerous articles in the popular press have touted the HGP as a commendable scientific endeavor that will result in new medical interventions that improve the quality and extend the length of life.

The positive public opinion surrounding the HGP has not deterred a vigorous debate about the ethical and moral concerns raised by genetics research. The concerns raised about the HGP are not significantly different in tenor from the concerns raised between the 1920s and 1950s, when genetics research first came to the public's attention. During both periods there were concerns about the misuse of genetic information and meddling with the natural course of human reproductive processes (i.e., inheritance). The two time periods have different foci, with much of the debate surrounding the HGP concerning employment and health care issues and the use of genetic information by individuals to control the genetic make-up of their offspring.

During the earlier period of genetics research, the primary focus of concern was government control of reproduction with the end goal of perfecting the human race, sometimes called "eugenics." In many ways, the goal was similar to the concepts applied to animal breeding. The HGP has changed the level of genetic knowledge available to the public. As well, the project has changed the level of medical intervention possible in the genetic process. The completion of the HGP means that once hypothetical concerns about genetic control of the human population are possible, thereby moving genetic manipulation of reproduction from the realm of science fiction to the realm of the possible.

The scientific process behind the HGP, with competing labs, one public and one private, each using a distinct methodology, is as interesting as the findings. The two labs pursued the same goal in parallel, which created an opportunity to test two significantly different methodologies in sequencing the human genome. The private lab used a shotgun approach and the public lab used a direct sequencing method, both of which are discussed later in the chapter. The separate funding streams for the labs also highlighted a long-held debate about whether research funding should come from private or public sources. Despite these differences, the conclusions varied insignificantly and just enough to keep the competition between the two labs interesting.

One less public outcome of the HGP is the intensive reexamination of the paradigm of evolution. A number of scientific fields, including biology and paleontology, rely on the paradigm of evolution to structure theory and therefore the direction of research questions. This means that the findings from the HGP may alter the knowledge that underpins a number of sciences, causing shifts in the fabric of scientific theory and, in turn, the direction of research questions. For example, the recent findings of the HGP alter the long-held theory that each gene produced one specific protein, which played a role in one identifiable trait. Now scientists theorize that one gene produces a number of different proteins. This finding has resulted in a growing interest in the functions of proteins, which appear to play a larger role in the development of traits than once thought. Later in the chapter the idea of significant shifts in our understanding of the roles genes play in inheritance, human biology, and the general quality of life experienced by human beings are explored.

ROLE OF GENES IN HUMAN INHERITANCE

To aid in the discussion about the HGP, a brief review of inheritance and the role of genes are covered in this section. A good starting place is with DNA (deoxyribonucleic acid), which is the genetic material we inherit from our biological parents. It is arranged by genes, which are located on 23 pairs of chromosomes, 46 in total, with one set from each biological parent. According to Terwilliger and Ott (1994, p. 2), specifically, DNA is "composed of a linear arrangement of similar molecules . . . whose sequence forms a code that contains information defining the structure of various protein molecules to be synthesized by the cell, the regulation of the production of these molecules, and a great many other functions, the entirety of which define much of what a person will become."

Alleles, which are mentioned throughout the chapter, are the different forms of a gene. Alleles produce structurally different proteins that affect how the protein functions. For example, in humans there are two forms of the gene that determines the shape of the earlobe, free from the head or attached to the head. These different forms of the gene are called alleles. When the alleles from the biological parents are the same it is referred to as a dominant trait, and when the two are different it is referred to as a recessive trait (Terwilliger & Ott, 1994). In the case of human earlobes, free ones are the dominant trait and attached are the recessive trait.

ADDITIONAL TERMS RELATED TO DNA AND GENES

Some terms associated with DNA and genes that are important to understanding the HGP include the following:

Exon: The region of a gene's DNA that encodes a portion of its protein. Exons are interspersed with noncoding introns.

Intron: The region of a gene's DNA that is not translated into a protein.

Homologous genes: Genes with similar structures and functions.

Coding DNA: Sequences transcribed into protein structures; also called exons.

Repetitive DNA: Sequences of varying lengths that occur in multiple copies in the genome; they represent much of the genome.

Pseudogene: A sequence of DNA similar to a gene but nonfunctional; probably the remnant of a once functional gene that accumulated mutations.

Polymorphism: A variation in DNA sequence within a population.

Regulatory region: A segment of DNA that controls whether a gene will be expressed and to what degree.

Parenthetically, it is interesting to note that one of the realizations of the HGP suggests that all members of a species have almost identical gene structures. That is, whether people are of one skin color or another, short or tall, or have other differences among them, the aggregate gene structures are almost the same—except for the small numbers of elements associated with the differences.

The end product of gene alleles, the protein process and the environment interacting is a phenotype. "Phenotype is the observed physical or functional traits that characterized an individual" (Johnson, 2001, p. 470). Specific phenotypes seen in individuals are thought to form through the interaction between their genotype and the environment. The next large frontier for research is to understand the interaction of genes in the environment in creating particular phenotypes. For most phenotypes this relationship will be complex and contain many factors but, for some, such as the earlobe example, genetics may play a large, almost singular role. Finally, when the word *genome* is used, it means the complete set of genes and alleles inherited from biological parents.

HISTORICAL HIGHLIGHTS
OF GENETICS RESEARCH

A number of notable researchers have laid the structural groundwork leading to the HGP. First is Gregor Mendel, who was briefly mentioned in Chapter 5. His genetic research published in 1866 was specifically aimed at studying several observable characteristics in pea plants through which he identified the fundamental principles of genetics. His methodology, which was both scientifically and mathematically rigorous, involved examining the results of cross-pollination on seven characteristics—flower color, flower position, seed color, seed shape, pod shape, pod color, and stem length—all of which had two distinct forms (Hawley & Mori, 1999). This method of studying genetics by examining the occurrence of the expressed forms of gene (i.e., phenotype) has been, until recently, the standard methodology for studying the influence of genetics upon inheritance, human biology, and behavior. There are two basic laws called Mendel's Laws of Genetics. The first law pertains to the purity and constancy of the gene. It states that genes are received from the parent and they will be passed on to the next generation in a precise and faithful fashion. The second law states that the offspring will receive one copy of each gene from the parent and will transmit only one copy to each gamete (sex cell) (Hawley & Mori, 1999).

Thomas Hunt Morgan in the early 1900s, using fruit flies, discovered the process of crossover between chromosomes, which results in recombinant chromosomes that are different from the chromosomes of the biological parents. This was a significant break from Mendel's Laws. The crossover effect creates diversity in offspring and confirms the relationship between chromosome behavior and inheritance. Morgan received the Nobel Prize in 1933 for his research. One of Morgan's students, Alfred H. Sturtevant, used the crossover data to develop one of the first methods for mapping the location of genes on chromosomes (Bodmer & McKie, 1997).

The next leap in genetics came in the 1920s when Frederick Griffith, a minister of health in London, discovered two forms of bacteria—smooth and rough. The rough bacteria were found to not be deadly whereas smooth bacteria were found to be deadly. When the smooth bacteria were heated they were rendered innocuous. This was demonstrated by injecting smooth bacteria that had been heated into mice without killing the mice. When heated smooth bacteria and live rough bacteria were injected together into a mouse, the bacteria killed the mouse. This experiment linked the death to a genetic transformation in the bacteria that resulted from combining the two types together (Bodmer & McKie, 1997).

Oswald Avery of the Rockefeller Institute of New York repeated Griffith's experiments in 1943 and discovered the "transforming principle" working in the bacteria. Avery named the transforming principle within the bacteria DNA. The methodology he used to identify DNA consisted of adding a drop of absolute ethyl alcohol to a solution that contained bacteria. The alcohol precipitated out "a fibrous substance" which, after stirring, wrapped itself around a glass rod, leaving behind the rest. The material that had wrapped itself around the glass rod was strands of DNA (Bodmer & McKie, 1997).

Alexander Todd in 1948 established how the chemical components of DNA were linked. His discovery led to identifying the backbone of DNA as being made of sugar and phosphate groups (sugar=deoxyribose). One of four possible bases is attached to each sugar on the opposite of the phosphate link: adenine (A) with thymine (T) and cytosine (C) with guanine (G). These pairs are known as pyrimidines. Todd received the Nobel Prize for his work in 1957 (Bodmer & McKie, 1997).

James D. Watson, Maurice H. Wilkins, and Francis H. C. Crick discovered the double-helix structure of DNA, publishing the information in the April 25, 1953, issue of the journal *Nature* (Bodmer & McKie, 1997). In 1972, Paul Berg and coworkers created the first recombinant DNA molecule. Five years later in 1977, Allan Maxam and Walter Gilbert at Harvard University and Fredrick Sanger from the United Kingdom Medical Research Council (MRC) invented the gel electrophoresis technique, which was used to sequence DNA. This process consists of subjecting a mixture of DNA molecules to an electrical charge that forces the strands through a jellylike material. When the charge is stopped, the strands of DNA molecules are trapped in the gel, with longer molecules toward the top of the gel, because they move slowly, and short molecules near the bottom. Paul Berger, Walter Gilbert, and Fredrick Sanger won the Nobel Prize in 1980 for developing methods to map the structure and function of DNA. By 1984, MRC scientists had identified the complete DNA sequence of a virus (1,700 genes) (Pennisi, 2001a). The completion of the virus DNA sequence led to discussions among researchers around the world who were interested in genetics and wanted to decipher the human genome.

The Human Genome Project's Development

The U.S. Human Genome Project began formally in 1990. Early discussions between the National Institute of Health (NIH), the Department of Energy (DOE), scientists from academia, and scientists working in the private sector resulted in disputes about credit, funding, patents, and methodology. Acrimony between the NIH and DOE was high as the two departments competed for control of the project.

During this period one of the central problems to completing the project was a lack of appropriate tools (Roberts, 2001). For example, the scientists that completed the 1,700-gene genome of a virus took 7 years using the current method of gel electrophoresis technique. The process of creating and reading the gels with DNA molecules is a labor-intensive and arduous process.

By October 1990, the groups and individuals that were to be involved in deciphering the human genome began the project. Initially, five labs were funded by streams of money from the NIH and DOE and through the National Center for Human Genome Research (NCHGR) were charged with sequencing different portions of the human genome. Because of the methodological limitations, scientists believed that a revolutionary technology was needed to sequence the human genome. Ultimately, the technology and methods evolved together over a relatively short period of time. Eventually, the HGP came to rely on a method called direct sequencing. The process of direct sequencing involves starting with small sections of DNA whose location on chromosomes is known, breaking them into pieces, and then successively sequencing the DNA from neighboring pieces of chromosome, thereby building larger pieces of known DNA. Originally the complete sequence of the human genome was planned to take 15 years, but rapid advances in sequencing and data storage technology have accelerated the expected completion date from 2005 to 2003, decreasing the expected time necessary to 13 years (Pennisi, 2001a).

Currently, sixteen labs conduct research on some part of the human genome for the public project. In 1997 the NCHGR became the National Human Genome Research Institute (NHGRI), and NIH took sole control over the Institute. At the same time, the DOE created the Joint Genome Institute (JGI). JGI and NHGRI provide the public funding for these centers through a grant process, which is similar to other federal entities that support research. There are ten other sequencing labs located in Eastern Europe, China, and Japan funded by their respective governments (Pennisi, 2001a).

In 1998, J. Craig Vente, one of the scientists involved in the early years of the HGP announced that he had opened a lab with private funding and planned to complete the human genome in 3 years. Celera, the private lab, started with 300 newly invented automated sequencers and a different sequencing methodology called shotgun sequencing. Shotgun sequencing starts with cutting up DNA into small fragments, sequencing the fragments, and reassembling them with a computer by searching for overlapping ends. This method was used in 1994–1995 to sequence the whole genome of a free living organism (*Haemophilus influenzae*, a bacteria) for the first time (Marshall, 2001a; Roberts, 2001). The public project had refused to fund research using the shotgun technique, claiming it would not work. However, the appearance of Celera and the jockeying between the two research teams is credited for the shorter time frame in completing a map by the public effort.

The research goal for both research teams was straightforward—to identify and sequence all the genes in human DNA. Identification means, in this case, to establish the various alleles associated with particular genes and sequencing refers to ascertaining the pinpoint location of genes along chromosomes. By accomplishing these tasks, the research teams hope to contribute significantly to the understanding of the specific roles that genes play in the biological functioning of human beings. Since the inception of genetics as a science, the relationship between genes, biology, heredity, and behavior has remained a central question. Findings from the HGP to date indicate that identifying the various alleles associated with genes will rely on determining the sequences of the three billion chemical bases that make up human DNA.

A timeline including the names and accomplishments of the many scientists involved in the HGP reprinted from *Science* follows. The timeline provides an in-depth review of significant dates and accomplishments associated with the HGP.

■ ■ ■ ■ ■ ▬▬▬▬▬▬▬▬▬▬▬▬▬▬▬▬▬▬▬▬▬▬▬▬▬▬▬▬▬▬▬▬▬▬▬

TIMELINE FOR THE HUMAN GENOME PROJECT

A History of the Human Genome Project 2001

(Reprinted with permission of *Science* [2001, Feb 9], *291*, p. 1195.)

1953

April	James Watson and Francis Crick discover the double helical structure of DNA (*Nature*).

1972

October	Paul Berg and co-workers create the first recombinant DNA molecule (*PNAS*).

1977

February	Allan Maxam and Walter Gilbert at Harvard University (*PNAS*) and
May	David Botstein of the Massachusetts Institute of Technology, Ronald Davis of Stanford University, and Mark Skolnick and Ray White of the University of Utah propose a method to map the entire human genome based on RFLPs (*American Journal of Human Genetics*).
December	Frederick Sanger at the U.K. Medical Research Council independently develop methods for sequencing DNA (*PNAS*).

1982

	Akiyoshi Wada, now at RIKEN in Japan, proposes automated sequencing and gets support to build robots from Hitachi.

1984

May	Charles Cantor and David Schwartz of Columbia University develop pulsed field electrophoresis (*Cell*).
July	MRC scientists decipher the complete DNA sequence of the Epstein-Barr virus, 170 kb (*Nature*).

(continued)

CONTINUED

1985

May   Robert Sinsheimer hosts a meeting at the University of California (UC), Santa Cruz, to discuss the feasibility of sequencing the human genome.

December   Kary Mullis and colleagues at Cetus Corp. develop PCR, a technique to replicate vast amounts of DNA (*Science*).

1986

February   Sydney Brenner of MRC urges the European Union to undertake a concerted program to map and sequence the human genome; Brenner also starts a small genome initiative at MRC.

March   The U.S. Department of Energy (DOE) hosts a meeting in Santa Fe, New Mexico, to discuss plans to sequence the human genome.

March   Renato Dulbecco of the Salk Institute promotes sequencing the human genome in a paper (*Science*).

June   Merits of a human genome project are hotly debated at a meeting at Cold Spring Harbor Laboratory in New York state, "The Molecular Biology of *Homo sapiens*."

June   Leroy Hood and Lloyd Smith of the California Institute of Technology (Caltech) and colleagues announce the first automated DNA sequencing machine (*Nature*).

September Charles Delisi begins genome studies at DOE, reallocating $5.3 million from the fiscal year 1987 budget.

1987

February   Walter Gilbert resigns from the U.S. National Research Council (NRC) genome panel and announces plan to start Genome Corp., with the goal of sequencing and copyrighting the human genome and selling data for profit.

April   An advisory panel suggests that DOE should spend $1 billion on mapping and sequencing the human genome over the next 7 years and that DOE should lead the U.S. effort. DOE's Human Genome initiative begins.

May   David Burke, Maynard Olson, and George Carle of Washington University in St. Louis develop YACs for cloning, increasing insert size 10-fold (*Science*).

October   Helen Donis-Keller and colleagues at Collaborative Research Inc. publish the "first" genetic map with 403 markers, sparking a fight over credit and priority (*Cell*).

October   DuPont scientists develop a system for rapid DNA sequencing with fluorescent chain-terminating dideoxynucleotides (*Science*).

October   Applied Biosystems Inc. puts the first automated sequencing machine, based on Hood's technology, on the market.

1988

February   In a pivotal report, the NRC endorses the Human Genome Project (HGP), calling for a phased approach and a rapid scale-up to $200 million a year of new money.

March   Prompted by advisers at a meeting in Reston, Virginia, James Wyngaarden, then director of the National Institutes of Health (NIH), decides that the agency should be a major player in the HGP, effectively seizing the lead from DOE.

June   The first annual genome meeting is held at Cold Spring Harbor Laboratory.

September   NIH establishes the Office of Human Genome Research and snags Watson as its head. Watson declares that 3% of the genome budget should be devoted to studies of social and ethical issues.

October   NIH and DOE sign a memorandum of understanding and agree to collaborate on the HGP.

1989

January   Norton Zinder of Rockefeller University chairs the first program advisory committee meeting for the HGP.

September   Olson, Hood, Botstein, and Cantor outline a new mapping strategy, using STSs (*Science*).

September   DOE and NIH start a joint committee on the ethical, legal, and social implications of the HGP.

October   NIH office is elevated to the National Center for Human Genome Research (NCHGR), with grant-awarding authority.

1990

                  Three groups develop capillary electrophoresis, one team led by Lloyd Smith (*Nucleic Acids Research*, August), the second by Barry Karger (*Analytical Chemistry*, January), and the third by Norman Dovichi (*Journal of Chromatography*, September).

April   NH and DOE publish a 5-year plan. Goals include a complete genetic map, a physical map with markers every 100 kb, and sequencing of an aggregate of 20 Mb of DNA in model organisms by 2005.

August   NIH begins large-scale sequencing trials on four model organisms: *Mycoplasma capricolum, Escherichia coli, Caenorhabditis elegans,* and *Saccharomyces cerevisiae*. Each research group agrees to sequence to 3 Mb at 75 cents a base within 3 years.

October   NIH and DOE restart the clock, declaring 1 October the official beginning of the HGP.

(continued)

CONTINUED

October	David Lipman, Eugene Myers, and colleagues at the National Center for Biotechnology Information (NCBI) publish the BLAST algorithm for aligning sequences (*Journal of Molecular Biology*).
June	NIH biologist J. Craig Venter announces a strategy to find expressed genes, using ESTs (*Science*). A fight erupts at a congressional hearing 1 month later, when Venter reveals that NIH if filing patent applications on thousands of these partial genes.
October	The Japanese rice genome sequencing effort begins.
December	Edward Uberbacher of Oak Ridge National Laboratory in Tennessee develops GRAIL, the first of many gene-finding programs (*PNAS*).

1992

April	After a dispute with then-NIH director Bernadine Healy over patenting partial genes, Watson resigns as head of NCHGR.
June	Venter leaves NIH to set up The Institute for Genomic Research (TIGR), a nonprofit in Rockville, Maryland. William Haseltine heads its sister company, Human Genome Sciences, to commercialize TIGR products.
July	Britain's Wellcome Trust enters the HGP with $95 million.
September	Mel Simon of Caltech and colleagues develop BAC's for cloning (*PNAS*).
October	U.S. and French teams complete the first physical maps of chromosomes.
October	David Page and colleagues of the Whitehead Institute map the Y chromosome (*Science*); Daniel Cohen of the Centre d'Etude du Polymophisme Humain (CEPH) and Génétheon and colleagues map chromosome 21 (*Nature*).
December	After lengthy debate, NIH and DOE release guidelines on sharing data and resources, encouraging rapid sharing and enabling researchers to keep data for 6 months.
December	U.S. and French teams complete the genetic maps of mouse and human: mouse, average marker spacing 4.3 cM, Eric Lander and colleagues at Whitehead (*Genetics*, June); human, average marker spacing 5 cM, Jean Weissenbach and colleagues at CEPH (*Nature*, October).

1993

April	Francis Collins of the University of Michigan is named director of NCHGR.
October	NIH and DOE publish a revised plan for 1993–98. The goals include sequencing 80 Mb of DNA by the end of 1998 and completing the human genome by 2005.

October   The Wellcome Trust and MRC open the Sanger Centre at Hinxton Hall, south of Cambridge, U.K. Led by John Sulston, the center becomes one of the major sequencing labs in the international consortium.

October   The GenBank database officially moves from Los Alamos to NCBI, ending NIH's and DOE's tussle over control.

1994

September   Jeffrey Murray of the University of Iowa, Cohen of Genethon, and colleagues publish a genetic linkage map of the human genome, with an average marker spacing of 0.7 cM (*Science*).

1995

May to   Richard Mathies and colleagues at UC Berkeley and Amersham
August   develop improved sequencing dyes (*PNAS*, May); Michael Reeve and Carl Fuller at Amersham develop thermostable polynerase (*Nature*, August).

July   Venter and Claire Frasier of TIGR and Hamilton Smith of Johns Hopkins publish the first sequence of a free-living organism, *Hamophilus influenzae*, 1.8 Mb (*Science*).

September   The Japanese government funds several sequencing groups for a total of $15.9 million over 5 years: Tokai University, University of Tokyo, and Keio University.

October   Patrick Brown of Stanford and colleagues publish first paper using a printed glass microarray of complimentary DNA (cDNA) probes (*Science*).

December   Researchers at Whitehead and Généthon (led by Lander and Thomas Hudson at Whitehead) publish a physical map of the human genome containing 15,000 markers (*Science*).

1996

February   At a meeting in Bermuda funded by the Wellcome Trust, international HGP partners agree to release sequence data into public databases within 24 hours.

April   NIH funds six groups to attempt large-scale sequencing of the human genome.

April   Affymetrix makes DNA chips commercially available.

September   DOE initiates 6 pilot projects, funded at $5 million total, to sequence the ends of BAC clones.

October   An international consortium publicly releases the complete genome sequence of the yeast *S. cerevisiae* (*Science*).

November   Yoshihide Hayashizaki's group at RIKEN completes the first set of full-length mouse cDNAs.

(continued)

CONTINUED

1997

January	NCHGR is promoted to the National Human Genome Research Institute; DOE creates the Joint Genome Institute.
September	Fred Blattner, Guy Plunkett, and University of Wisconsin, Madison, colleagues complete the DNA sequence of *E. coli*, 5 Mb (Science).
September	Molecular Dynamics introduces the MegaBACE, a capillary sequencing machine.

1998

January	NIH announces a new project to find SNPs.
February	Representatives of Japan, the U.S., the E.U., China, and South Korea meet in Tsukuba, Japan, to establish guidelines for an international collaboration to sequence the rice genome.
March	Phil Green and Brent Ewing of Washington University and colleagues publish a program called phred for automatically interpreting sequencer data (*Genetic Research*). Both phred and its sister program phrap (used for assembling sequences) had been in wide use since 1995.
May	PE Biosystems Inc. introduces the PE Prism 3700 capillary sequencing machine.
May	Venter announces a new company named Celera and declares that it will sequence the human genome within 3 years for $300 million.
May	In response, the Wellcome Trust doubles its support for the HGP to $330 million, taking on responsibility for one-third of the sequencing.
October	NIH and DOE throw HGP into overdrive with a new goal of creating "working draft" of the human genome by 2001, and they move the completion date for the finished draft from 2005 to 2003.
December	Sulston of the Sanger Centre and Robert Waterston of Washington University and colleagues complete the genomic sequence of *C. elegans* (*Science*).

1999

March	NIH again moves up the completion date for the rough draft, to spring 2000. Large-scale sequencing efforts are concentrated in centers at Whitehead, Washington University, Baylor, Sanger, and DOE's Joint Genome Institute.
April	Ten companies and the Wellcome Trust launch the SNP consortium, with plans to publicly release data quarterly.
September	NIH launches a project to sequence the mouse genome, devoting $130 million over 3 years.
December	British, Japanese, and U.S. researchers complete the first sequence of a human chromosome, number 22 (*Nature*).

2000

March	Celera and academic collaborators sequence the 180 Mb genome of the fruit fly, *Drosophilia melanogaster,* the largest genome yet sequenced and a validation of Venter's controversial whole-genome shotgun method (*Science*).
March	Because of disagreement over a data-release policy, plans for HGP and Celera to collaborate disintegrate amid considerable sniping.
May	HGP consortium led by German and Japanese researchers publishes the complete sequence of chromosome 21 (*Nature*).
June	At a White House ceremony, HGP and Celera jointly announce working drafts of the human genome sequence, declare their feud at an end, and promise simultaneous publication.
October	DOE and MRC launch a collaborative project to sequence the genome of the puffer fish, *Fugu rubripes,* by March 2001.
December	An international consortium completes the sequencing of the first plant *Arabidopsis thaliana,* 125 Mb.
December	HGP and Celera's plans for joint publication in *Science* collapse; HGP sends its paper to *Nature.*

2001

February	The HGP consortium publishes its working draft in *Nature* (15 February), and Celera publishes its draft in *Science* (16 February).

Findings from the Human Genome Project

At the beginning of the HGP, the theorized number of genes in the human genome ranged between 80,000 and 100,000. Findings from the HGP suggest that this range is nearly three times the number of genes found in the human genome. The public research team has identified a rough draft of the human genome by comparing unknown portions of the gene sequence to high-resolution maps of chromosome 16 and 19 developed at the DOE Lab at Los Alamos (direct sequencing). The public effort as of 2001 predicts there are 31,780 genes contained in the human genome. Celera, the private lab, also has a rough draft of the human genome that suggests there are 39,114 genes, using a shotgun method (Baltimore, 2001). The differences between the two research teams' findings highlight the ambiguity of pinning down details of this subject. Both research teams have stated that the precise gene count may not be known for years to come.

The two research teams have rough sequences for 90 percent of the chromosome areas that contain high concentrations of genes. The estimated size of the human genome, in terms of the chemical bases that determine protein structures, is 3.2 gigabases (Gb) or 3.2 billion chemical bases (Baltimore, 2001). Comparatively, the first free-living organism mapped, *Haemophilus influenzae,* a bacterium, has

1.8 megabases (Mb) or 1.8 million chemical bases. Surprisingly, only between 1.1 percent and 1.5 percent of the gene-rich regions actually encode proteins, which are control cell development (Baltimore, 2001). More than half of DNA is made up of various types of repeated sequences including four classes of elements from parasitic DNA, repeats of just a few bases, and recent duplications of large segments of DNA (Baltimore, 2001). Some scientists predict that these large areas, once thought of as desolate, will yield interesting functions such as the on/off switch that tells genes when to perform their functions.

Since the inception of the HGP, approximately 200 disease-related genes have been identified, including the gene responsible for cystic fibrosis (Chakravarti, 2001; Jimeniz-Sanchez, Childs, & Valle, 2001; Peltonen & McKusick, 2001). For 7 years researchers sought to identify the gene associated with cystic fibrosis because it is a known monogenetic disorder. This means the relationship between the gene involved and the phenotype is simple and direct, unlike most gene–phenotype relationships. Cystic fibrosis affects some 30,000 people in the United States; about 1 in every 29 people carry the allele that leads to it. The average age of death for people who have cystic fibrosis is 31. The genetic underpinning of other monogenic disorders included Huntington's disease, early-onset Alzheimer's disease, and Fragile X, a form of mental retardation, has progressed quickly as the human genome is sequenced. There has also been movement toward understanding the genetic role in multifaceted disorders such as late onset Alzheimer's disease, attention deficit hyperactivity disorder, dyslexia, and schizophrenia. Beyond diseases and disorders, there has been interest in the relationship between genetics and behavior. For example, genetic components are identified as one of many factors that cause aggression and homosexuality.

Some long-held theories about the functioning of genes have been altered due to findings from the HGP. For example, how scientists view the architecture of chromosomes and distributions of genes and geneless areas along chromosomes is significantly different than before the HGP. Scientists are particularly fascinated by the aforementioned low percentage of the genes that actually code for proteins, the occurrence of massive chromosome sections where there are repeated sequences, and the fact that the human genome seems to share 223 genes with bacteria, that do not exist in the other genomes sequenced (Baltimore, 2001; Galas, 2001).

Previous to the HGP, biologists believed that genes came in sets of various alleles, all of which produced one specific protein that resulted in an expressed trait. Using the earlobe example from earlier in the chapter, if a person received two genes, one from each parent, with the recessive allele for attached earlobes, the alleles would produce the specific protein that resulted in the expressed form of attached earlobes. Now the various alleles associated with a gene are believed to produce a wide array of proteins. Specifically, splicer proteins rearrange RNA transcripts, resulting in hundreds of different possible proteins from a single gene. Beyond the sheer number of proteins, one protein may play a role in several expressed traits, and, conversely, more than one protein may be involved in an expressed trait. Furthermore, the relationship between the genes and proteins may be influenced by the larger cellular structure in which it is embedded (Commoner,

2002; Fields, 2001). This makes the goal of identifying all possible alleles of genes a difficult and elusive task that is likely to take a significant number of years despite the aforementioned methodological advances.

The role of proteins as mediators in the process of genes acting on the molecular process in a way that controls the occurrence of inherited traits has become an area of research that some predict will surpass the field of genetics in the quest to understand human biological functioning. For example, in 1997 Stanley B. Prusiner won the Nobel Prize for his work concerning the role of nucleic-acid-free proteins, or "prions," in how disease infects living organisms. The finding helps explain why normal sterilization methods do not protect against mad cow disease (bovine spongiform encephalopathy) (Commoner, 2002).

Of equal importance are the technological developments that resulted from the HGP. In fact, the study of genetic and biological data with statistical techniques and computers is now known as bioinformatics. Because of the data storage and data analysis needs associated with sequencing process, the HGP developed faster, more efficient computer technologies that expanded data analysis methods and storage beyond frontiers thought not possible. For example, BLAST is a computer program that was created to find genes that are shared by different organisms (Roos, 2001). The process of analyzing numerous identifiers to make comparisons between objects like genes has applications in other sciences that would like to expand the number and complexity of factors involved in understanding an object, interaction, or phenomenon under study. The goal of creating databases to store the massive amount of data gathered by the HGP has pushed computer scientists to create complex databases that allow the public to access the data collected by the HGP. The improvements in database technology have also resulted in wide, sweeping improvements for other scientific endeavors.

Beyond data analysis and storage methods, the introduction of automated sequencers by the company Molecular Dynamics in 1997 removed much of the tedious, labor-intensive work involved in sequencing from human beings (i.e., lab technicians) to machines. In 1998, a competing automated sequencing machine was introduced by PE Biosystems. The machines created by PE Biosystems are used by Celera. The success of both research teams, particularly in the improvement of speed, is directly linked to the development of these machines. The sequencing of genomes as a result of these machines has grown at exponential rates (Marshall, 2001b; Roberts, 2001).

Finally, since 1990 when the HGP began, the methodologies used to decipher the human genome have also been used to understand other genomes that were presumably less complex. As mentioned earlier, the first free-living genome was sequenced in 1995. The genome of yeast with one nuclide was completed in 1997 and the first animal (mouse) genome was completed in 1998. By 2000, approximately two dozen genomes were completed, including those of the fruit fly, the nematode, *Caenorhabditis elegans,* a simple worm, and prokaryotes like *E coli.* Deciphering these genomes has helped refine the methodology used to read the human genome as well as provide comparison points (Rubin, 2001; Stoneking, 2001).

As a result of comparing genomes, scientists have discovered that many of the genes identified in the human genome are similar to genes identified in other organisms. The number of chemical bases associated with the genes is smaller in less complex organisms, indicating that what differentiates humans from fruit flies is the complexity in how genes function. Complex organisms, such as the mouse, which is a mammal long known to share a significant number of biological traits with humans, share not only similar genomes, but the same number of chemical bases (approximately 3 Gb) (Rubin, 2001).

Future of the Human Genome Project

For the immediate future, both research teams are working on finishing the rough draft of the human genome. As the sixteen labs charged with conducting the research for the public project start to differentiate themselves in focus, there is concern that some may turn to more profitable genomic research before the sequence is complete (Pennisi, 2001b). The smaller labs, which have limited sequencing capacity in comparison to some of the ever-growing larger labs like the one at Whitehead/MIT Genome Center and Sanger Centre in England, are interested in developing the tools necessary to interpret the finds from the HGP (Pennisi, 2001b). The tools developed by these labs will be used to study the role genes play in human development, human behavior, as well as the occurrence of disease. The larger labs, which have made huge investments in sequencing tools, remain focused on the process of sequencing genomes. The goal of sequencing other living organisms is also considered a useful tool in building a better understanding of gene functioning.

Researchers are already examining other genomes as a method of elucidating the relationship between genes, the environment, and the final expressed trait seen in individuals (i.e., phenotype). Researchers have also begun comparing genomes from different organisms in an attempt to clarify the exact processes involved in evolution. For example, the growing interest to sequence the genomes of primates resulted in the chimpanzee genome being sequenced in 2002. Only about 1.3 percent of the chimpanzee genome is different from the human genome, but this difference in genes results in over 50 million different chemical bases, meaning that the genetic difference accounts for a significant level of developmental variation. Initial indications show that the primary difference between humans and chimpanzees is linked to the proteins associated with brain development (Kotulak, 2002).

Once the immediate goal of completing a finished sequence of the human genome is accomplished, the task of interpreting the human genome will require decades of research. The immediate questions of interest are not as lofty as understanding gene functioning or the process of evolution. The initial building blocks to the process of understanding gene functioning include answering the following questions: (1) When and how are genes turned on? (2) How do chromosomes work generationally? (3) What parts of the human genome produce proteins?

Because of the financial and humanitarian issues associated with identifying the genetic underpinnings of the diseases that afflict human kind, the research teams will continue to work in this area. As a result, the findings from the HGP are expected to create a significant shift in biomedical research. To date, the focus of biomedical research has been on structural genomics, monogenetic disorders, and analysis of single genes. The future of biomedical research is likely to be focused on functional genomics, proteomics, multifactor disorders, and analysis of multi-gene interactions (Chakravarti, 2001). These shifts in research focus represent a significant leap forward in biomedical approaches to combating human disorders and diseases.

ETHICAL ISSUES

The findings from the HGP indicate that the genetic differences between individuals represent less than 1 percent of the total human genome, as mentioned earlier in this chapter. Little seems to distinguish one individual human being from another, genetically. Based on this information, researchers believe that the findings from the HGP are difficult to use in support of racism as has sometimes been the case in the past with other genetics research. Beyond the finding that there is little variation in individual human genetics, future findings are likely to indicate that everyone carries both harmful and beneficial alleles (Pääbo, 2001). In this scenario, no one race, culture, or ethnic group can be viewed as containing genetic material that makes them inferior or superior. Instead, groups and individuals will be viewed as containing a number of genetic strengths and weaknesses (Pääbo, 2001).

However, with the daunting possibility of genetic discrimination, researchers involved in the HGP have had to publicly confront the specters of eugenics, social Darwinism, the Holocaust during World War II, and ongoing ethnic cleansing around the world. Five percent of the total budget for the HGP was spent on examining the ethical issues associated with the research. This was initially proposed in 1988 by Nobel Prize winner James Watson, 2 years before the HGP officially began. To direct the process of examining the ethical issues involved in the HGP, the DOE and NIH created the Ethical, Legal, and Social Implications of the HGP (ELSI) group. The group has set two overarching goals: (1) to help understand the ethical, legal, and social implications of the HGP; and (2) to identify and define the major issues of concern and begin to develop policies to address these issues. The group has also identified four additional issues of importance (Pääbo, 2001):

1. Issues surrounding genetic research mimic those of standard human subject concerns (informed consent, privacy) as well as commercialization, and patenting of genetic material. Who owns the data?
2. Clinical integration of new technologies.
3. Privacy and nondiscriminatory use and interpretation of genetic information.
4. Genetic education for professionals.

Most of the ELSI goals are related to an issue familiar to social work—confidentiality. The gathering of genetic material for analysis exposes research participants to a number of confidentiality issues. Researchers from the HGP insured the protection of research participants' genetic information from public access by giving the participants total control over the information. Research participants who did not want their genetic information used in the HGP were allowed to withdraw their participation. For the individuals who did participate, a number of steps were used to insure their privacy. Other entities and institutions are gathering genetic information, including blood banks, hospitals, the United States Armed Forces, and forensic DNA banks (Jeffords & Daschle, 2001). How this information is protected is of great concern. Beyond the issues associated with individual confidentiality are those issues raised by research that focuses on studying small identifiable groups such as the Amish (Jeffords & Daschle, 2001; Pääbo, 2001). Does this kind of research expose individuals in these groups to undue stigmatization?

Because more individuals over time will have their genetic information revealed, controlling who has access to the information is one solution to public concerns related to employment and health insurance issues. Already a small number of employers have said that in some instances they will use genetic testing to screen potential employees for a number of genetic predispositions. For example, in 2000, a railroad company wanted to screen its employees for the genetic predisposition to carpel tunnel syndrome. The tasks performed by employees were known to potentially lead to carpel tunnel syndrome and the company had experienced a high number of workers' compensation claims involving the syndrome. Nothing came of this situation, but similar situations will develop over time as access to genetic information becomes increasingly feasible. The concept of health insurance and how the United States funds the provision of health care may also be impacted by the findings from the HGP (Jeffords & Daschle, 2001). Many in the public worry about whether or not individuals with a genetic predisposition to diseases like schizophrenia or late-onset Alzheimer's will be denied access to reasonable health insurance or will be expected to carry an unwarranted amount of the risk for something that may never occur.

There are already some policies in place that address the public's concerns surrounding employment and health insurance issues. For example, in response to the concerns surrounding employment discrimination, President Clinton in 1999 put into place precedent-setting administrative policy stating that the federal executive departments and agencies cannot discriminate against employees based on genetics (Jeffords & Daschle, 2001). The Health Insurance Portability and Accountability Act of 1996 provides some protection against individuals being denied access to health insurance based on genetics (Jeffords & Daschle, 2001). According to the act, for individuals participating in group plans, eligibility and premiums cannot be based on genetic information. Besides the federal government, as of 2001, thirty-seven states had laws concerning genetic discrimination and health insurance and twenty-four states had laws concerning genetic discrimination and employment (Jeffords & Daschle, 2001).

The most controversial aspect of genetic research has always pertained to issues related to reproduction. Between the 1920s and 1960s, this concern was linked primarily to government intervention in reproduction. The eugenics movement, Nazism, and Social Darwinism espoused ideas pertaining to perfecting the human race through the process of controlled breeding. In the United States, this took the form of sterilizing people who were mentally retarded and the criminally insane to prevent them from reproducing. The theory was that by sterilizing these groups the occurrence of mental retardation and criminal insanity in the general population would decline. Today, reproduction concerns focus on individual choice. A growing variety of genetics tests are available to pregnant women wanting to screen their fetuses for various inherited problems. *In vitro* fertilization methods offer an opportunity for women to screen and choose fertilized eggs for particular genetic traits. For example, in 2002 a woman using *in vitro* fertilization identified the fertilized eggs that would result in a child that had a specific bone marrow type. The identified bone marrow type genetically matched the woman's other child who needed a bone marrow transplant. In this case, no child was harmed, and the genetic identification of the inseminated egg may have saved another child's life. But for some critics of genetics research this kind of manipulation of reproduction harkens back to Social Darwinism and the eugenics movement.

HUMAN GENOME PROJECT AND SOCIAL WORK

The findings from the HGP are likely to change the theories of human behavior and disease. For example, the etiology and mechanisms behind the occurrence of mental health and health problems, aging, aggressive behavior, and substance abuse will be understood more fully. Theories about human development are also likely to change dramatically as we begin to understand the intricate relationship between genetics and human biology. These changes to theory will come slowly over the course of many years and how future findings from the HGP will impact these areas of theory is difficult to estimate.

For the profession of social work, the effect on theoretical bases is particularly important because of the current debate within the profession about the importance of theory in directing practice. Much of the current human behavior theory used to underpin social work practice is outdated and heavily reliant on a perspective that discounts the importance of genetics and human biology. Findings from the HGP may revitalize human behavior theories by helping researchers develop accurate understandings of the etiology of human behavior and disorder.

One of the significant professional roles that social workers can play today is in the area of genetic counseling. A growing number of individuals and families are going to be confronted with troubling genetic information. Helping these individuals and families understand the meaning that genetic information carries as well as how to proceed with interventions is a role that clinical social workers could develop. Counseling about hereditary conditions and family planning is also an area where professional social workers work can make a significant contribution. The counseling services that social workers already provide in the area of reproduction and family planning are an important starting place for the practice of genetic counseling.

Social work should remain an advocate for the voiceless in society around the issue of confidentiality, taking a strong stance on how and why genetic material is gathered. Insuring confidentiality of genetic information, protecting access to health care, and advocating for the employment rights of vulnerable groups is congruent with social work's value system. Pursuing these areas of concern provides practice opportunities for students interested in policy advocacy as well as an opportunity for social work to enhance its work as a voice in the public policy arena for underrepresented groups of people.

CONCLUSIONS

The HGP has been equated with splitting the atom and the manned moon missions. The findings from the HGP are expected to change the way we think about ourselves as human beings. Theories of biology, behavior, and development are going to be significantly altered in ways that are hard to predict. Questions such as what the relationship between genes and proteins means for understanding the relationship between genes and expressed traits (i.e., phenotypes) are already beginning to shape this new vision of humanity. In answering the aforementioned question, the HGP has confirmed that the relationship between genes and expressed traits is rarely direct. Instead, there are numerous variables intervening and interacting with genes to create expressed traits.

Science itself is going to change in ways never before imagined. Already there is serious talk among researchers that proteomics "the large scale analysis of a cell's proteins has supplanted genetics as the focus of biology" (Jasny & Szuromi, 2001, p. 1155). As well, the findings from HGP will have a significant impact on the practice of medicine and other allied health fields, including social work. For example, some theorists are beginning to question the long-term viability of some interventions currently used with individuals experiencing mental illness. Others talk about understanding the biological process so well that medication and medical procedures are individualized to the point that they are tailored to a specific individual's biology. In the area of disease, improved understanding of the cell life cycle and the role that DNA plays may contribute to improved treatments for cancer as well as slow down the aging process. Needless to say, the possible applications of the knowledge gained from the HGP seem far reaching, and social work should not only be prepared to adapt these changes but actively participate in their development.

The knowledge gained by the HGP also carries risks worth considering. The moral and ethical issues that confront the researchers working on the HGP are long-standing. Concerns about reproduction, genetic discrimination, and confidentiality of genetic information raise questions that relate to our perceptions of individual rights and the relationship of the individual to the greater society. How insurance companies, employers, and the government will use the findings from the HGP is hard to estimate, but history indicates that care must be taken—particularly when vulnerable groups of people are involved. Social work, a long-time ally of vulnerable groups, should actively engage the government in developing policy that addresses these ethical and moral concerns now, before policy is set in place.

For now, the HGP has a draft of the human genome and the complete genomes for a number of other organisms. From this perspective, what meaning is derived from knowing the genetic sequences of all living organisms is difficult to estimate. Humanity is likely to learn much about itself and its relationship to the other living organisms that share this world.

DISCUSSION QUESTIONS

1. Identify one finding from the Human Genome Project and discuss how it might impact our understanding of human behavior.

2. What distinguished the public lab from the private lab in methods and findings?

3. What are the two overarching goals and four additional issues identified by the Ethical, Legal, and Social Implications of the HGP group?

4. Discuss what the HGP means for professional social workers.

5. Identify three key figures from the history of genetics research and discuss how their research findings contributed to our understanding of genetics.

■ ■ ■ ■ ■ ■

HUMAN PROBLEMS, ISSUES, AND BIOLOGY

The four chapters that comprise Part III of the text deal with some of the specific impacts of biology on human conduct, human growth, and human problems. Chapter 8 describes, in some detail, the biological bases for human disability, health, illness, and the treatment of diseases. Although the chapter is not a full tracing of all of these issues, it provides some basics from which readers can move forward in better understanding the ways in which biology is a source of disability, health, and illness.

The materials also focus on the biology of health and illness, and include discussions of many of the most significant health conditions for social workers. They also provide information on the treatment of health problems, something in which social workers are very often engaged.

Chapter 9 looks at the biological bases for understanding mental health and mental illness. Although the treatments social workers use in the mental health field are largely social and psychological, there are also many dimensions of mental health and mental illness that are biological in nature. Psychopharmaceutical preparations are widely used in the treatment of mental illness. And the biological resources can be used in identifying and diagnosing specific mental health problems.

Chapter 10 provides information on some of the biological elements of drugs and alcohol, major issues for the practice of social work in the current era. Some of the ways in which drugs and alcohol affect the human body, especially the brain, are discussed. The chapter also includes discussions of smoking, the use and misuse of legal pharmaceutical drugs, and, of course, lengthy discussions of the treatment for the use and misuse of legal substances, which may also have significant effects on the functioning of individuals.

The last chapter in Part III discusses sexuality and sexual orientation, which are critical issues in human biology. Many of those who are served by social workers may have, as the bases of their problems, difficulties with their sexual functioning and their sexual orientation. Therefore, this chapter is an essential part of the text and may be one of the most useful in developing plans for serving clients.

CHAPTER EIGHT

THE BIOLOGY OF DISABILITY, HEALTH, ILLNESS, AND TREATMENT

With health, everything is a source of pleasure; without it,
nothing else, whatever it may be, is enjoyable. . . . Health is
by far the most important element in human happiness.

—Arthur Schopenhauer

Perhaps the most important biological concern of social workers and others in the human services is disease and its treatment. Many people who face social and personal problems have them because of illness. Therefore, helping people deal with the social consequences of illness is often a major challenge for social workers. In addition, many social agencies as well as other human services programs are directly associated with the prevention of illness through the promotion of healthy lifestyles, health screening, and immunizations. Therefore, health and illness are major biological issues for those who work with people in social agencies and other systems.

This chapter discusses several diseases and groups of diseases. Of course, not all health conditions are mentioned. Some of the primary diseases and causes of death are discussed along with many others that often come to the attention of social workers. For information on the thousands of disease conditions that humans encounter, readers may want to consult a general medical manual such as the *American Medical Association Encyclopedia* (Clayman, 1989) or the *Merck Manual* (Beers & Berkow, 1999). Both of these resources provide detailed information on a large number of health conditions.

Diseases may be caused in a number of ways. Some are caused by bacteria, which are treatable with antibiotics and other substances. Viruses cause other illnesses, such as colds, influenza, and other conditions. Generally, virus-caused illnesses cannot be treated with antibiotics, but some forms of them can be prevented with immunizations. The length of their courses and severity can also be treated early with medicines after they are contracted. But the most severe must be dealt with through prevention. A good example is polio, which can be prevented with injections or orally taking vaccines, as can measles, whooping cough, and small-pox, which was the first illness prevented with a vaccine.

Viruses and bacterial illnesses can be contracted through contact with others who have the disease by breathing or ingesting body secretions or by direct contact with the infected person's blood or blood products (such as semen in the case of the virus-caused condition, AIDS) or can come genetically through inheritance. Cystic fibrosis; hemophilia, which is excessive bleeding following injury; and Hunting-ton's disease, which causes deterioration of the nervous system, are examples along with many others of genetically based conditions (Clayman, 1989). Allergies, which are sensitivities to specific allergens, are another example. Allergies can lead to death when there is a severe reaction called anaphylactic shock to insect bites, foods such as shellfish and peanuts, molds, and plants. Some people are allergic to such substances, whereas most are not.

Illness can also result from abnormal cell growth and reproduction such as in cancer. Diseases such as cancer, heart disease, and stroke can also result from bodily changes that may result from uses of substances such as alcohol and tobacco; overeat-ing and the consequent obesity; lack of exercise; high blood cholesterol, resulting from an individual's physiology or from dietary choices; and other "lifestyle" factors.

TYPES OF MEDICINE

For the treatment of illnesses, there is a range of healing professions, some more widely recognized and accepted than others. There are several different kinds of medicine, although that which is best known by most Americans is *allopathic medi-cine,* which is the term used to describe conventional medicine as practiced by a graduate of a medical school or a college that grants the MD degree (Clayman, 1989).

Osteopathic medicine is now recognized by most state licensing boards as a practice that is comparable to allopathic medicine. Osteopaths graduate from schools called schools of osteopathic medicine and they prescribe drugs and are qualified and licensed to practice all forms of medicine and surgery. That practice was founded in 1874 and focused primarily on the roles of the musculoskeletal sys-tem in the functioning of the human body. Although there is still that sort of emphasis and concern about disturbances in one body system affecting other body systems, much of the current theory of osteopathic medicine is similar to that of the allopathic physician. Osteopathic physicians also have training in body manipula-tion of various kinds.

Another well-known health practice field is chiropractic. The American Med-ical Association and most physicians reject chiropractic as a scientifically based form of healing. The *AMA Encyclopedia of Medicine* (Clayman, 1989, p. 270) describes chiropractic as

> A theory of healing based on the belief that disease results from a lack of normal nerve function. Chiropractic relies on physical manipulation and adjustment of the

spine for therapy, rather than on drugs or surgery. Physicians believe that no scientific basis for chiropractic theory has ever been established and that it is ineffective in the treatment of such common ailments as hypertension, heart disease, stroke, cancer, diabetes, and infectious diseases.

That denial of effectiveness is to counter claims made in some chiropractic advertising that manipulation of the spinal cord and the like can cure illnesses. Some chiropractors and chiropractic advertising make claims only for relieving pains in the back and other parts of the skeletal system and do not make the claims for cures of more systemic conditions that are the basis of the denial of effectiveness by the American Medical Association.

Naturopathic and homeopathic are other examples of philosophies of healing, which rely on specific theories that are discussed in Chapter 1.

HEART DISEASE

Of all the illnesses, heart disease is probably the best known. Coronary heart disease is America's number one killer. Taken with stroke or cerebral hemorrhage, which is related to some of the same problems, heart disease is a major health problem—really *the* major health problem—faced by Americans. There are some risk factors that can increase an individual's risk of developing heart disease. The controllable factors are high blood pressure, high blood cholesterol, smoking, obesity, physical inactivity, diabetes, and stress. The uncontrollable risk factors are gender, heredity, and age. Coronary heart disease occurs when the coronary arteries become narrowed and enough blood cannot be supplied to the heart. A heart attack occurs when the blood supply is cut off completely. The tests that can be used to detect coronary heart disease are the electrocardiogram, a stress test, nuclear scanning, and coronary angiography. Coronary heart disease can be treated with lifestyle changes and medications, and, in more severe cases, surgery.

In early 2002, The Associated Press (Nano, 2002) reported on research that was published in *The New England Journal of Medicine* that suggested the human heart regenerates and repairs itself after it is damaged by heart attacks or repaired with surgery. Researchers in New York and Italy discovered evidence that the heart has stem cells which, like other stem cells, transform themselves into many kinds of tissue such as muscle. The researchers planned to further study the phenomenon with the hope that they might be able to isolate the stem cells and use them in treating patients with failing hearts.

More and more, it appears possible to correct serious health problems while still working with fetal organisms (Park, 2002a). In 2002, surgeons were able to repair a heart valve defect in a 23-week-old fetus by using needles and small balloons to open the heart valve and make the blood flow. The balloon appeared to be doing its job for the fetus.

New surgical procedures such as heart transplants and heart bypasses and medicines have also played major roles in reducing heart disease and stroke.

Defibrillation

One of the most dramatic and severe heart disturbances is fibrillation, which causes the heart to stop pumping blood. The lack of blood can cause the heart to stop beating, which is called cardiac arrest, and can also lead to brain damage, because of the lack of blood to the brain. The primary solution to the problem of fibrillation is defibrillation, which is a process that uses an electronic device to send an electric shock to the heart so as to stop a very rapid, irregular heartbeat, and restore the regular heart rhythm (De Milto, 2002).

Usually, defibrillation is achieved with a device that is carried on emergency vehicles and available in hospitals. Some airplanes also carry the devices. Paddle-like objects are placed on the patient's chest and an electric shock passes through them to shock the heart and achieve defibrillation. Speed is important in the procedure. For every minute that the heart is in fibrillation, 10 percent of the ability to restart the heart is lost. Death from fibrillation can occur in a matter of minutes (De Milto, 2002).

The Food and Drug Administration approved a wearable defibrillator in 2002. Persons with high risk of cardiac arrest can wear the lightweight machines, which detect abnormal heart rhythms in the patient and carry out defibrillation (*Popular Science*, 2002). Those who perform defibrillation are cautious about applying the procedure to patients who are alert or have pulses because defibrillation can cause lethal heart rhythm disturbances. The paddles are also not used on a woman's breasts or over a heart pacemaker (De Milto, 2002).

Blood Pressure

A familiar measure of heart functioning is the blood pressure test. Two different kinds of pressure are tested. The higher number, systolic, is the pressure that is created when the heart muscle contracts and the large blood vessel, the aorta, recoils from the pressure when blood comes through it. Diastolic, the lower number, pressure is when the ventricles relax between beats. It measures the resistance of the small arteries and is an indicator of how hard the heart has to pump (Clayman, 1989). Most readers will be familiar with blood pressure tests. A young person who is healthy has a blood pressure reading of about 110 systolic and 75 diastolic, which may increase to about 130 and 90 for a person age 60 or older.

The pulse, which is counted by touching the wrist or neck and which should reflect the heart rate, is another measurement of the cardiovascular system. According to Clayman (1989), most people have a heart rate between 60 and 100 beats per minute at rest. Exercise increases the heart rate and decreases the resting rate, and for this reason some top athletes have resting heart rates under 60 beats per minute. Irregular heart beats as well as rates in most people below 60 or over 100 are considered signs of possible problems with the nervous system, which controls the rate of the heart.

Some people use regular doses of aspirin as a preventive of heart problems. Aspirin thins the blood and could help overcome the problems of arteries narrowed by cholesterol and blood clots. Some health specialists recommend aspirin therapy for people who have recovered from heart attacks—to prevent others. It is also a common recommendation that persons who appear to be having heart attacks immediately chew aspirins, which can limit the damage caused by the attack.

As suggested, for a long time, risk of heart disease and stroke was evaluated in terms of blood cholesterol levels as well as other factors. However, in mid-2002, researchers began to report that heart attacks could also be associated with inflammation in the body (Haney, 2002c). This finding appeared to be an answer to the puzzle of why some half of heart attack victims have normal or low cholesterol. Those who have inflammation, which can occur in any part of the body, may be at equal or greater risk than those who have high cholesterol readings. The inflammations are associated with the same kinds of body functions that cause swelling, heat, and redness when people experience infections or allergic rashes. The plaque in the bloodstream, which is associated with heart attacks, can become inflamed and lead to heart attacks. People who are overweight are more likely to have fat cells with inflammatory proteins. High blood pressure, low-level infections, smoking, and chronic gum disease are also possible sources of the kinds of inflammation that can cause heart attacks.

Persons with suspected inflammation can be evaluated with a test for the C-reactive protein, which is a symptom of inflammation. Apparently, the test is fairly simple but can reveal a propensity to have heart attacks, which is a strong indicator of the inflammation problem, according to Haney (2002c).

The treatments for inflammation include many of those that are also recommended for people who are possibly subject to heart attacks, such as weight loss, exercise, moderate use of alcohol, giving up smoking, and lowering blood pressure. Heart medicines such as aspirin, ACE inhibitors, and statin drugs, which are used in treating heart disease, also appear to have an ability to help reduce susceptibility to heart attacks from inflammation.

PARKINSON'S DISEASE

Parkinson's is a neurological disease that causes tremors and other bodily changes. Although it largely occurs in older adults, many young people also contract it (Rosenbaum, 1989). It can be treated with surgery and with some medicines such as L-Dopa. Although its origins are not fully known and its symptoms may result, in some cases, from traumatic brain injury, there are some who believe it is a product of environmental pollution of various kinds.

DIABETES

Diabetes, the seventh leading cause of death in America (Reagan & Brookins-Fisher, 2002), is a disease characterized by high levels of blood glucose that result from defects in insulin secretion. Insulin is a hormone and diabetes is an illness that can be attributed to problems with that hormone. There are approximately 16 million Americans living with diabetes and about 800,000 new cases are diagnosed every year.

According to Atkinson (2002), the increase in diabetes cases represents a 50 percent rise among Americans aged 30 to 50 and a tenfold increase among adolescents. The disease is also the leading cause of new cases of blindness and limb amputations that are not related to trauma such as accidents.

Western Europeans and North Americans appear to be the groups most susceptible to the disease. There are four types of diabetes: Type 1, Type 2, gestational, and other specific types. Type 1 diabetes is juvenile diabetes and classified as insulin dependent. It constitutes 5–10 percent of diabetes cases. Type 2 diabetes is classified as noninsulin dependent and makes up about 90–95 percent of people living with diabetes. Gestational diabetes occurs in 2–5 percent of pregnancies but goes away after the pregnancy. The "other specific types" of diabetes result from specific genetic syndromes, surgeries, etc., and account for 1–2 percent of diabetes cases.

Diabetes is diagnosed by either the fasting plasma glucose test or the oral glucose test, in which patients take glucose and have their blood sugar level tested several times after consuming the substance. Treatment for diabetes is aimed at keeping the blood glucose level near normal at all times. The type of diabetes will impact the treatment. The most common treatments are diet control, exercise, home blood glucose testing, and, in more serious cases such as those that are insulin dependent, oral medication or insulin injections (www.niddk.nih.gov).

ALZHEIMER'S DISEASE

Although Alzheimer's may be genetic in nature, Alzheimer's disease, the symptoms of which are forgetfulness and other brain-based dysfunctions, is not a single-gene disorder. More than one gene mutation can cause Alzheimer's. According to Dr. George T. Grossberg (2002), Alzheimer's is caused by an excess of amyloid, a brain protein. It forms a kind of plaque in the brains of patients who have the disease.

The two basic types of Alzheimer's disease are familial and sporadic. Familial is rare and associated with gene mutations on chromosomes 1, 14, and 21. It is the result of a certain inheritance pattern called autosomal dominant. With this pattern, all offspring have a 50 percent chance of developing Alzheimer's if one of their parents had it, and it normally occurs earlier in life. Sporadic Alzheimer's disease occurs later in life and is more common. It appears to be related to a gene found on chromosome 19. However, the cause of Alzheimer's—why some people develop it and others do not—is not yet known.

People with Alzheimer's do not just experience memory loss but also a decline in cognitive functioning and changes in behavior. There are also some physical problems associated with the condition for some patients. The condition can be detected with some methods of tracing brain activity.

As suggested, Alzheimer's is a progressive, degenerative disease of the brain. There are some 4 million Americans with Alzheimer's disease. The average lifetime cost per patient is $175,000. Currently four medications are approved by the FDA for Alzheimer's: Cognex, Aricept, Reminyl, and Exelon. A recent study (Grossberg, 2002; Tanner, 2002) found that older women who used cholesterol-reducing drugs such as Lipitor, Zacor, and Mevacor had less mental impairment than those who did not use the drugs. Apparently, high cholesterol levels harm the brain and can lead to the kinds of mental problems associated with Alzheimer's.

In addition to the people living with Alzheimer's, caregivers are also impacted directly by the disease. More than 80 percent of caregivers experience high levels of stress and suffer from depression, which can be unhealthy for both the caregiver and the patient.

The Forgetting (Shenk, 2001) is a book about how people's view of Alzheimer's has changed the human condition throughout time, today, and in the future. Shenk also shows the mechanics of the disease and how it affects a person and his or her family. To him, it is not an alien condition, but a human one. Throughout time, Alzheimer's was considered a normal part of aging. When a person became old, they had trouble learning, and they easily forgot information. Poets, playwrights, and philosophers wrote of different occurrences of this throughout time. Even Ralph Waldo Emerson had all of the symptoms of Alzheimer's, but it was not diagnosed in his time.

Alois Alzheimer, a German physician, was the first to realize that it was different from dementia. He realized this through a woman named Auguste D., who was only 51. Her husband had brought her to the Frankfurt hospital in 1951. She was disoriented and unable to write her name without losing track of her intentions. When she died 4 years later, she was mute and incontinent. After examining her brain tissue, he realized the cortex had clumps of brown plaque, and a third of the neurons were filled with tangled filaments. These became the physical signs of the disease, which is diagnosed with certainty through an autopsy.

In the past, many people acquired the disease after 65, but many people did not live that long, so the number of people who had the disease was small. Today, many people live longer because of modern health care, so many more people are seen with the disease. Shenk says this is the irony of modern technology. The number of people who have this disease will only increase in the future because of this technology. Even though foundations, governments, and drug companies are spending billions to search for effective treatments, families in the near future will still face this disease with panic.

Many people have learned to live with their disease and have tried to find the brighter side of it. For example, the painter Willim de Kooning thought his work became lighter after he was diagnosed with Alzheimer's. Shenk (2001) says until we learn to prevent or treat Alzheimer's, the challenge is to find the meaning it communicates.

Jonathan Franzen (2001) wrote about his father, who was a patient with Alzheimer's disease. He describes the deterioration in his father's memory and his understanding of events around him. Franzen notes that senile dementia has been around for a long time but life in the past was relatively short and old age was also rare. What is now known as Alzheimer's was considered a natural byproduct of aging.

For a long time, Alzheimer's was considered a rare medical disease much like Huntington's. However, in the 1950s, another physician, according to Franzen, conducted autopsies of the brains of 210 victims of senile dementia and found the plaques and tangles that Alzheimer had discovered in most of them.

It took a while for medicine to determine that senile dementia was not simply a byproduct of aging and was, in fact, a neurological condition. There is some evidence that Alzheimer's extends life even while it is voiding the personality of the patient.

Genes have been identified that lead to early-onset Alzheimer's (Tanner, 2002c). According to one news article, a woman who wanted to become pregnant also had siblings who had developed early-onset Alzheimer's. She became pregnant through *in vitro* fertilization, in which some of her eggs were fertilized. However, the eggs that were implanted after sterilization were screened for the early Alzheimer's gene and those that had it were not implanted. A new method can detect the early-onset gene as well as other conditions such as Tay-Sachs and sickle cell anemia. The test is not readily available, according to Tanner (2002c), because it is primarily used to screen for fairly rare conditions.

According to Grossberg (2002), injecting a radioactive substance into a patient and then examining the patient's brain can reveal minor decreases in brain-cell activity, and that analysis can predict Alzheimer's 10 years before the patient develops clinical symptoms.

Scientists are reporting that a blood test can identify people with Alzheimer's disease before they have symptoms of the disease (Recer, 2002). That early knowledge will help enable them be treated for the condition before it affects their bodies. Thus far, the test has been effective only with animals, but it may be applicable to humans soon. Of course, this is not the test for the early onset of Alzheimer's discussed previously. This is a test that will apply to people who develop the condition later in life.

Better diagnostic procedures through electronic scanners such as positron-emission tomography and imaging equipment are helping, and numerous medicines are being studied that can reduce the effects of the disease or even prevent its development (Cowley, 2002). Although there are currently no specific treatments for Alzheimer's, there seems to be evidence that folic acid and drugs that lower cholesterol can have a positive effect on delaying the onset of the condition.

About 4 million Americans currently have Alzheimer's disease (Recer, 2002). It is expected that there will be 14 million people with the disease by 2050.

News reports (Test Vaccine, 2002) in 2002 said that twelve volunteer patients who had been inoculated with an experimental vaccine to reverse the effects of Alzheimer's disease have become seriously ill with brain inflammation. The vaccine, which was developed in Ireland, had been considered effective and safe, but the latest use of it with patients suggested it could harm Alzheimer's patients rather than reverse or cure the illness. The inoculations were being stopped. Additional information on Alzheimer's can be found in Chapter 12.

THE COMMON COLD

Of all the illnesses encountered by humans, the "cold" is the virus that affects the most individuals in the most ways, most often. However, as Gawande (2002) points out, little is known about the nature of the virus, the means of transmission, the cure, or even the prevention of the illness. It is pervasive but something of a mystery.

A new pill developed to relieve the common cold has not yet been proven safe enough for Americans to take. The pills that have been developed seem to reduce the effectiveness of birth control pills and also do not prevent or cure colds but appear to shorten their duration. Some of those who studied the pill (Neergaard, 2002c) were concerned that the cold viruses, which the pills attack, could perhaps mutate and cause more serious health problems than the cold.

GENETIC CONDITIONS

The chapters on genetics and the Human Genome Project help explain the ways in which health conditions are inherited. Many health conditions are partly or largely inherited from parents.

One of the significant roles that social workers play is in genetic counseling. They help families understand the possible hereditary conditions, if any, that their children might experience. In some cases, families choose to abort their fetuses rather than deliver children with some of the kinds of severe hereditary deficiencies or conditions that they might encounter. In other cases, they are simply informed of the possible outcomes of the pregnancy and choose to go ahead with the birth.

As the human genome becomes better understood, more and more health issues are being evaluated genetically. For example, a new study (Neergaard, 2002b) found that many women have an X chromosome that may be lethal to male fetuses. It is possible, based on the research of Eric Hoffman, an expert on the genetics of some forms of inherited muscular dystrophy, that some multiple miscarriages are a product of these genetic issues.

MULTIPLE SCLEROSIS

Multiple sclerosis (MS) is a chronic, potentially disabling disease of the central nervous system. People are normally diagnosed between the ages of 20 and 40. The symptoms come and go without warning and can range from paralysis, numbness, blurred or double vision, to blindness. Every week about 200 people are diagnosed with MS. Currently there are a third of a million people living with MS in the United States.

There are four types of multiple sclerosis: relapsing remitting, primary progressive, secondary progressive, and progressive relapsing. Eighty percent of people diagnosed have relapsing remitting MS. MS is not a fatal disease. However, it can change an individual's quality of life. The risk for the general population to have MS is one in one thousand. In a family where one person has MS, the risk is about two to five in one thousand so there may be some genetic basis to the condition. To date, there is no test available to determine if one is genetically susceptible to MS.

The cause of MS is not known. There are currently three drug therapies approved by the Food and Drug Administration—Avonex, Betaseron, and Copaxone—to slow down the progression of the disease for people with relapsing forms of MS.

The disease is diagnosed by ruling out other diseases, and through a medical history, MRI tests, spinal taps, and various physical examinations.

New research suggests (Tanner, 2001) that multiple sclerosis may result from the same virus that is associated with another disease, mononucleosis. The common virus is Epstein-Barr, which has also been linked to forms of cancer and other nerve disorders.

Obviously, one of the social consequences of multiple sclerosis is disability. Some persons who have the condition lose their capacity to work and to engage fully in family life. Social workers often deal with those phenomena, and doing so with a sound knowledge of the biology of the condition increases their ability to serve such clients effectively. They can know the prognosis and likely course of the condition as well as the ways in which they can best guide clients for long-term employment and other plans.

CYSTIC FIBROSIS

Among the hereditary, genetic illnesses is cystic fibrosis, which Johnson (2001) calls the most fatal genetic disease in North America. About one of every 3,300 children born has the disease and about one in every twenty-nine people carry the altered gene that leads to it. It is such a serious problem that the average age of death for people who have the illness is 31 as discussed in Chapter 7.

The symptoms of the disease are coughing, wheezing, lack of weight gain, and others. The symptoms are what cause the fatality. Vigorous physical therapy, medicine to reduce mucous and dislodge it, and careful attention to vitamins and enzymes can help. There is also a drug called Pulmozyme that thins the mucous and cuts the number of respiratory infections. There is also an inhalant antibiotic that helps control the effects of cystic fibrosis.

ARTHRITIS AND OSTEOARTHRITIS

One of the nation's most pervasive diseases is arthritis, of which there are some 100 different types. However, the most common is osteoarthritis, which, as Chapter 4 mentions, has its most significant effects on older people—people over 50. As previously mentioned, the condition begins much earlier for many sufferers, as young as their 20s. However, the effects do not show up dramatically until the later years (Gorman & Park, 2002). The most serious consequences of arthritis are the loss of mobility and pain.

The basic theory of osteoarthritis is that it is a result of degeneration of the cartilage, which is the shock absorber in the joints, cushioning them. Although experts still believe that cartilage problems are fundamental to osteoarthritis, it is also clear that the bones, tendons, and ligaments are also involved. Each individual's biochemistry makes their cartilage's ability to resist damage and degeneration different (Gorman & Park, 2002).

Injuries, including broken bones, and wearing poorly fitted shoes can exacerbate the problems of osteoarthritis or cause its earlier onset. However, those biochemical differences mentioned above may be more significant indicators of who will and who will not develop the disease. The disease usually affects a single joint such as the knee or hip, the back, or several joints.

Preventing the condition is different for each person but generally keeping one's weight down, exercising, and building one's muscles seem to be associated with the prevention of osteoarthritis (Gorman & Park, 2002). Treatment for the condition includes over the counter medicines such as acetaminophen and aspirin as well as some prescription treatments including corticosteroids and some antibiotics, which can inhibit the loss of cartilage. Exercise also seems to help patients cope with the disease and prevents further deterioration. Some surgical procedures are also used including the fusion of bones and the replacement of major joints such as the hip or knee (Gorman & Park, 2002).

Rheumatoid Arthritis

Unlike the slow development of osteoarthritis, rheumatoid arthritis may develop overnight and cause crippling. It is a systemic disease, an autoimmune disorder. The system attacks the body's joints. Patients with the condition suffer from swollen joints and stiffness, often of the hands or feet. But, according the Bjerklie (2002), it can also cause loss of appetite, fatigue, and some generally immobilizing physical consequences. Although it usually attacks adults, it may cause these problems in children. Women are more susceptible to the disease than men (Bjerklie, 2002).

Some prescription medicines help control the effects of the disease and can prevent the frequent almost total debilitation that victims of the condition may have experienced in the past.

Fibromyalgia

A condition that is sometimes considered part of the overall group of arthritic conditions is fibromyalgia. According to Thomas (1993, p. 728), it constitutes "chronic pain in muscles and soft tissues surrounding joints."

The condition is one that has been difficult to classify or treat, although it is increasingly given as a diagnosis for persons who suffer from otherwise unexplained pain.

CANCER

Overview of Cancer

As discussed earlier, cancer is one of the major causes of disability and death in the United States. According to the American Cancer Society, cancer is defined as a group of diseases that are characterized by an uncontrolled growth and spread of abnormal cells. "There are an estimated 200 different kinds of cancer. They can cause uncontrolled growth of cells derived from normal tissues, and of being able to kill the host by the spread of cells from the site of origin to distant sites or by local spread" (Thomas, 1993, p. 297).

Each year, the American Cancer Society publishes a report on the incidence of cancer and the percentage of cases found at various sites in the body. According to Thomas (1993), 32 percent of cancer is at the breast and 23 percent in the prostate. Lung cancer contributes 18 percent of all cases. Colon and rectum cancer is found in about 14 percent of men and women. Both genders have skin cancer in about 3 percent of reported cases. In women, 8 percent of cancer begins in the uterus and 4 percent in the ovaries. Less than 5 percent of cancers are in the mouth. Nine percent of men with cancer have leukemia or lymphomas, which are in the blood, compared to 7 percent of women with cancer.

Cancer deaths also vary by site. Only 1 percent of cancer deaths are from skin cancer, for example, whereas only 2 percent of men and only 1 percent of women with cancer die from oral cancer. Thirty-four percent of cancer deaths in males are from lung cancer compared to 22 percent of women, although the difference is growing smaller because of the increased use of cigarettes by women. Twelve percent of men who die of cancer die from prostate cancer and 19 percent of female deaths are from breast cancer. Five percent of women die from ovarian cancer and 4 percent from cancer of the uterus. Colon and rectal cancer kills 11 percent of men with the disease, and 12 percent of women die from cancer at those sites. Nine percent of both male and female cancer deaths result from leukemia and lymphomas. Nineteen percent of all deaths are scattered through the remaining cancer sites.

Cancer can be caused by both internal and external factors, such as hormones, the immune system, chemicals, and radiation. It is treated with radiation, chemotherapy, hormones, surgery, and immunotherapy. Different types of cancer vary in their rates of growth, patterns of spread, and their response to different types of treatment. Because of that, it is difficult to generalize about cancer. Leading forms of cancer, such as breast cancer in women and prostate cancer in men, differ significantly from other common forms of the disease.

Anyone is at risk for developing cancer. In the United States, the American Cancer Society says that men have a one in two lifetime risk of developing cancer and women have a one in three risk (lifetime risk is defined as the probability that an individual over their lifetime will develop cancer). The risk of developing most types of cancer can be reduced by changing one's lifestyle. Examples are stopping smoking or eating a better diet.

Cancer is the second leading cause of death in the United States. Regular screening examinations can lead to early detection of cancer, which is when cancer is in the early stages and treatment is most successful. The National Institutes of Health estimates that the overall annual cost for treating cancer is $107 billion.

Some students of physiology have developed new approaches to understanding the immune system and its relationship to cancer. According to Ryan (2002), Polly Matzinger has studied the immune system and discovered that it does not drive away foreign substances immediately after they are introduced. Instead, the immune cells respond only when the healthy cells signal that they are in danger. To the immune system, cancer cells appear to be healthy, normal cells. So one solution to the problem of cancer may be to inject toxins into tumors so that the immune system recognizes that it is under threat.

Cancer and Genetic Testing

Genetic testing identifies the ways that traits are passed from parents to their children. It has been discovered that genetics may be an important factor in the development of cancer. The Human Genome Project, which is discussed in detail in Chapter 7, is a program whose goal is to determine the complete DNA sequence. In June 2000, scientists completed mapping the DNA sequence of the human genome. Now the goal of the HGP is to determine how to use this information. Scientists may be able to find ways to detect diseases earlier by genetic testing and find out if one is at risk for developing disease. However, with this new form of genetic testing, there is also a negative side to finding out what diseases one may have or is likely to have. Insurance companies and potential employers could use this information to discriminate against individuals (U.S. National Cancer Institute, 2001).

Breast Cancer

Breast cancer is a form of the disease that affects many Americans, almost all of whom are women, and is said to be a result of one's gene susceptibility and environmental factors. Hereditary breast cancer accounts for 5–10 percent of women's cases. Two classes of genes play roles in the development of cancer: the oncogenes and the tumor-suppressor genes. Oncogenes control cell growth, which, when activated by mutation, can trigger cancerous cell growth. Tumor-suppressor genes prevent uncontrolled cell growth and are able to keep cancer from forming.

There are both benign and malignant breast tumors. Benign tumors are abnormal growths that do not spread outside of the breast and that are not life threatening. Malignant tumors, which can spread to other parts of the body, are identified as cancer. The most common types of breast cancer are ductal carcinoma *in situ,* infiltrating ductal carcinoma, infiltrating lobular carcinoma, and lobular carcinoma in situ. Breast cancer is the most common cancer among women and the second leading cause of death in women. However, death rates have declined as a result of better detection and improved treatment. There are certain risk factors linked to the disease. Risk factors that cannot be influenced are gender, age, genetics, family history, personal history, race, and menstrual periods. The risk factors that can be controlled are one's diet, exercise, and alcohol intake. According to Haney (2002b), women who gain large amounts of weight during pregnancy place themselves at special risk for the disease.

The three tools used to detect breast cancer are mammograms, clinical breast examinations, and breast self-examinations. The most common sign of breast cancer is a new lump or mass found in the breast area. It is important to have anything unusual checked by a physician. The most common treatments for breast cancer are surgery, radiation therapy, hormone therapy, and chemotherapy (U.S. National Cancer Institute, 2001; U.S. National Institute of Environmental Health Sciences, 2001).

Despite some research questioning the value of mammograms for all women, the U.S. government has reaffirmed its belief in the procedure as a way of early diagnosis of breast cancer. Several published studies questioned the value of mammograms in detecting breast cancer early, but the U.S. Preventive Health Service (Neergaard, 2002a) decided that there was fair evidence that regularly getting a mammogram could reduce the possibilities of dying from breast cancer by 20 percent over a period of 10 years. The benefits are greatest for older women, between 50 and 69, and it may be just as useful for any woman to have the exam every other year as it is to have it every year.

Prostate Cancer

Prostate cancer, a men's disease, begins in the prostate gland. Men of any age can develop prostate cancer, but it is found most often in men over 50. Prostate cancer is about twice as common among African American men as it is with white American men. Prostate cancer is the most common type of cancer in men in the United States. Currently the cause of prostate cancer is not known. It is said that there may be a link to a certain gene that causes some men to develop prostate cancer. The risk factors identified for prostate cancer are age, race, diet, and family history. There are two tests used to detect prostate cancer: the PSA blood test and the digital rectal exam. The PSA blood test measures a protein made by prostate cells. The digital rectal exam is a physical exam that searches for lumps on the prostate. All men at the age of 50 should begin having both the PSA and digital rectal exam to screen for prostate cancer. The most common treatments for prostate cancer are surgery, radiation, and hormone treatment. Age, overall health, and the stage and grade of cancer are factors that will determine what treatment is the best choice for individuals.

It is possible that diet and lifestyle may be major factors in treating prostate cancer, according to Noonan and Springen (2002). The writers for *Newsweek* report that Dr. Dean Ornish has been treating prostate cancer patients by prescribing vegan vegetarian diets with only 10 percent fat, the elimination of alcohol, 3 hours of exercise per week, as well as meditation, stress reduction exercises, and participation in a support group. The patients he has treated and studied had an average 6.5 percent decrease in their PSAs and those who were most compliant had 9 percent decreases. The treatment appears to arrest the growth of the cancer and begin the body on the way to a cure. Ornish has used similar treatments for heart disease patients with equally encouraging results.

Colon Cancer

One common and growing form of cancer is that of the colon. The colon is a part of the large intestine and its function is to remove waste material in the anus and to adsorb salt and water (Cheers, 2001). Several other health conditions are associated with the colon, such as ulcerative colitis. Because of the high incidence of colon cancer, there is a heavy focus on educating Americans about the need for examinations of the colon through laboratory tests of a patient's waste materials, and the administration of sigmoidoscopy and colonoscopy, which are procedures conducted by physicians to examine the intestine for polyps and other lesions that might lead to colon cancer.

According to a study published in the *Journal of the National Cancer Institute* (Recer, 2002a), the diet histories of 135,000 male and female colon cancer patients could be changed by the ingestion of 700 to 800 mg of calcium daily. Doing so seemed to reduce their risk of cancer by almost half. Although the researchers were not willing to make a specific recommendation, there is some hope that treatment with calcium could prevent the 90,000 annually diagnosed cases of colon cancer in the United States.

A recent study (Haney, 2002a) found that taking a baby aspirin daily reduces the risk of colon cancer by preventing the growth of polyps in the colon. The study was conducted by John A. Baron of Dartmouth Medical School and presented at a meeting of the American Association of Cancer Research. Parenthetically, it was reported (Adler & Underwood, 2002) that aspirin may also be an effective treatment for infertility, Alzheimer's disease, gum disease, and eye disease, which are also discussed in this text. Some studies have shown that regular, low doses of the drug may double the likelihood of women becoming pregnant, prevent serious visual problems, and cut the risk of developing Alzheimer's by half.

Curtis Pesmen (July, 2001), an author, contributed a first-person account of colorectal cancer treatment, which included surgery, to *Esquire* magazine. He describes the destructive treatment, which includes chemotherapy, radiation, and surgery, the trio of measures used in dealing with many cancers, although not all are possible in all cases.

Colorectal cancer strikes some 130,000 Americans every year and is one of the most difficult to arrest. Pesmen writes of the sexual dysfunction associated with the treatments for the cancer and also suggests rules for dealing with persons who have the disease. He says people should avoid offering to help if they are not told what help is needed. Instead, he suggests, friends and family of cancer patients should think of any good ideas and just do them—without being asked and without asking. Entertaining children, caring for pets, assisting with transportation, and caring for a lawn or other parts of a household are examples of ways that patients and their families might be assisted. And do not ask, "Is he going to make it?" Good wishes are helpful as is useful information, but counseling about sound lifestyles or attitudes are usually too late once the patient has the condition.

Cancer Summary

Cancer is one of the more complicated of all life-threatening illnesses. In fact, many scientists doubt that cancer is a single disease. Jerome Groopman (2001), writing in the *New Yorker*, suggests that although government foundations have attempted to reduce cancer deaths by half, the fact is that there has been a slow and steady increase in deaths from cancer since the nation began dedicating itself to eradicating the disease. Targeted efforts to eradicate cancer by identifying it as a result of viruses and by developing new medicines have been only sporadically successful. Groopman points out that chemotherapy, one of the more commonly used methods of treating cancer, perhaps destroys the cancer tissue but also destroys much of the healthy tissue and cells surrounding the cancer. Although Hodgkin's lymphoma, a disease of the lymph system, and testicular cancer can now almost always be cured, many other cancers cannot.

There have been some reductions in cancer of about a quarter percent annually, but those changes are attributed to a decline in cigarette smoking and improved screening with mammograms, examinations of the colon and intestines to detect colon cancer, and pap smears to detect uterine cancer. In fact, the best solution for cancer appears to be early detection and early therapy. Many of those who treat cancer patients, a medical specialty called oncology, say that they rarely see patients until they are very sick and sometimes near death.

There is some evidence that the risks of smoking have been underestimated. According to Ross (2002), smoking tobacco causes cancer in many more parts of the body than originally believed. Researchers meeting in London in 2002 noted that the much larger group of cancers are associated with smoking and with secondhand smoke. Only two cancers that were thought to be possibly related to tobacco use—breast cancer and cancer of the endometrium, or lining of the womb—were found not to be associated with the use of the substance.

Some of the developed cancer treatments cause significant side effects and sometimes the treatments are fatal. This is all despite the news media carrying information regularly on what are purported to be major breakthroughs in the treatment of cancer. However, many of those treatments are usually only effective in dealing with one type of cancer and one body site rather than a major breakthrough in treating all cancers.

According to Groopman (2001), about 550,000 Americans die of cancer every year, which is an average of 15,000 each day. In many ways, cancer is an illness of the elderly, but even considering that, the overall increase in cancer deaths continues.

Groopman believes that much of cancer research has been built on a false premise—that cancers are caused by viruses, which is true for some but not for anywhere near all. Some of the treatments that have been developed for cancer have been useful in treatments of other conditions such as AIDS. However, the success in treating cancer, itself, has not been as dramatic as the efforts to eliminate cancer has been suggested.

It is particularly important for social workers to help clients understand the importance of regular screening for cancerous conditions and to work for the development of programs, especially for low-income people, to screen for cancer and to obtain early treatment for it.

Social workers and others who work in the field of health services have to use special approaches in dealing with cancer patients. According to Thomas (1993, p. 299),

> It is important when working with the patient with cancer that all members of the health team work in collaboration with each other as well as with the patient and family. Provide knowledge of the disease process, its progress, treatment, and outcome for the patient and family. Identify and support patient and family coping mechanisms and allow for and encourage verbalization of feelings and fears, particularly with relation to death and dying . . . also strive to decrease the patient's fears of helplessness, avoid giving false hope, and provide the patient and family with realistic reassurance about pain control.

AIDS

One of the diseases of special interest and concern to social workers is AIDS. It and other sexually transmitted diseases are discussed in detail in Chapter 13, focused on public health and biology. AIDS is one of the most serious of all current health problems. It is also especially significant because it is so likely to affect vulnerable groups in the population. The condition disproportionately affects people of minority sexual orientation, especially gay men. It is also more likely to strike minorities of color more than white people. The condition is also closely tied to the use of intravenous drugs because of its transmission through the exchange of bodily fluids, especially blood. Because AIDS is a fatal illness, the basic strategy for dealing with it has to be prevention, although, as the chapter on public health explains, there are drugs that mitigate against its most devastating effects and, in some cases, prolong the lives of those who have it.

Other sexually transmitted diseases are also serious problems and are typically viewed as public health problems because they are transmitted through human contact. They also require education about safe practices, such as using condoms and following up with treatment if the condition is contracted and identified. There are cures for most sexually transmitted diseases, often through the use of antibiotic medicines.

LEPROSY

Leprosy is one of the most feared and best known of diseases. It is frequently mentioned in the Bible, according to Gutfeld (2001). The biblical cases were probably all kinds of skin conditions and probably not all the leprosy that they may have been called.

According to Gutfeld (2001), leprosy is communicable and is caused by a bacterium that is in the same family as the tuberculosis germ. The bacteria live inside the cells of the skin and nerves and cause cells to malfunction. The disease causes people to lose the sense of touch. In recent years, there has been a resistance developed to dapsone, the most pervasive leprosy drug; therefore, other curative drugs, which are much more expensive, may have to be used for many patients.

There is no vaccine against the disease, and because it appears to be primarily a disease of poor people in poor countries, it is especially difficult to believe that one will contract it in the United States. Patients lose the ability to feel things, including pain. So people who suffer from leprosy knock their hands and feet against things more often than they should, which causes many fractures and leads to the damaged limbs being absorbed into the body.

Only a few cases are diagnosed in America every year and most of those are among immigrants. Most of the cases are in Hawaii, Louisiana, California, New York, and Texas. There were only 102 new cases in 1998. There are some 2 million cases worldwide and most of those are in Africa, India, and Brazil.

The more correct name of the disease is Hansen's disease, named for the discoverer of the bacterium. In the United States in the past, most of those who suffered from the disease were treated at the Hansen's Disease Center in Carville, Louisiana. Those with the condition are treated under the auspices of the U.S. Public Health Service. Ninety-five percent of people have a natural immunity to the illness (Gutfeld, 2001).

The disease primarily damages the nerves and the limbs and facial area and leads to skin damage, but there can also be severe complications such as blindness and disfigurement. However, it is not highly contagious (Clayman, 1989). The bacterium causing the disease is *Mycobacterium leprae,* and it is spread in droplets of nasal mucus. Persons with the disease are infectious only during the early stages. The disease is confirmed by a biopsy. There are about 20 million people who have the disease in Asia, Central and South America, and Africa, and fewer than 20 percent have access to treatment. The known cases in the United States are about 4,000, and three-fourths of those who have the disease were born in places other than the United States.

UNDERSTANDING ILLNESS
AND PREVENTING DISEASE

Perhaps one of the most significant difficulties in understanding illness is the suggestion that all the major conditions of illness are similar. In fact, there has been significant progress in reducing and treating heart disease and stroke. In some ways, that has resulted from better education about diet and exercise as well as such associated factors as alcohol use and cigarette smoking, which is a primary culprit in both heart disease and stroke.

Healthy Living

But, generally, the social worker's role in illness and prevention of illness is often in helping people understand the rules for healthy living and ensuring that health education is made available to clients as well as treatment as discussed earlier. It has been confirmed over and over again that there are six or seven basic rules for healthy living and most of them are not very complicated. They deal with lifestyles, diet, and other choices readily available to everyone. They include eating breakfast, not eating between meals, keeping one's weight down, not smoking cigarettes, drinking alcohol only moderately, and exercising regularly. People who follow those rules or most of them have much healthier lives than those who follow only one or two or none of them.

Exercise, in particular, is coming to be understood as a major factor in preventing illness. A study conducted by Veterans Affairs professionals and Stanford University (McConnaughey, 2002) found that fitness, often achieved with exercise, is a major factor in preventing death. The researchers studied 6,200 men who were referred for testing on treadmills. Some had heart disease and others did not. Of the 6,200 men, 1,256 died within the next decade. Those who were most fit, as measured by the number of METs (an abbreviation for metabolic functioning) they produced, had the lower death rates. Exercise to the extent of two METs was roughly equivalent to walking less than 2 miles per hour. Five METs was equal to walking at 4 miles per hour and eight METs to jogging at 6 miles per hour. The death rates of those who could not get beyond four METs was more than double the death rates of people who could exercise past eight METs.

Pesmen (2002) reports that people can cut their age-related health declines in half by regular exercise. Seriously working out for a decade or more has that sort of result. Blood vessels can be added through exercise, for example, making the circulatory system more efficient.

Of course, health risks still abound and accidents, deadly viruses, and other kinds of phenomena can cause serious illness and end the lives of even people who follow the rules carefully. But for most people, staying healthy involves doing the kinds of things suggested by the rules.

An illustration of the issues associated with health and lifestyles is the recent discussions of what is called "metabolic syndrome," a condition that has been recognized since the 1920s (Tanner, 2002). The *Journal of the American Medical Association* reported on the condition, which may have some genetic or viral sources, but which is primarily a condition caused by lifestyles. People who have the condition often have large amounts of abdominal fat, high blood pressure, poor cholesterol readings, and high blood sugar. Most who have it also have low levels of HDLs (high density lipoproteins), a blood substance that tends to protect health. The more LDLs (low density lipoproteins) and the less HDLs in a person's system, the more prone they are to heart attacks, diabetes, and strokes. The condition greatly increases the possibility that those who have it will suffer from diabetes, strokes, and heart attacks. The solution to the problem, for many of those who have it, is to eat less, exercise more, and, generally, follow the health rules suggested here.

DISABILITIES

The federal definition of a disability states:

> A person is considered to have a disability if he or she has difficulty performing certain functions (seeing, hearing, talking, walking, climbing stairs, and lifting and carrying), or has difficulties performing activities of daily living, or has difficulty with certain social roles (doing school work for children, working at a job and around the house for adults). A person who is unable to perform one or more activities or uses an assistive device to get around, or who needs assistance from another person to perform basic activities is considered to have a severe disability. (U.S. Department of Commerce, 1997, p. 2)

About 9 million people of all ages have disabilities that are so severe that they require the personal assistance of others to carry out their activities. Those who are primary helpers are relatives in about 80 percent of the cases, and half of the helpers live with the person who has the disability (U.S. Department of Commerce, 1997).

About one person in every five in the United States has some kind of disability and one in ten has a severe disability. Those figures are expected to increase with the aging of the population. People 65 and older will make up one-fifth of the population by 2030. Over half of the people 65 and older in 1995 had some level of disability (U.S. Department of Commerce, 1997).

Disability and Employment

In terms of employment, according to the U.S. Department of Commerce (1997), among those aged 21–64, 82 percent of people without disabilities had jobs or businesses compared to 77 percent of those with nonsevere disabilities and 26 percent with severe disabilities. There have been some gains in employment for people with severe disabilities in recent years.

Although they may be underemployed, people with disabilities are largely employed to some extent, as indicated. Over 64 percent of people who have hearing disabilities are employed. Nearly 48 percent of people who have seeing difficulties are employed and 41.3 percent of people with mental disabilities are employed. However, only 33.5 percent of those who have difficulty walking are employed. These figures are based on a survey conducted in 1991 (U.S. Department of Commerce, 1997).

The *Social Work Dictionary* defines disability as "temporary or permanent ability to perform the activities that most others can perform, usually as a result of a physical or mental condition or infirmity" (Barker, 1999, p. 130), and developmental disability as "a condition that produces functional impairment as a result of disease, genetic disorder, or impaired growth pattern manifested before adulthood, likely to continue indefinitely, and requiring specific and lifelong or extended care" (Barker, 1999, p. 126).

More than three-fourths of Americans aged 22 to 64 who have disabilities do not receive public assistance. However, among those who do receive public assistance such as Supplemental Security Income and Temporary Assistance for Needy Families, disability is relatively common. About half the people who receive assistance from those programs have severe or nonsevere disabilities (U.S. Department of Commerce, 1997).

Disability is closely connected with age. More than half of the people who had any disability were 65 and older in 1995. About 19 percent were 15–65 years of age and 9.1 percent were under 14. Those with severe disabilities were about one-third 65 and older, 8.7 percent were between 15 and 64, and 1.1 percent under 14 years of age.

There are also differences in disability by ethnic group. Age is not the only factor that makes a difference in the incidence of disability. Severe disability occurs among 20 percent of whites who are not of Hispanic origin, 34 percent among African Americans, and 28 percent among people of Hispanic origin (U.S. Department of Commerce, 1997).

Many disabilities occur together. That is, someone may be deaf, blind, and also have autism or cerebral palsy. According to Reagan and Brookins-Fisher (2002, pp. 335–337), the following are the leading disabilities in the United States, with the percentages of Americans affected given in parentheses: arthritis/rheumatism (27 percent), back/spinal injury (21 percent), heart problems (17 percent), respiratory problems (10 percent). In addition, 10 percent or more of the population faces visual impairments, diabetes, hearing loss, hypertension, and orthopedic impairments.

Many disabilities are biological in nature. In some cases, as described in other sections of the book, they are hereditary or genetic in nature. Others may result from the blood incompatibilities of the mother and the fetus (Rathus, Nevid, & Fichner-Rathus, 2002). The mother may lack the Rh factor, whereas the fetus may have it, because the father may be Rh positive. The mother's antibodies attack the fetus's red blood cells, which may lead to brain damage or even death. Screening and medical treatments can prevent the problem in subsequent pregnancies (the first pregnancy usually does not result in these incompatibilities), which demonstrates the importance of genetic counseling for couples who intend to have children.

A woman's syphilis can cause a miscarriage or lead to the child being stillborn or born with syphilis (Rathus et al., 2002). The same authors say that mothers who have rubella, also known as German measles, during the early months of pregnancy, may give birth to children who are deaf, have heart disease, mental retardation, or cataracts. The fact that many women have had the disease or been inoculated against it has reduced the numbers of cases of children born with disabilities because of it.

Another common congenital abnormality is cleft palate or cleft lip (Cheers, 2001). This occurs when the tissues of the upper lip and upper jaw do not fuse during the development of the fetus. The gap can be closed by surgery, but many operations are required to completely overcome the problem. In some cases, the conditions may be hereditary and occur among members of the same family. Sometimes the problem is also associated with heart defects.

According to Rathus et al. (2002), several other conditions can lead to disabilities at birth. Mothers who have AIDS may pass elements of that condition to their children. Tobacco and marijuana smoke can harm a fetus. So can prescription drugs such as antihistamines, acne drugs, antibiotics, and others. The consumption of hormones, excessive vitamins, narcotics, tranquilizers and sedatives as well as alcohol and hallucinogens, can all lead to children being born with many different kinds of disabilities.

Other kinds of childhood disabilities may result from genetic and chromosomal factors. Neural tube defects such as anencephaly, in which part of the brain is missing, and spina bifida, in which part of the spine is exposed or missing, may occur. Although children born with anencephaly die shortly after birth, many children with spina bifida live into adulthood with near-normal lifespans. Phenylketonuria is a disease in which the child cannot metabolize phenylalanine, which can lead to mental retardation. Retinoblastoma is a genetic condition that causes blindness (Rathus et al., 2002).

Cerebral Palsy

Other disabling conditions that become apparent at birth are not specifically hereditary or genetic. Cerebral palsy is caused by damage to the brain before, during, or shortly after birth (National Information Center for Children and Youth with Disabilities [NICHCY], 1992). It may result from illnesses during pregnancy, lack of oxygen supply to the baby, accidents, poisoning, child abuse, and other factors.

Cerebral palsy is the developmental disability that more people have than any other. About two children of every 4,000 born in the United States have some type of cerebral palsy. At least 5,000 toddlers and 1,200–1,500 preschoolers are diagnosed with cerebral palsy each year. In all, some 500,000 people in the United States have some degree of cerebral palsy. The numbers with cerebral palsy are larger than any other developmental disability, including Down syndrome, epilepsy, and autism (*Ask the Doctor,* 2002). According to the "Ask the Doctor" Web page (2002), children with very mild cerebral palsy sometimes recover from the condition before they reach school age. But for most, cerebral palsy is a lifetime disability. There are also varying degrees and types of cerebral palsy. There is spastic cerebral palsy, which is stiff and difficult movement; athetoid cerebral palsy, which is involuntary and uncontrolled movement; ataxic cerebral palsy, which is a disturbed sense of balance and depth perception; and mixed cerebral palsy, which may be a combination of those types for any one person. As indicated in this chapter, many people with cerebral palsy also have other disabilities such as autism, deafness, or blindness.

All people who have cerebral palsy have damage to the area of the brain that controls muscle tone. Therefore, they may have an increased level of muscle tone, reduced muscle tone, or a combination of the two, which leads to fluctuations in muscle tone. The parts of the body affected by cerebral palsy depends on where in the brain the damage occurred (*Ask the Doctor,* 2002).

Down Syndrome

The health condition or developmental disability called Down syndrome is the result of the presence of an extra chromosome, number 21. There appears to be one Down syndrome birth in every 1,000 to 1,100 live births. Therefore, every year, 3,000–5,000 children are born with this disorder. About 250,000 families in the United States are affected by Down syndrome (Pueschel, 2002).

Children who have Down syndrome are generally smaller, and their physical and mental developments are slower than in children who do not have the condition. The intelligence quotient of children with Down syndrome is from mild to moderate mental retardation. However, not all children with the condition are mentally retarded. Some may be borderline to low average in intelligence.

Motor development of children with Down syndrome is slow. Many do not begin to walk until they are 15 to 36 months old, as compared to the 12–14-month age at which most children learn to walk.

As suggested earlier, instead of the normal number of 46 chromosomes in each cell, the individual with Down syndrome has 47 chromosomes, and that is called the trisomyate 21. There is also a second type of Down syndrome called "translocation," in which the extra chromosome is attached to or translocated onto another chromosome, usually 14, 21, or 22. Many times, the parents of a child with Down syndrome are the carriers of the translocation.

There is another chromosome problem called mosaicism, which is found in about 1 percent of individuals with Down syndrome. In that case, some cells have

47 chromosomes and others have 46 chromosomes. Mosaicism is thought to be the result of a cell division error soon after conception.

Pueschel (2002) says that no one really knows the cause of Down syndrome. Beliefs include that it results from hormonal abnormalities, X-rays, viral infections, genetic issues, and immunologic problems. With the advancing age of the mother, the possibility of having a child with Down syndrome increases. However, more than 85 percent of children with Down syndrome are born to mothers who are younger than age 35. Some researchers think that older fathers may be a risk factor for Down syndrome.

The disabilities associated with Down syndrome are much more than the mental retardation, speech deficits, and mobility delays described earlier. About 60 to 85 percent of children with Down syndrome have hearing problems and 40 to 45 percent have congenital heart disease. There is also a high incidence of intestinal abnormalities such as in the esophagus and the small bowel. Many infants require surgical correction of problems in the intestinal track and the anus.

Children with Down syndrome have more eye problems than children who do not have the disorder. Two percent of infants with Down syndrome have cataracts which need to be removed. Cross-eyedness, near-sightedness, and far-sightedness are also more common with children who have Down syndrome.

Many children with Down syndrome fail to thrive in infancy because of eating problems, especially if they have serious heart disease. Obesity is often noted, however, during adolescence and early adulthood.

Children with Down syndrome also are more likely to have thyroid disfunctions. Between 15 and 20 percent of children with Down syndrome have hypothyroidism, and that condition may affect the central nervous system functioning.

Children may also experience dislocation of the kneecap, hip dislocation, and other skeletal system problems. In addition, children with Down syndrome are more susceptible to immunologic concerns, leukemia, Alzheimer's disease (which affects large numbers of people with Down syndrome as they grow older), seizure disorder, skin disorder, and sleep apnea.

However, there is no specific medical treatment for Down syndrome. The symptoms and disabilities discussed have to be treated as they would be treated in a person who does not have the condition.

Hydrocephalus

Another illness associated with early disabilities is hydrocephalus, which is a result of the increased accumulation of cerebrospinal fluid within the ventricles of the brain. The condition may result from developmental problems, infections, brain tumors, or injuries. Many children are born with the condition and there are treatments involving the installation of a "shunt," which allows cerebrospinal fluid to flow out of the head (Thomas, 1993).

Children may also be born with seizure disorders, some of which are classified as epilepsy. The conditions may result from injuries or any number of other factors that are not always known.

Mental retardation other than Down syndrome may also result from genetic factors. The condition may also arise from a lack of oxygen, accidents of the mother or the mother's illnesses such as rubella or meningitis, before, during, or shortly after birth, which result in brain damage (NICHCY, 2002).

Social Workers and Disabilities

Social workers are especially concerned with services for people who have disabilities, who constitute a vulnerable population, for a variety of reasons. One of those reasons is that disabilities have major social consequences. They can interfere with the ability of a person to succeed in school, with the capacity of an individual to marry and participate effectively in family life, and disabilities may also require extensive and constant health care services.

Social workers work in many kinds of settings that provide help to assist people with disabilities in their capacity to function effectively in social situations. In many cases, social workers are employed in disability centers such as those operated by vocational rehabilitation agencies and which are designed to help people with disabilities learn vocational skills and to achieve adequate functioning in activities of daily living such as household maintenance, child rearing, and food preparation. Social workers also serve people with disabilities through counseling programs and also often work in education programs for people with disabilities, including public schools.

Since the passage of the Americans with Disabilities Act in 1990 (P. L. 101–336), people with disabilities have enjoyed greater protections and guarantees of services than they had in the past. Children in schools are "mainstreamed" instead of being separated into special education classes. Public transportation and public accommodations must be made accessible to people with disabilities through the use of specially designed buses and trains, through the required installation of elevators in governmental and other public facilities, and, in some cases, the provision of aides or attendants for children with disabilities in public schools.

As some of the material in this section suggests, there are many examples that indicate that people with disabilities are among the most vulnerable in the United States. They are vulnerable to abuse, neglect, and deprivation, including unemployment.

Disabilities are also referred to in other sections of this text, including Chapter 2, on the basics of biology, anatomy, and physiology, as well as Chapter 4 on lifespan development.

ENVIRONMENTAL ILLNESS

Some health problems are also often associated with the environment. Conditions such as asthma, especially among adults, have increased as air pollution has become more severe. According to Reagan and Brookins-Fisher (2002), about 20 percent of the U.S. population suffers from asthma. The effects of the water supply, the impact of allergens on people who have allergic conditions, and the intensity of the sun are potential causes of illness that are directly associated with the environment. Some additional discussion of environmental health issues can be found in Chapter 13 on public health and biology.

Emphysema is a severe lung illness that limits the ability to breathe. It is often related to air pollution, but the best understood precursor to the disease is cigarette smoking (Reagan & Brookins-Fisher, 2002).

PERSONAL CHOICES, HEALTH, AND ILLNESS

Chapter 13, dealing with public health and biology, provides information on the preventive aspects of health and illness. As the chapter suggests, healthy living choices—especially careful attention to diet, avoiding obesity, exercising regularly, and avoiding some of the toxic substances that are causes of ill health such as alcohol and tobacco—can have a great deal to do with illness prevention. In some ways, social work roles include educating clients about the avoidance of behaviors that cause disease and pursuing behaviors that enhance health.

Perhaps the most important lesson that can be conveyed to clients is that people are often their own best health advocates. Knowing when to see a physician, knowing what to ask, being certain one understands, seeking second opinions before embarking on potentially dangerous treatments, and working to improve and maintain one's own health are critical issues in health preservation. And we are often our best health care "providers" simply by staying alert and concerned about our condition.

Perhaps this point is best made by columnist Anna Quindlen (2002), who writes that it is time to question the one-size fits all approach to health care. She was writing about the controversy over hormone replacement therapy mentioned earlier in this chapter. Her view is that physicians prescribed such therapy without considering the individual needs of patients. She says, "The day of the MDeity should be over; doctors have acted like little gods because patients have treated them as though they were" (Quindlen, 2002, p. 64). The import of her statement is that patients—the consumers of health care—must study their own health and involve themselves in decisions about their health.

SUMMARY

This chapter identifies some of the major health problems facing Americans, their nature, treatments that are used for them, and some of the roles social workers play in dealing with them. Although, obviously, not all health problems and diseases are discussed, some of those that are implicated in ending large numbers of lives are explicated in some detail. In addition, hereditary and developmental conditions are discussed. Clearly, human biology is, in some of the most important and practical ways, a factor in determining health and illness. For social workers, abstract knowledge of human biology is important but never quite so important as it is in understanding the health and well-being of those whom social workers serve.

There are many other health conditions that affect thousands or even millions of people that are not discussed in this chapter. To discuss all of them would require a volume as large as Clayman's (1989) encyclopedia or Beers and Berkow's (1999) manual. Those as well as standard medical dictionaries such as Thomas's (1993) can help shed light on the conditions discussed in this chapter as well as those that are not. Information from the Internet, as discussed in Chapter 1, is also available on most health problems and illnesses, often in great detail.

Of course, other chapters in this text also address some of the important issues of health and illness associated with other phenomena such as aging, the use and misuse of substances such as alcohol and drugs, as well as the genetic bases of some disease conditions. The basic information in this chapter should assist in better understanding the materials in other parts of the text.

DISCUSSION QUESTIONS

1. AIDS and cancer are both potentially fatal conditions. What might be some of the similarities and differences between a capable social worker's approach to working with two groups of people, one of which was suffering from cancer and the other of which was suffering from AIDS?

2. Describe some of the roles that lifestyles or personal choices about behavior, diet, and chemical ingestion play in illnesses among people. Be as specific as possible about the way in which such personal choices contribute to developing specific health conditions.

3. Discuss what you believe might be the social and emotional differences in a client's reactions to having a genetic health condition and one that is contracted through contact with others or through lifestyle choices about diet, exercise, and habits such as smoking. Do you believe there are qualitative differences in those reactions? In what ways could a social worker be helpful to a client who is reacting emotionally to health conditions? How might a client be served differently who is facing a life-long health problem as opposed to one who has a time-limited condition?

4. Select four of the conditions described in this chapter and search for information about them on the Internet, using one of the available Web browsers and an appropriate search engine such as Google or Yahoo!. What do you find? How reliable do you believe the information to be? How, in your opinion, can Internet information best be evaluated for accuracy and reliability?

CHAPTER NINE

BIOLOGY AND MENTAL ILLNESS

> *Mental health problems do not affect three or four*
> *out of every five persons but one out of one.*
> —William Menninger (1957)

> *The precise causes (etiology) of most mental disorders are not known.*
> *But the key word in this statement is* precise. *The* precise *causes of most*
> *mental disorders—or, indeed, of mental health—may not be known,*
> *but the broad forces that shape them* are *known: these are biological,*
> *psychological, and social/culture factors.*
> *What is most important to reiterate is that the causes of health and*
> *disease are generally viewed as a product of the* interplay *or* interaction
> *between biological, psychological, and sociocultural factors. This is true for*
> *all health and illness, including mental health and mental illness.*
> —U.S. Department of Health and Human Services (1999)

> *The dogma that "mental diseases are diseases of the brain" is*
> *a hangover from the materialism of the 1870s. It has become*
> *a prejudice which hinders all progress, with nothing to justify it.*
> —Carl G. Jung (1916)

An unsettled area of interest for social workers is the relationship between biology and mental illness. There has been a slow but perceptible shift in the theories concerning the origins of mental health problems that have been based on a complex and evolving understanding of the causes underlying human behavior. Willard Gaylin, a physician and psychotherapist who has written eleven books, captures this shift in the title of his latest book, *Talk Is Not Enough* (2000). The growth in understanding the biological factors associated with mental health disorders has called into question some of the techniques used by social workers in helping people with mental health problems. In the rest of the chapter the latest research concerning genetics, brain structure and functioning, and pharmacological interventions are examined with an eye toward how these new findings can be integrated with our present understanding of mental health. In fact, we argue strongly that the underpinnings of mental health disorders are best seen as an intertwined relationship between environment and biology.

From the 1950s to the late 1980s, many theories of mental health problems (psychoanalytic theory, family dynamics theory, systems theory, cognitive behavior) were dominated by a bias toward culturally determined explanations—ones that place the causality for mental health problems almost solely on the environment (family and other human relationships, neighborhood, culture, socioeconomic status) surrounding the person experiencing the mental health problems. The shift toward a more integrated approach to understanding the origins of mental health problems can be seen in the growing number of medically based interventions used. Increasingly, mental health disorders are treated by physicians with medicine and other physical approaches. Of course, some of the primary means of dealing with mental illness in the United States continue to involve community resources, community services, case management, counseling, and a number of other approaches that are outside the scope of this book.

The influence of medical approaches on the types of interventions used with people experiencing mental health disorders does, however, have a long history. Before much of the history of mental health and mental illness, which replaced insanity and other pejorative concepts in understanding those whose behavior was unacceptable, there has been an effort to demonstrate the ways in which mental illness results from physiological conditions. There is a strong desire to equate mental illness with physical illness in the sense that mental illness is simply another form of health problem. However, the evidence that mental illness is like physical illness is not as certain as some might hope, and the debate about the extent of biological or physiological bases for mental illness as well as the degree of acceptance of various kinds of treatments continues.

Of course, there are some biological, physical problems that lead to emotional difficulties and problematic behavior. Brain diseases such as Alzheimer's and other neurological conditions lead to behavior that is not socially acceptable. Clearly, however, these are physical diseases with psychological and behavioral consequences rather than general categories of functioning such as mental illness or emotional difficulty.

Mohr and Mohr (2001) state that there are three aspects of biology that are important to future discussions about the role of biology in mental health. First is the concept of neuroplasticity or the idea of how the brain "kindles" and "sensitizes." Little is currently understood about normal brain development and how the brain functions on a daily basis. The second aspect of biology important to understanding mental health disorders is the effects of "life events on brain and behavior." An example of this relationship is found in post-traumatic stress disorder (PTSD), which is discussed later in the chapter. Research shows that horrific events (environment) actually change the brain's chemistry (biology) in a way that causes the symptomatology associated with PTSD. The third area that is worth exploring is the understanding of the interactions between genes and the environment.

GENETIC AND BIOLOGICAL UNDERPINNINGS
OF MENTAL HEALTH DISORDERS

The history of genetics research concerning the origins of mental health problems is rife with attempts to study single-gene inheritance for schizophrenia, bipolar disorder, and depression, to name a few mental health disorders. These studies have ultimately shown that genes play a weak role in the complex behaviors associated with mental health problems. In fact, the underlying genetic predisposition for schizophrenia and bipolar disorder may actually consist of a number of genes that are triggered by certain environmental cues. Therefore, the idea of finding single-gene relationships to mental health problems has long since been abandoned as a rational explanation for mental illnesses. However, being able to test people for a weak genetic predisposition to certain mental health problems will help in developing interventions that are based on preventing the necessary environmental cues that trigger the underlying biology of mental health disorders. To pinpoint the environmental cues necessary to put together a prevention intervention requires an understanding of how the genes that induce the biological aspect of the disorder function.

Research surrounding schizophrenia serves as an example of a weak genetic approach. According to Begley (2002), in a popular magazine cover story on schizophrenia, there are some genetic predispositions to the condition. However, it is not a direct or perfect relationship. An identical twin may have the condition but the twin's sibling may have it in fewer than half the cases. Of course, schizophrenia is the most prevalent of the psychoses and is characterized by symptoms such as delusions, hallucinations, odd behavior and body postures, and sometimes the absence of feelings or incoherent speech. For more information, the weak biological approach is discussed in Chapter 5.

In contrast, there are mental health disorders that have clear biological underpinnings and appear to have few genetic links. PTSD is one of the psychological conditions that also involves some neurobiological and physiological changes, but little grounding in genetics. People with PTSD have alterations in the central and autonomic nervous system, including altered brainwave activity. Sleep abnormalities are also associated with PTSD as is some elevation of thyroid functions and higher than normal levels of natural opiates in the brain (Davidson & Foa, 1993; Kessler, Sonnega, Bromet, Hughes, & Nelson, 1996). These changes appear to be the result of exposure to severe and/or repeated trauma, which has no relationship to genetic inheritance. Both kinds of biological underpinnings are discussed in this chapter.

Other mental health and developmental disabilities such as autism, attention-deficit hyperactivity disorder (ADHD), reading disability, and mild mental impairment also show a tendency toward weak inheritance factors. Asherson and Curran (2001, p. 123) state that in fact most mental health disorders "do not conform to Mendelian patterns of segregation and are thought to result from the combined effects of several genes (oligogenic) or perhaps many genes (polygenic), each of which, on its own, has only a small effect. In these cases, variations of single genes are neither sufficient nor necessary to cause the disorder, but such genes act as susceptibility genes, increasing risk for the disorder." Asherson and Curran (2001, p. 123) go on to state that "mapping and identifying the genes responsible for such complex disorders represents a greater challenge than that posed by rare Mendelian diseases, but one that is becoming rapidly more tractable."

Clearly, genes and the environment play roles in the development of mental health disorders; however, the extent of each and the relationship both have with the ultimate realization of a mental health disorder remain unknown. The first step in gaining this knowledge is the identification of the genes involved in the biological portion of the equation. After identification, the greatest challenge for researchers and practitioners will be "describing the molecular mechanisms involved and their relationship to biological and behavioural function. Bridges will need to be built between structure and function, between molecular mechanisms and behaviours, and between social, genetic and developmental psychiatry. This area of functional genomics will be the real challenge in the post-genomic era if we are to see tangible benefits from current progress in mapping out the genetic and environmental influences" (Asherson & Curran, 2001, p. 126).

THE BRAIN AND MENTAL ILLNESS

Psychological illness may be identified as dysfunctions of the mind or diseases of the brain. The problem with this simplistic model is that the total functioning of the brain is poorly understood. The brain appears to develop under two significant influences. The first influence is the genetic underpinning to brain development. The second influence is the impact of environmental cues on sculpting the brain's functioning and in turn the processes of thinking, emotions, and behavior. The evidence therefore indicates that the brain's functioning and structure are defined by both biology and the environment.

See Figure 9.1 for identification of the brain's regions and their general functioning.

Neuroimaging the Brain

One of the interesting ways of measuring the relationship between biology and mental health disorders is the use of neuroimaging machines such as magnetic resonance imaging (MRI), proton spectroscopy (MRS), and positron emission tomography (PET) to examine the physical features and functioning of the brain. These neuroimaging machines have contributed significantly to the improved understanding of the brain's structure and function. Using these machines, which create highly detailed and precise images of the brain, has not only improved understanding of general functioning of the brain but also the etiology of mental health disorders as related to the brain's possible role in these disorders (Callicott & Weinberger, 1999). Neuroimaging has been used to also examine the influence of environment by examining how environmental cues cause functional changes in the brain.

Neuroimaging machines typically perform one of two types of functions. One type of machine is used for structural analysis of the brain and the other exam-

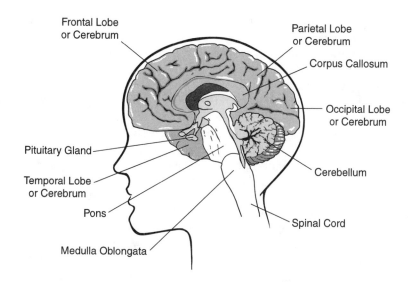

Frontal Lobe
or Cerebrum

Parietal Lobe
or Cerebrum

Corpus Callosum

Occipital Lobe
or Cerebrum

Pituitary Gland

Cerebellum

Temporal Lobe
or Cerebrum

Pons

Medulla Oblongata

Spinal Cord

Cerebellum—the part of the brain below the back of the cerebrum. It regulates balance, posture, movement, and muscle coordination.

Corpus Callosum—a large bundle of nerve fibers that connect the left and right cerebral hemispheres. In the lateral section, it looks a bit like a "C" on its side.

Frontal Lobe of the Cerebrum—the top, front regions of each of the cerebral hemispheres. They are used for reasoning, emotions, judgment, and voluntary movement.

Medulla Oblongata—the lowest section of the brainstem (at the top end of the spinal cord); it controls automatic functions including heartbeat, breathing, etc.

Occipital Lobe of the Cerebrum—the region at the back of each cerebral hemisphere that contains the centers of vision and reading ability (located at the back of the head).

Parietal Lobe of the Cerebrum—the middle lobe of each cerebral hemisphere between the frontal and occipital lobes; it contains important sensory centers (located at the upper rear of the head).

Pituitary Gland—a gland attached to the base of the brain (located between the Pons and the Corpus Callosum) that secretes hormones.

Pons—the part of the brainstem that joins the hemispheres of the cerebellum and connects the cerebrum with the cerebellum. It is located just above the Medulla Oblongata.

Spinal Cord—a thick bundle of nerve fibers that runs from the base of the brain to the hip area, running through the spine (vertebrae).

Temporal Lobe of the Cerebrum—the region at the lower side of each cerebral hemisphere; contains centers of hearing and memory (located at the sides of the head).

FIGURE 9.1   Lateral View of the Brain

Reprinted with permission from enchantedlearning.com

ines the ongoing functioning of the brain. MRI is an example of neuroimaging that is used to examine the structure of the brain. By examining the structure, researchers look for abnormalities in the anatomy of the brain. PET and MRS are neuroimaging machines used to examine the functioning of the brain. These machines provide researchers with an opportunity to examine abnormalities in ongoing activity (Lilienfeld, 1998). For example, PETs measure the flow of blood in the brain and allow observers to identify what parts of the brain are active during mental activities.

Callicott and Weinberger (1999, p. 127) in their analysis of neuroimaging state that no "gross structural lesions are associated with the most prevalent mental illnesses." Neuroimaging has shown that the abnormalities in the brains of individuals experiencing a mental illness are "subtle or affect complex functional dynamics, perhaps at the intricate level of cortical process." Because neuroimaging allows for the study of brain functioning, it offers the possibility of examining these subtle and complex functional dynamics.

Callicott and Weinberger (1999) ask the interesting question of whether there is a clinical value to neuroimaging. First, the question of whether symptoms of mental health—their severity, duration, and frequency—are reflected in the neuroimaging needs to be answered. Evidence from a MRI, MRS, PET, and other neuroimaging techniques indicates that there are particular deviations in quantifiable measures of brain function in specific areas of the brain that give regular insight into the severity, duration, and frequency of symptomatology. An example cited by Callicott and Weinberger (1999, p. 112) is that a finding from a PET "suggested abnormalities in orbitofrontal cortex and caudat nucleus/basal ganglia in obsessive compulsive disorder (OCD)." Given that there is some possibility of measuring changes in brain functioning, Callicott and Weinberger (1999) suggest that neuroimaging has the possibility for monitoring and adjusting pharmacological interventions in a way that is much more refined than present methods.

Currently there are few clinical applications for neuroimaging. Part of the problem with developing clinical applications for neuroimaging is the lack of a broad-based understanding of how the brain functions under normal conditions during various developmental stages. Without a full image of the brain functioning under normal circumstances, there is not a baseline from which to judge functioning that is not normal. As a result of this, there continue to be problems with identifying distinctions between state and trait characteristics, the effects of medication, the reliability of findings, the plasticity of the brain, and the long-term development of the brain (Callicott & Weinberger, 1999). Callicott and Weinberger suggest that the study of children and the developing brain is one method that may help provide a better understanding of brain functioning and ultimately the clinical usefulness of neuroimaging.

The Brain and Post-Traumatic Stress Disorder (PTSD)

During the 1970s and 1980s, many of the Vietnam veterans seeking relief from PTSD were treated using a talk therapy approach. Talk therapy, based on the work done with Vietnam veterans, has also been used as the primary intervention with people that experience PTSD because of childhood abuse, torture, and other types of trauma. Research has shown that talk-based intervention has not proven as effective as initially thought (Butler, 1996). Butler cites research by psychiatrists at the West Haven Veterans Administration, Yale, Harvard, UCLA, and Dartmouth indicating strongly that PTSD is not only an emotional response to trauma but also elicits a change in brain chemistry (Butler, 1996, p. 40).

Some of the features of PTSD, such as "almost unbearable states of physiological arousal: a hypersensitive emotional tripwire, an exaggerated startle response and profound distortions of memory," sleep disorders, and "wildly swinging inner states" have underpinnings in altered brain chemistry (Butler, 1996, p. 40). Butler (1996) cites research and advances in endocrinology, animal behavior, neurochemistry, and neuroimaging as contributing to increased understanding of the biological underpinnings of PTSD. As a result of this, researchers suspect that individuals with the most serious forms of PTSD—created by particularly dramatic incidents and/or long ongoing trauma—may never be the same again biologically (Butler, 1996).

Butler (1996), citing the *Neurobiological and Clinical Consequences of Stress* (Friedman, Charney, & Deutch, 1995), states that "the body responds to extreme stress by releasing a cascade of cortisol, adrenaline and other hormones that can damage brain cells, impair memory and set in motion a long-lasting and worsening disregulation of the body's complex biochemistry." The result is a "breakdown of the normal stress response because the system is overtaxed" (p. 40).

The two primary fight-or-flight hormones are adrenaline and noradrenaline. When stress or a sense of danger is present, people will often feel what is commonly referred to as a "rush of adrenaline." This increase in hormones quickens our senses, increases our heartbeat, and enhances our memory and clarity. These are all good effects of an adrenaline rush and they serve a purpose related to survival. When stress that elicits these responses in the brain is continuous, causing prolonged exposure of the brain to these chemicals, there are immediate and long-term changes. "Repeated adrenaline rushes seem to progressively sensitize brain chemistry, provoking ever-greater floods of adrenaline at lower thresholds" (Butler, 1996, p. 41). This results in hyperactive fight-or-flight responses. "Floods of adrenaline and noradrenaline not only increase and accompany emotional and neurobiological arousal, they also can trigger the seizure-like cinematic relivings of trauma known as flashbacks" (Butler, 1996, p. 42).

Beyond what appear to be long-term alterations to brain chemistry, recent research suggests that severe and prolonged trauma may have long-term impacts on the hippocampus, the "seahorse-shaped structure deep in the brain" that is "crucial to short-term memory and may play a role in the sorting and storing of long-term memories (Butler, 1996, p. 43). MRI studies have indicated that the size of the hippocampus is reduced in trauma victims when compared to individuals who are not traumatized. Whether people with small hippocampi are more susceptible to PTSD or if PTSD alters the size of the hippocampus is not yet known.

Schizophrenia and the Brain

Phyllis A. Brown in a 1994 article describes the symptomatology associated with schizophrenia as having difficulty communicating in language or facial expression, a lack of empathy, and an inability to judge others' intentions toward them.

These problems are coupled with a breakdown in the processing and filtering of information taken in by the senses. The result is an overwhelming of the mind that is unable to shut out the many environmental cues it takes in coupled with an inability to relate to other human beings.

A mounting quantity of research indicates that brain abnormalities associated with schizophrenia arise very early in life, probably before birth, which disrupt the normal development of the brain. Brown (1994) states that "the challenge facing scientists is not only to uncover the precise nature of those abnormalities and devise methods of treating them, but also to show how they relate to the disturbances of mind suffered by schizophrenics" (p. 26).

Initial research points to an association between schizophrenia and overactivity in the part of the brain that is involved in arousal and motivation (Begley, 2002). People with schizophrenia also appear to have an excessive amount of the neuroprocessor dopamine. In healthy people, the dopamine flow between brain cells is carefully controlled, but in people with schizophrenia the substance surges out of control and disrupts the usual relationships between brain cells.

Much like PTSD, the specific cause for chemical differences in the brains of individuals experiencing schizophrenia is unknown. The most significant has to do with dopamine, "a neurotransmitter, that ferries impulses between nerve cells" (Brown, 1994, p. 27). Researchers suspect that "imbalances in constituents of fatty substances called phospholipids that make up the cell membranes of neurons" disrupt the neurotransimission processes performed by dopamine. "The strongest evidence to support the involvement of dopamine in schizophrenia is that drugs which block certain dopamine receptors in the basal ganglia reduce the symptoms of the disease, while other drugs that stimulate the dopamine system, such as amphetamines can produce schizophrenia-like symptoms even in healthy people" (Brown, 1994, p. 129).

The structural differences observed in the brains of people experiencing schizophrenia by using neuroimaging include lateral ventricles that "tend to be significantly larger than normal brains" and "a smaller volume of tissue in the left temporal lobe than in normal brains" (Brown, 1994, p. 27). Neuroimaging also suggests that there are possible structural abnormalities in the hippocampus of individuals experiencing schizophrenia, which is the part of the brain that processes learning and memory. None of these features is shared by all individuals experiencing schizophrenia, and no one particular structural abnormality appears to be significant in and of itself.

In the two examples discussed—PTSD and schizophrenia—a significant amount of evidence suggests that people who experience these disorders have both structural and functional differences in their brain. Evidence also suggests that depression, learning disorders, eating disorders, and a host of other problems that fall under the rubric of mental health have some relationship to structural and/or functional abnormalities in the brain. What these brain differences actually mean is still undetermined. Furthermore, which came first—the abnormal brain structure or function or the mental health disorder (i.e., which was the causal agent)—has yet to be determined, leaving the question of which caused which open to debate. Other biological determining factors that may have yet undetermined influence on the brain development of people with schizophrenia include the age of the father—the older he is, the more likely the child is to develop schizophrenia; viruses that cause difficulty with the fetal brain development; mothers who suffer from rubella or malnutrition while pregnant; and having a family member who has schizophrenia (Begley, 2002).

PHARMACOLOGICAL INTERVENTIONS

The profession of social work in general and medical social work in particular have been influenced significantly by the medical model. Therefore, the mixing of pharmacological interventions with more traditional social work approaches such as community-based services and talk therapy is not surprising. In fact, Gaylin (2000) points out that in recent years, the trend has been toward a primary use of psychotropic drugs to treat mental health disorders. As a result of this increased use of pharmacological interventions, there has been a revolution in the care of people with the severe mental health problem of psychosis because of drugs.

For example, the drugs used for schizophrenia block dopamine. Early drugs blocked the substance in the whole set of brain pathways, but new drugs focus their effects on the brain pathways that control the thoughts and behaviors associated with schizophrenia and leave the rest of the brain's functions alone. These new drugs include Clozaril, Risperdal, Zyprexa, Geodon, and Seroquel. According to W. Alexander Morton (2002), a professor of pharmacy practice, the daily cost of these antipsychotic medications, which are called "atypicals," ranges from about $7 to $12 per day per patient. Another new drug, aripiprazole, is supposed to have even fewer side effects than other atypicals. The reason for the decrease in side effects is that aripiprazole does not entirely shut off or turn on receptors for dopamine. Instead, it does a little of both, acting more as a monitor of the dopamine flow. Because of this refinement, there is less chance of tremors, stiffness, weight gain, sexual dysfunction, and risk of diabetes, which are associated with some antipsychotic drugs. Specificity has not increased the apparent positive impact of the previous generations of drugs for schizophrenia, but instead decreased significantly the amount of undesirable side effects (Anand, 2002).

When studying pharmacological interventions for mental health disorders, one should understand the basic processes of pharmacokinetics, pharmacodynamics, and neurotransmission (Farmer & Bentley, 2001). These are the three processes that underlie the manner in which medication works for people experiencing mental health disorders. Each process provides practitioners with quantification of how medication is impacting on a person's health.

Pharmacokinetics is the study of how a person's body responds (physically) to taking medication. Farmer and Bentley state there are four biological processes associated with pharmacokinetics—absorption, distribution, metabolism, and excretion—studied in pharmacokinetics: (1) Absorption is the process of medication moving from its intake point to the bloodstream, (2) distribution is the process of medication moving from the bloodstream to its intended point of intervention in the brain, (3) metabolism is the process of the medication breaking down to inactive ingredients that the body can remove, and (4) excretion is the process of removing medication from the body "mainly via the kidneys, through bile, feces, and urine, and also through sweat, saliva, tears, and breast milk" (Farmer & Bentley, 2001, p. 214).

One of the most important information items used to understand the process of pharmacokinetics is the level of medication in the blood stream. Blood levels, which is what the measure is commonly called, represent how much of the medication is active in a person's bloodstream. This gives social workers, clients, and their psychiatrists information useful in setting appropriate medication levels. Blood levels can also give insight into whether or not clients are complying with the medication regime laid out in treatment plans.

Understanding the pharmacodynamics of medication informs social workers of how medication impacts on the client's body. One of the most straightforward quantifications of measuring this impact is the *therapeutic index*. The index shows medications' level of toxicity, thereby providing a range of possible blood levels in which medications can be prescribed. In correspondence with blood levels, the therapeutic index helps social workers monitor the overall impact and general effectiveness of medicine interventions.

Finally, neurotransmission is important for social workers to understand when working with clients taking medication. The rationale for medications is often understood by knowing their effect on the process of transmission of chemicals in the brain. Typically, medications raise or decrease the levels of neurotransmitters such as serotonin and dopamine, which naturally occur in the human brain. These neurotransmitters often play key roles in determining emotion and behavior, as discussed earlier. Beyond providing the rationale for why a medication should be prescribed, understanding neurotransmission and how medication influences that transmission also gives insight into why adverse side effects occur, how they are manifested, and how they can be controlled (Farmer & Bentley, 2001).

Pharmacological Interventions and Depression

"Currently available antidepressants act primarily by blocking the reuptake of monoamines, inhibiting their degradation, or interfering with their binding to specific receptors. (To date, treatment of depression has revolved around agents that exert effects on monamine reuptake or receptor activity. Many of the current medications are agents within one class and are remarkably similar to each other in both therapeutic and side effects.) The introduction of selective serotonin reuptake inhibitors (SSRIs) in 1988 into the United States revolutionized pharmacological therapy for a number of depressive, anxiety, and eating disorders. There are now five SSRIs on the U.S. market—fluoxetine, paroxetine, sertraline, fluvoxamine, and citalopram. These drugs differ from their predecessor tricyclic antidepressants (TCAs) by selectively and potentially inhibiting the uptake of serotonin into presynaptic neurons with little effect on blocking norepinephrine reuptake. The TCAs are primarily noradrenergic in their effect. Moreover, the SSRIs exert virtually no effect on blocking muscarinic acetylcholine or histamine-1 receptors and thus do not produce the panoply of side effects that are seen commonly with the TCAs, for example, dry mouth, constipation, orthostatic hypotension, or sedation. These pharmacological differences have accounted for efficacy of the SSRIs over a wider range of conditions (major depression, dysthymia, obsessive-compulsive disorder, premenstrual dysphoria, etc.) as well as a more favorable side-effect profile" (Schatzberg, 1999, pp. 179–180).

An example of how brain development interacts with medication effectiveness is the debate about whether SSRIs are as effective as TCAs in geriatric patients. Improved knowledge concerning brain development and how changes created by aging influence the brain's functioning will help improve the accuracy of medication interventions. The same debate also surrounds the effectiveness of SSRIs for people experiencing severe depression compared to those with mild depression. "At this time there is an intense debate as to whether SSRIs produce as much effect as do the older TCAs in geriatric and severely depressed patients." Schatzberg (1999, p. 181) states that

> the psychopharmacologist of the twenty-first century will have a better understanding of the maximal gain to be expected from SSRIs versus that from TCAs or other noradrenergic agents in more severely depressed or elderly patients. We may then have a hierarchy of treatments based on severity of depression. For example, a particular SSRI might be used preferentially in a patient with mild-to-moderate depression, whereas a TCA-like agent might be prescribed for a more severely depressed patient.

What is missing from pharmacological interventions is effective, nonaddictive, dopaminergic agents (combining the norepinephrine/dopamine uptake blocker) for antidepressant therapy.

Pharmacological Interventions and Bipolar Disorder

Research pertaining to the effectiveness of drug interventions with individuals experiencing bipolar disorder highlights the relationship between biology and personality. A popular medication intervention is the use of mood stabilizers (e.g., lithium), which work by penetrating cells via sodium. (However, they do not leave the body as effectively as sodium.) Once in the cell, mood stabilizers interact with cell systems involved with the transmitter release and second-message systems in a way that blocks the particular transmitters and hormones associated with mood. However, this process does not have the same outcome for all forms of bipolar disorder. For example, people who respond best to lithium are individuals with classical mania rather than the mixed or schizoaffective form. People with elated-grandiose mania showed a better response to lithium than people with the destructive-paranoid type. Dysphoric mania was also less likely to improve. (Murashita, Kato, Shioiri, Inubushi, & Kato, 2000).

Pharmacological Interventions and Gender

Until recently, the medical community assumed that psychotropic agents had the same pharmacokinetic and pharmacodynamic processes for men and women. Most of the animal and human research concerning psychotropic agents has been conducted with male research participants. Schatzberg (1999) points to the passage of the Women's Health Equity Act in 1993 as playing an important role in encouraging more research in this area. He shows that differences in how men and women respond to antidepressants may exist, with women being more tolerant of SSRIs than men. Schatzberg (1999) also touches on the idea that race, ethnicity, and culture may have an influence on how medications work.

Summary

Although psychotherapy, which might broadly but not quite accurately be described as counseling, is considered by some in mental health to be inadequate without the addition of medicines, many mental health practitioners consider medicine, alone, without psychotherapy to also be inadequate. The medicines can calm the agitated mental health patient. Other drugs may help the depressed person overcome that depression. There are medicines that treat severe, psychotic mental health problems; others that treat obsessive and compulsive behavior; and many others.

In general, Morton (2002) reports that many of the psychoactive medicines have "broad-spectrum" effects. That is, drugs designed to deal with depression, of which there are many, may also function as antianxiety preparations. They may also be effective in helping patients deal with anger, impulse control, and premenstrual emotional problems. The antidepression medicines generally have some adverse consequences such as headaches, gastrointestinal discomfort, weight gain, and sexual dysfunction.

MENTAL ILLNESS AND PHYSICAL FACTORS

The major sources of information on mental health and mental illness suggest a variety of ways in which physical or biological processes and factors are involved in mental functioning. Although they may be associated, it is difficult to determine if the physical factors predate and bring on the mental problems or if the physical factors are manifestations of the mental condition.

The Diagnostic and Statistical Manual of Mental Disorders (DSM-IV) (Frances, 1994), which is the most authoritative source on mental illness and which is used in diagnosing mental conditions in psychiatric practice and in most mental health services, describes a number of physical features that are associated with mental illnesses. The manual does not cite studies that demonstrate that mental illnesses are "caused" by physical factors because no such studies, to date, have been definitive. However, the DSM-IV reports that associations are identified between physiological

■ ■ ■ ■ ■ ▬▬▬

ELECTROCONVULSIVE THERAPIES

One of the complicated and controversial biological issues associated with mental ill-ness is the use of ECT or electroconvulsive therapy. Historically, the concept has also been defined as shock treatments, and it has been used in treating mental illness since the 1930s (Smith, 2001).

A magazine editor, Daniel Smith of the *Atlantic* (2001), traces the use of electro-convulsive therapy from its beginnings to its current uses, which Smith says are quite effective with people who are suffering from severe depression. Clearly, many mental health experts, particularly psychiatrists, are enthusiastic users of ECT and insist that some earlier difficulties with the treatment have been overcome by careful use of anesthetics and muscle relaxants. The problems associated with the use of ECT include broken limbs and other kinds of physical problems. However, Smith (2001) suggests that those have been overcome.

Objections to ECT by patients and by mental health reformers are that if not used properly it can cause death, and that ECT is really a form of closed-head brain injury. Even advocates, however, agree that ECT causes memory loss among most of those who are treated with it. Smith (2001) also notes that much of the criticism of ECT is political rather than medically oriented. He notes that the Church of Scientology is one of the strongest critics of the treatment.

One may conclude that the use of ECT is effective in the treatment of certain kinds of mental illness, such as depression—especially severe depression. However, it has its critics, and even its advocates are not certain exactly why and how ECT works to help patients overcome depression. That alone does not invalidate the use of the treatment. There are other medicines and procedures that have positive effects for patients but are not fully understood in terms of their biology and biochemistry.

Smith (2001) points out that some advocates also view ECT as an effective antipsychotic and anticatatonic drug. Psychosis is, of course, severe mental illness such as schizophrenia, and catatonia is a mental condition that immobilizes patients and removes them from any significant involvement with others. For much of psychiatric practice, the psychotrophic drugs favored by Gaylin (2001) are the treatment of choice. But, as Smith notes, such drugs are "a frustratingly inexact method of treatment—with a long wait between the first pill and any sign of relief. Often though they don't work at all. This can be fatal for a patient who is suicidally depressed. Moreover, some patients prove resistant to medication" (Smith, 2001, p. 82).

Daniel Smith's article on ECT encouraged several letters to the editor in the May 2001 issue. Michael M. Faenza (May 2001), representing the National Association of Mental Health, disagreed with the characterization of those who opposed ECT as just a few former patients, dissenting psychiatrists, and the Church of Scientology. Faenza says that many established organizations, such as his own, which is the largest non-profit organization dealing with mental health from the United States, say that ECT should be used with extreme caution and that other treatment approaches should be used first and only if they have failed or been carefully evaluated and rejected should ECT be used. Many people are injured by ECT in various ways, he points out, and there is no way of knowing who will be most injured in the process.

Perhaps the most crucial was a letter from Dr. Thomas A. Preston, a professor of medicine at the University of Washington (Preston, 2002). He points out that Smith's

(continued)

CONTINUED

article focused on testimonials and anecdotes, which any therapy can often engender. However, there was no evidence in the Smith article, the physician points out, of carefully evaluated treatments, experimental evaluations, or other reliable means of determining the efficacy of ECT. He wonders if it is not just a high-powered form of placebo.

In a rejoinder, Daniel Smith responded to those writers and others who wondered why Smith failed to say that little had been done to scientifically test the safety of ECT as well as its efficacy (Smith, 2001). He does not respond to the lack of scientific evaluation of the process. He says he was reporting the use of it by many psychiatry experts and many patients who said that the procedure does not injure the brain or otherwise injure patients. He says that as it is now administered, the procedure is safe and useful for people with severe mental illnesses and with failures in treatment of other kinds. However, he agrees that some people lose memory and have other negative effects, but he says that these problems are minimal.

Electroconvulsive therapy is, according to Hales and Hales (1996), the treatment of choice for people who have very severe depressions and who are suicidal, delusional, or whose disorders are otherwise life threatening. People who have to have rapid improvement or whose lives are threatened because of their emotional problems are good candidates, according to Hales and Hales (1995), for ECT.

---

factors and mental illnesses. The DSM-IV actually denies that physical findings are always associated with the condition called schizophrenia, perhaps the most commonly diagnosed major mental illness. "No laboratory findings have been identified that are diagnostic of schizophrenia" (Frances, 1994, p. 280). The DSM-IV points out, however, that specific laboratory findings have been shown to be abnormal in groups of people with schizophrenia, compared to control groups. And, the DSM-IV reports, structural brain abnormalities seem to occur in people with schizophrenia. Some of the abnormalities found are decreased size of various parts of the brain and of the brain itself. Some people with schizophrenia have abnormal brain blood flow. Some people with the condition drink very large amounts of water and may have electrolyte imbalances (Frances, 1994).

The DSM-IV goes on to say that many persons with schizophrenia are sometimes physically awkward, may have poor coordination, and may confuse left and right. Some also have small physical abnormalities such as a highly arched palate, narrow- or wide-set eyes, or subtle malformations of the ear (Frances, 1994, p. 280). However, these physical indicators are not part of the "diagnostic criteria" the DSM-IV uses to confirm or deny a diagnosis of schizophrenia.

Part of the problem with tying mental illnesses to physical conditions is that it is difficult to determine which came first. Do the substances in the brain result from the schizophrenia, do the two occur together, or is schizophrenia a product of physical substances and factors?

Many psychiatric conditions have physical manifestations. Those who suffer from major depression, in addition to the emotional factors in their feelings and behavior, may also demonstrate slow speech, thinking, and body movements, according to the DSM-IV (Frances, 1994). Schizophrenia also may decrease energy, make the patient especially tired, and cause fatigue. Small tasks may require substantial effort and exhaustion may result from ordinary physical activity. However, there are no specific laboratory findings that are associated with depression. There are, however, some laboratory findings that seem to occur in groups of people who have major depression.

Electroencephalogram (EEG) abnormalities may occur in large proportions of patients who suffer from depression. Neurotransmitters, such as serotonin, dopamine, and acetylcholine, may be found in larger quantities than in people who are not depressed. Those substances are found in the blood, spinal fluid, and perhaps urine. These kinds of findings suggest that depression causes physiological changes, and physiological changes may also cause mental illnesses.

The DSM-IV also specifies a large number of pain disorders. These might be significantly uncomfortable for the patient, but their origins may be from psychological factors. One may also encounter pain disorders that have psychological as well as general medical conditions as causes. Pain that is strictly based on a general medical condition is not considered a mental disorder, but many times, pain disorders can be associated with herniated disks and other physical problems. These kinds of disorders are not to be confused with somatization disorders, which are physical pains that have their origins in psychological problems.

The *Diagnostic and Statistical Manual* has a set of conditions called disorders due to a general medical condition (Frances, 1994). It lists the following conditions that may be due to general medical conditions: delirium, dementia, amnestic disorder (a variety of memory problems that are more commonly called forms of "amnesia"), psychotic disorder, mood disorder, anxiety disorder, sexual dysfunction, and sleep disorder. For a condition to be classified as one that is a result of a general medical condition, a physical examination or laboratory findings has to show that the disturbance is a direct physiological consequence of a general medical condition.

Diagnosticians may also find that there are features in the disorder that are different than the usual features one finds with the problem. For example, a person who has schizophrenia or symptoms that are associated with schizophrenia but who has the condition the first time at advanced age would indicate a disease that is usually a medical disorder rather than a mental illness alone. Diagnosticians are urged to find evidence in the literature establishing the relationship between the physiological medical condition and the illness. They are also urged to be sure that the disturbance is not likely to be the product of another medical mental disorder. The disturbance should also be one that is not found exclusively during the course of a patient's delirium.

There are also other categories such as catatonic disorders and personality changes that can be associated with general medical conditions. It is clear that many mental illnesses have some association with physical conditions. The exact relationship between physical and mental conditions is basically not known. Whether illnesses have their genesis in the body or the mind is not fully understood, but there are characteristics of both that are affected by both; that is, some conditions have both physical and mental manifestations and it is not completely understood in which realm they began.

BIOLOGY AND FACIAL EXPRESSIONS

One of the more remarkable discoveries about the associations between biology and physiology with human behavior is the study of facial expressions and the ways in which they communicate emotions, which is also discussed in the descriptions of some mental health conditions. Such knowledge is especially important in diagnosing and treating mental illness. Gladwell (2002), writing in the *New Yorker*, describes the work of Paul Ekman, a psychologist at the University of California at San Francisco, who has devoted decades to the study of facial expressions, facial muscles, and the display of emotions through those facial expressions.

Gladwell (2002) points out that Darwin, in some of his later writings, particularly the book he wrote in 1872 called *The Expression of the Emotions in Animals,* said that all mammals show emotions in their faces. The study of facial expressions and their association with emotions has proceeded since that time.

Ekman traveled throughout the world to determine exactly how facial expressions communicate emotions. He discovered that in places as varied as New Guinea, Japan, and South America, there were almost universal interpretations of the same facial expressions.

Gladwell (2002) writes that Ekman worked with Silvan Tomkins, another psychologist who taught at Rutgers and Princeton and studied at Harvard, who was Ekman's partner in developing the facial expression theories. Ekman, along with Tomkins, used a variety of films and photographs to examine the bulges and wrinkles in the face and to associate particular forms of facial expressions with behavior.

Following up on the work of Tomkins, Ekman and his colleague Wallace Friesen (Gladwell, 2002) worked to create a taxonomy of facial expressions. They sat across from each other for hours, day after day, and made every face they could think of. They went further and learned the anatomy of facial muscles. From those studies, they were able to identify every distinct movement that the face was able to make. Ekman and Friesen categorized those facial movements into forty-three "action units" (Gladwell, 2002) and began attempting to display to one another each of the "action units" that were possible. They then began analyzing the "action units" in combination and decided, over a period of 7 years, that there were 300 combinations of two muscles, and when a third was added, 4,000 possible combinations. When five facial muscles are used at one time, they decided that there were 10,000 visible facial expressions. Most of the expressions do not mean anything or very much, but about 3,000 do. Ekman, according to Gladwell (2002), has specific identifications for each of those "action units" and each seems to mean something different. Gladwell (2002, p. 63) writes,

> Happiness, for instance, is essentially A.U. (action unit) six and twelve—contracting the muscles that raise the cheek . . . in combination with the zygomatic major, which pulls up the corners of the lips. Fear is A.U. one, two, and four, or, more fully, one, two, four, five, and twenty, with or without action units twenty-five, twenty-six, or twenty-seven.

Perhaps most remarkable was the discovery that when people consciously forced their faces into the action units that were identified, they felt the emotions that the facial expressions communicated; that is, if they forced their faces into sad expressions, they felt sad, happy expressions led to happy feelings, etc.

Police officers have found knowledge of these facial expressions helpful in determining whether or not they were in danger from a criminal. Those who understand the system are also able to make psychiatric diagnoses of patients by determining not only what they say but also the facial expressions they display. They are able to detect hostility, depression, and any number of kinds of feelings as well as feelings that could be turned into actions, from simply observing and pinpointing facial expressions.

Ekman, according to Gladwell (2002), developed many of his concepts, especially those of understanding the ability to diagnose and fully comprehend human emotions, from the works of the late sociologist Erving Goffman. Goffman theorized that people use words to communicate information that they are willing to have others know about themselves. But he pointed out that we tend to look away when people use gestures that may be revealing of one thing or another but that they would not want others to know about, such as picking their noses or cleaning their ears. People probably have the same kinds of feelings about their facial expressions, which often contradict their words.

Genuinely understanding human behavior and emotions is critical to social workers, particularly when they work with those who are experiencing mental illness, with children, and with violators of the law. Therefore, using some of the techniques that Ekman has developed can be an important dimension to assessment, diagnosis, and treatment. Of course, there are many other uses for the knowledge that Gladwell (2002) describes. For example, the movies *Toy Story* and *Shrek* drew on the detailed facial expression information that Ekman developed.

SUBSTANCE ABUSE

A whole class of mental disorders is attributed to the abuse of substances, particularly intoxicating or other mind-altering products. The *Diagnostic and Statistical Manual of Mental Disorders* (Frances, 1994) also speaks of substance abuse phenomena such as alcohol abuse and drug abuse. Patients may suffer from substance abuse with or without physiological dependence on drugs or alcohol.

Many specific illnesses are associated with substance use. These include substance-induced delirium, substance-induced illness persisting dementia, substance-induced persisting amnestic disorder, or, as is often used as the terminology, amnesia, substance abuse psychotic disorder, substance-induced mood disorder, anxiety disorder, sexual dysfunction, and sleep disorder. In other words, the biological effects of some substances, including alcohol, may cause individuals to exhibit psychiatric symptoms.

The DSM-IV provides detailed information on the effects of amphetamines, caffeine, cannabis, and cocaine. Hallucinogens such as LSD, which are also covered in the DSM-IV, have a particularly powerful relationship with psychiatric symptomatology because of their mind-altering influence on individuals' perceptions. Cocaine is also associated with a variety of mental disorders. For the more powerful of substances, withdrawal is also a category of illness. Hallucinogens are also causes of some mental illnesses such as dependence on the substance, flashbacks, and other behavioral disorders. Inhalants may contribute to mental illness. The hydrocarbons in gasoline, glue, paint thinners, and spray paints are all causes of a variety of intoxications, deliriums, and disorders. Nicotine is a source of dependence and disorders, including problems associated with withdrawal from the substance. People are also physically affected by opiates, which include opium, heroin, and other substances obtained from the opium plant. A variety of other substances such as sedatives, hypnotic drugs, and anxiolytics are also sources of possible mental disorders. Generally, one may conclude that a whole range of mental disorders arises from the use of various substances, many of them illegal, which affect the mind. More information on drugs and alcohol is provided in Chapter 10.

DEVELOPMENTAL DISABILITIES

Some developmental disabilities also have mental health components and it is difficult to classify them as biological or mental conditions. Some, of course, qualify for both designations. One condition that is associated with brain dysfunctions is autism, which the DSM-IV (Frances, 1994, p. 66) describes as "the presence of markedly abnormal or impaired development in social interaction and communication and a markedly restricted repertoire of activity and interests." The publication also says that the characteristics of the condition are quite varied and may include inability to sustain eye contact, unusual body posture, and misuse or lack of use of gestures. The condition is usually diagnosed before age 3.

People with autism may have restricted use of language, a strong desire to maintain certain rituals such as taking the same route to school every day as well as similar insistence on avoiding change, and unusual body movements or habits such as tapping on objects, clapping hands, rocking, and swaying. In many cases, there is also a diagnosis of mental retardation. Abnormal eating patterns, strong connections to objects such as a piece of string are common, and, generally, the condition is associated with what appear to others as non-normal behaviors and perhaps obsessions. About one-third of people with autism may grow into reasonably well-functioning adults, but even the most successful continue to exhibit problematic behavior in relation to other people.

One of the lingering issues in understanding autism and some other developmental disorders is that some of those with the conditions also display artistic brilliance and remarkable memories, as is often seen on television and in the theatrical movie *Rain Man*. Treffert and Wallace (2002), writing in *Scientific American*, describe several cases of what is now called "savant syndrome," a term that replaced the demeaning "idiot savant." J. Langdon Down, who identified the form of developmental disability or mental retardation known as Down syndrome, first identified savant syndrome. In 1887, Treffert and Wallace (2002) write, Down described ten individuals with the condition who he had met while serving as superintendent of the Earlswood Asylum in London.

Treffert and Wallace (2002) say that some 100 cases have been described in the scientific literature. The phenomenon of savant syndrome usually occurs among people with IQs of 40–70 but sometimes with IQs as high as 114. It also affects males more than females. There are four to six male savants for every female. It can be inborn or congenital, but it also may develop after a brain trauma or injury such as the brain disease of encephalitis.

Described in Treffert and Wallace's (2002) article is a man who is blind and who never studied piano and who has cerebral palsy and other developmental disabilities who plays thousands of music pieces flawlessly (after hearing them only once) and even composes music. Many musical savants have perfect pitch and can perform with ease and great skill, especially on the piano. They also discuss a man named Kim Peek, who was the inspiration for the lead character in *Rain Man*. He is developmentally disabled but knows more than 7,600 books by heart as well as every area code, highway, zip code, and TV station in the United States. He can tell a person, once he knows the person's date of birth, the day of the week on which the person was born, and the day of the week when that person will turn age 65. Yet he depends on his father for meeting his basic living needs. Another of their examples is a savant artist who can see a fleeting picture of an animal and sculpt in 20 minutes a perfect replica of what he saw, down to the exact muscles and fibers.

All savants have remarkable memories that are based on habitual repetition. They may not understand what they have memorized, however. Some savants have great talents that would be noteworthy even among people who are not savants. Treffert and Wallace (2002) call such people "prodigious savants," but they suggest that there are probably fewer than 50 alive at any time.

Efforts to understand the biology of the savant syndrome have led many researchers to suggest that problems in the left brain hemisphere, either before or during birth or as a result of injury, cause the right hemisphere to develop powerfully. One researcher, Bernard Rimland of the Autism Research Institute in San Diego, who has data on more than 34,000 individuals (Treffert & Wallace, 2002) believes that the skills displayed in those with the syndrome are associated with right brain hemisphere functions while their most deficient abilities are associated with left brain hemisphere functions.

With regard to the development of the savant syndrome, one researcher studied five elderly people with "frontotemporal dementia," a form of deteriorating memory and understanding. All had developed art skills with which they were able to copy artworks and paint beautifully. Their conditions had caused damage in the left brain hemisphere, which supports the idea that the right brain compensates, in unusually strong patterns, for losses in the left, among those with savant syndrome.

Experimental electrical stimulation of the brains of some people who did not have autism led to the development, often for short periods of time, of great skills. However, it is likely that the savant skills are limited to only a portion of the normal population, just as they are limited to only a portion of the population who have autism.

■ ■ ■ ■ ■

SLEEP RESEARCH

Although more of a physical issue than mental, sleep patterns are also biologically important and may usefully be discussed in this chapter. There is actually less known about sleep and the human body's need for it than would ordinarily be assumed. Some new studies are beginning to suggest that the normally accepted one-third of each day for sleep may not be valid or appropriate—or even healthy.

Vedantam (2002) reported that sleeping six or seven hours a night is perhaps healthier than the usually recommended eight hours. A professor of psychiatry at the University of California at San Diego, Daniel Kripke, led a study of one million Americans for six years from a massive survey conducted by the American Cancer Society between 1982 and 1988. "Women sleeping eight, nine and 10 hours a night had 13 percent, 23 percent and 41 percent higher risk of dying, respectively, than those who slept seven hours, the study found. Men sleeping eight, nine and 10 hours a night had 12 percent, 17 percent and 34 percent greater risk of dying within the study period" (Vedantam, 2002, p. A10). The study also found that sleeping five hours increased the risk of death by five percent for women and 11 percent for men but that women who slept only three hours had a 33 percent increase in death whereas men who slept three hours had a 19 percent increase, compared to those who slept seven hours. Of course, the data are based on self-reports and may not fully represent sleep patterns. It may also be true that those who have underlying illnesses are more tired and sleep more than healthier people.

Treffert and Wallace (2002) say that there is more to be learned about the human development of those with savant syndrome than can be understood with brain function alone. Caretakers, families, teachers, and therapists of those who have the syndrome have obviously made major contributions to the talents of these individuals.

CRITICAL ANALYSIS OF BIOLOGY AND MENTAL HEALTH

Critics of the biological approach to mental illness suggest that treating emotional problems biologically can have a positive effect but that does not mean that the problems are themselves biological. Gaylin (2000) says that science lacks understanding of the functioning of the brain—at least of the brain insofar as it is associated with mental and emotional problems. He notes that some may call mental illness a brain disease but he thinks it is more appropriate to talk about emotional illnesses rather than diseases. Brain researchers would agree that our understanding of the brain's functioning is still growing. However, that does not mean we should not consider its possible importance.

Gaylin (2000) also says that psychotherapists tend to believe that behavior is the result of many forces and counter forces, and the evidence presented in this chapter supports this contention. What is functional and what is dysfunctional is something of a set of social constructs rather than specific pathologies as one encounters with physical problems such as high blood pressure or heart disease.

Gaylin (2000) asserts that the talking kinds of treatment that are afforded people with emotional problems such as counseling and psychotherapy are difficult to evaluate. Compared to physical medicine, he notes, the quality of service and the recovery rate of patients is less well known in the mental health fields. He says, "With psychotherapy who knows who gets better?" (Gaylin, 2000, p. 6). However, a recent study conducted by the National Institute of Mental Health compared cognitive therapy (talk-related intervention focused on learning new behaviors and thought patterns) with pharmacological interventions. The findings indicate that cognitive therapy is as successful at treating clients experiencing depression as the sole use of SSRIs. The significant difference between cognitive therapy and medication was the speed at which the intervention worked. Medication typically had an immediate impact, whereas cognitive therapy took several weeks before achieving similar results. The other difference was in cost: 4 months of cognitive therapy cost $2,250 compared to 16 months of medication for $2,590 (Begley, 2002).

CONCLUSIONS

Mental health direct practice interventions and policy have been significantly influenced by the strongly held belief that mental health problems are caused predominantly by environmental factors such as relationships with the family of origin, access to resources, and the way we perceive our environment and learn from it. Although these represent factors worth consideration, the biology issues associated with mental illness need to be better integrated into social workers' understanding of mental disorders. From a policy standpoint, in a 1975 article in *Science* Franklyn N. Arnhoff states: "The major public policy decisions, however, have tended to ignore substantive issues and developments in biological psychiatry and the behavioral sciences" (p. 1277). The profession of social work and the public in general have adopted simplistic explanations for human behavior that are overly reliant on either environmental or biological explanations.

"Understanding mental disorders, discovering more effective treatments, and possessing, eventually, effective approaches to prevention demand that we learn from molecular biology and genetics. The pathophysiology of mental disorders depends on the complex interaction of genetic and environmental factors affecting the development and subsequent function of the brain, and hence our mental lives and behavior. Identification of disease vulnerability genes will provide important clues not only to neuroscientists trying to understand pathophysiology, but also to behavioral scientists and others trying to identify environmental factors that lead to illness or resilience" (Hyman, 1999, p. 97).

"Very often people have these simplistic explanations in which they say someone is bad because he grew up in a ghetto, that is not true because you can live in a ghetto and come out a saint and likewise you can have a wonderful supporting environment and become a completely awful person" (Kotulak, 2002, p. 97).

Behavior is not simply the result of a bad environment or bad genes but a complex, and at this stage little understood, interaction between the two.

The biological underpinnings examined and outlined in this chapter point to the necessity of social workers integrating them into our theories of human behavior. The strength of the evidence suggests that holding onto understandings of mental health that derive sole explanation from cultural and environmental factors may result in applying interventions that are not as effective as possible. Many of the researchers and scientists working on understanding the biological underpinning of mental health are unsure of the clinical meaning for their findings. As well, there is no sense at this stage of what kind of policy changes will occur as our understanding of the etiology of mental health disorders grows. These gaps in understanding and the fact that applications have not moved beyond the research lab do not mean that social workers can afford to ignore the trends.

The chemical changes in the brains of people experiencing PTSD suggest that talk therapy of any sort may fall short of offering conclusive cures. In fact, one of the central features of talk therapy with victims of PTSD is to relive the experience. This, given the research pertaining to brain chemistry, may continue the process of crystalizing the experience within the person's brain. This process means there are currently limitations to interventions (medication and relearning how to respond to stress). Equally so, future interventions may be able to correct the changes in brain chemistry caused by traumatic incidents. Even if this is the case, clearly, traditional talk therapy will play a role in helping people with PTSD regain their former lives.

There has been a recent concerted effort to understand the extent of biological and physiological bases for mental illness. Levin and Petrila (1996) point out that starting in the late 1980s the application of public health methodologies to understanding the distribution and extent of mental health problems contributed significantly to the advancement of knowledge concerning them. This growing body of research findings is causing the reevaluation of the role of genes and other biological factors in shaping people's behavior. Therefore, mental health social workers who want to remain current with interventions known to have positive impacts and the changing theories of human behavior need to educate themselves about emerging research in the biological sciences, medicine, behavior, genetics, and molecular biology (Efan & Greene, 2000).

DISCUSSION QUESTIONS

1. Discuss three aspects of biology that are important to future discussions about the role of biology in mental health.

2. Discuss the role of genetics in mental health disorders and cite two examples.

3. Identify the biological aspects of PTSD and discuss the treatment implications of these aspects.

4. What are some of the physical attributes associated with schizophrenia and major depression?

CHAPTER TEN

BIOLOGICAL ELEMENTS OF TOBACCO, DRUGS, AND ALCOHOL

Drug misuse is not a disease. It is a decision, like the decision to step out in front of a moving car. You would call that not a disease but an error of judgment.

—Philip K. Dick

First you take a drink, then the drink takes a drink, then the drink takes you.

—F. Scott Fitzgerald

Among the many issues that cross over between understanding human behavior and determining effective social policies is the social reaction to the use of psychoactive drugs and alcohol. Drugs are introduced into the body to cause physiological change, according to Johnson (2001). Psychoactive drugs, including alcohol and nicotine, which is a property of tobacco, affect the brain and nervous system and the higher order functions of the human being such as consciousness, emotions, and behavior, which are among the higher brain functions (Johnson, 2001). Of course, a sophisticated approach to the problem, which is a constant subject of public discussion, is to classify these issues into a larger rubric of "substance abuse." That is, people have problems, many of them, initially at least, biological in nature, with substances that affect the brain and personal behavior. Although the current emphasis is on concerns about psychoactive substances such as amphetamines, cocaine, and heroin that can have profound effects on human behavior, those who work with substance abusers and substance abuse programs also recognize marijuana, a less powerful substance, as well as legal substances such as some prescription medicines and alcohol as both biologically and socially important.

Not only academic but also popular writers and public figures deal with the issues of drug and alcohol. The problems associated with them are long-term subjects of magazine articles, books, TV programs, movies, and other popular media, including music. These popular representations of substance abuse have significant effects on public attitudes about the issues.

It is difficult to separate human behavior from social policy issues about these substances. According to one popular journalist and television personality (O'Reilly, 2000), between 50 and 75 percent of men who are arrested test positively for drugs. He says that the rate for women arrestees is even higher. He also notes that inebriated adults commit some 75 percent of child physical abuse. The same author notes that $30 billion is spent annually by local, state, and federal agencies to deal with drug problems.

Federal crime statistics show the same kinds of problems and also document the extent of arrests for substance abuse violations. In 1995, over 1 million men and women were arrested on drug charges and another half million for drunkenness (Brunner, 1997). Thus, the scope of the public issues surrounding drug and alcohol abuse, not including the mental and physical health issues associated with the misuse of and addiction to legal drugs, is immense.

O'Reilly also asserts that the misuse of drugs and the abuse of alcohol have permanent consequences for the individual. Changes in the brain are such that they permanently affect the capacities of the user.

He is also skeptical about treatment programs. He claims that 60 to 80 percent of addicts want nothing to do with treatment efforts and that only 13 percent of those who go through treatment remain free of substance abuse. His solution is a combination of the law enforcement efforts that currently dominate the problem and treatment. O'Reilly proposes that a plan used in Alabama be adopted nationally. It gives those convicted of drug use a choice—either forced rehabilitation in a prison drug facility or a longer sentence in a correctional institution. All but a few choose the rehabilitation. Twice as many of those who experience rehabilitation remain free of drugs than those who do not.

The secret of the success of the program is that it removes those who use drugs from the environment where substances are available, which has the additional benefit of protecting the public. He also believes that public policy alone will not solve the drug problem—the only solution is to reduce the demand, which can only be done by reducing the numbers of users. If there is no demand, the vendors of illegal drugs would have less motivation to make a business out of importing and selling illegal substances.

O'Reilly does not deal with legal drugs (although those who might use them under illegal circumstances such as forging prescriptions could, one supposes, also be convicted and forced into rehabilitation). He also says he knows little about solutions to the problems of alcoholism because alcohol is a legal substance.

Another popular writer (Gladwell, 2000) takes a more biological approach to understanding issues of addiction and substance abuse. Gladwell writes primarily about cigarette use among young people and attributes its persistence to social factors—the "coolness" of cigarette smokers, the desire to fit in, and the contagiousness of the habit. However, whether or not one becomes a heavy smoker or an addict is highly individualized and probably related to genetic differences among people.

He notes that federal surveys about drug abuse show that a little over 1 percent of those polled acknowledge having used heroin at least once. However, only a few (18 percent) of those who had used it had also used it in the past year and only 9 percent in the past month. And less than 1 percent of those who have used cocaine at any time become regular users. His belief is that experimentation is normal for teenagers. Experimentation is socially induced, but addiction is likely to be biological—not every experimenter with cigarettes or other substances becomes a heavy user or addict.

Although discussions of drugs often talk about their negative consequences, the fact is that many drugs have maintained the lives and well-being of humans. One of the most important drugs used in the world is caffeine, which is found in coffee, chocolate, tea, and many soft drinks. According to Weinberg and Dealer (2001), caffeine is a stimulant and the rise of the use of coffee made many social changes possible. They attribute the industrial revolution, in part, to the discovery and use of caffeine. Drinking coffee enables people to awaken in the morning and work on similar schedules. Some authors (Gladwell, 2001) say that the modern human personality is a synthetic creation that is regulated and medicated in dose of caffeine to make it possible for us to be focused, awake, and alert when we need to be. He suggests that coffee is a source of modern productivity and is relied on by many people to make them successful. Of course, caffeine from all products, soft drinks, tea, and coffee, all contribute to the capacity of people to be awake.

Caffeine also has some problematic side effects. In some cases, caffeine can cause tumors and cysts, especially in breast tissue. It can also lead to neural damage in infants, high startle responses in adults, and general nervousness or "jitteriness" among those who use excessive quantities of the substance.

Similar kinds of comments may be made about other kinds of drugs, particularly psychoactive medicines. Such medicines can be abused and dangerous, and the abuse of tranquilizers and antidepressants is very likely to be the source of more substance abuse problems than are all the illegal drugs. On the other hand, when properly used, psychoactive drugs have made it possible for people to function and to cope with their emotional problems.

One of the issues associated with drugs is identifying ways in which drug use can be discovered among school children. In 2002, the U.S. Supreme Court was determining whether or not required drug testing for students who wanted to participate in after-school activities would deny them their privacy rights. Random or not, voluntary testing violates rights is a major issue of dispute (Gearan, 2002).

Not all illegal drug use is related to psychoactive drugs. Athletes may become involved in the use of anabolic steroids, which are synthetic derivatives of testosterone, the male sex hormone. According to Beers and Berkow (1999), steroids have androgenic as well as anabolic consequences. The androgenic effects include increases in sex drive, changes in hair growth, and increased aggressiveness. The anabolic effects include growth of muscle mass and building of tissues. There are efforts to emphasize the anabolic effects and minimize the androgenic in the production of the steroids. However, not all the results can be free of the androgenic effects.

Steroids are used in some medical treatments. However, the greatest concern is their use by athletes to develop strength and size. Bodybuilders are frequent users of the substances. Some athletes use multiple drugs to improve their bodies and their athletic abilities. Although there have been few detailed studies of the effects of these drugs, there is evidence that they can cause atrophy of the testicles among men, increase hairiness in bodies of women, increase aggression, and have other less than desirable outcomes.

In a symposium, *Rolling Stone* magazine published interviews with a broad range of influential Americans who have a variety of positions on drugs and on the national response to them. Participants ranging from Dan Rather of CBS News to many members of Congress, one governor, a variety of musicians, and many other important public figures spoke out on the subject. *Rolling Stone* seems to take a generally tolerant position on drug use, and the majority of the comments were more along the lines of the virtues of legalizing drugs than on decrying their dangers to users.

Traditional controlled substances are drugs that are illegal, including cocaine, heroin, and marijuana. In addition, newer substances such as LSD, ecstasy, and others, along with herbal drugs such as mescaline, are also controlled. All these drugs are potentially dangerous to individuals. There are many prominent deaths annually from the use of the substances or the use of them in combination with other legal and illegal drugs, including alcohol.

New synthetic drugs are also developed all the time. One that has become prominent is 2C-T-7, nicknamed T-7 or tripstasy, which was developed by a professor at the University of California (Brown, 2002). The drug has caused several deaths, one of which was reported in a national magazine. Apparently the Internet is a major source of information about new drugs and their effects. It is possible that more and more dangerous substances will be developed during the current century, each of which is a potential cause of illness and, in extreme cases, death. This drug entered the commercial market in Amsterdam in 1999 but was removed on government demand after the first deaths were recorded (Brown, 2002). It went underground but resurfaced on the illicit drug market and was publicized on the Internet.

The developer of the drug, Alexander Shulgin, who had taught forensic chemistry at the University of California at Berkeley (Brown, 2002), regretted that T-7, one of 120 new compounds he developed, was in the illicit drug market. For the subjects with whom he tried the compound, including himself, people felt peaceful after 5 days. He sought improvement of the spiritual aspect of the psyche, not of a recreational substance.

Shulgin was, according to Brown (2002b), the popularizer of Ecstasy, a hallucinogenic drug that has gained high degrees of popularity in the United States and Europe. He synthesized the drug in 1976. It is called, more officially, MDMA, which stands for 3,4–methylenedioxymethamphetamine. Shulgin is something of an expert on the creation of hallucinogenic drugs, including DOM and STP, and has written books on the subject.

PRESCRIPTION MEDICINES

It is not only illegal drugs that pose a problem in human health. The misuse or abuse of prescription medicines, especially psychoactive medicines such as tranquilizers and stimulants, can pose health risks too. Some of those prescription substances are described later in this chapter.

Another new drug issue is the misuse of the prescription painkiller Oxy-Contin (Rosenberg, 2002). The drug, which was designed to treat severe, chronic pain, is a synthetic form of heroin. It has become a street drug, purchased and used illegally in some parts of the United States and in England. Rosenberg (2002) reports that there has been an increase of 1,000 percent in prescriptions for the medicine since 1996 and that 5,261 emergency room incidents involving the drug were reported in the first half of 2000. The pills sell on the street for $20 to $40. The drug is a particular problem for children born to mothers who use it. Some fetuses die before they are born. Others are born with low weights and other physical and mental difficulties.

One study (Casriel, 2002) conducted at the University of Miami and funded by the Robert Wood Johnson Foundation found that occasional drug users are no less reliable as employees and, generally, as citizens than those who use no illicit drugs. For long periods of time, Americans have dipped into the drug culture and used any of a number of illegal substances without becoming ill, dying, or becoming addicted. In other words, it appears possible for some people to use illicit drugs without it becoming a huge personal or social problem. Of course, that calls into question the testing used by many companies to screen potential employees. An employee might fail a drug test but that same employee might be an effective and reliable worker for the employer.

PHYSIOLOGY OF DRUGS

Regan (2001) wrote about the physiology of drugs. The author, who is a professor in Dublin, Ireland, provides information on the brain chemistry of drugs that are psychoactive. He points out that Prozac and probably most other antidepressants prevent the serotonin transmitted from being conserved by the presynapse and that enhances their action and lifts moods. He points out that consciousness is a chemical process just as are the results of psychoactive drugs. He also says that substances that alter minds have a major impact on the evolution of human society and that the introduction of such substances as coffee, tea, chocolate, and nicotine to Europe moved many Europeans from the haze of alcohol use. It is interesting that there was, during the 1990s, a time of great economic and great technological development, a major increase in coffee as a product in the United States and much of Europe, which might be associated with economic development and the increase in productivity.

He also suggests that humans have been using drugs throughout history and before history was recorded and it is likely that modern human physiology could be a result of the impact of drugs on the body—that mind-altering substances not only impacted what we thought and how we operated but may be an influence on who we are, what we think, and how we live.

SUBSTANCE USE DATA

According to Johnson (2001), whose statements about the blood-brain barrier and the physiology of psychoactive drugs are discussed in Chapter 3, these are the psychoactive substances that affect people and the percentage uses of them by 18- to 25-year-olds, during their lifetimes, as reported by the U.S. Department of Health and Human Services in 1996 appear in Table 10.1. Data were not available for some of the newer substances described in this chapter or of ecstasy, which is reputed to be fairly widely used by young people in the United States.

There appear to be a variety of opinions and demographic differences about drug use. For example, surveys of high school seniors show that White students use cocaine at seven or eight times the rate of African American students, and somewhat similar figures have been obtained for heroin use. Whites are a third more likely to sell drugs than African Americans. However, African American youth are in prison for drugs at a rate of 510 per 100,000 people compared to whites, who are incarcerated at a rate of only 30 per 100,000 people.

Kay Redfield Jamison, professor of psychiatry at Johns Hopkins University (Wenner, 2001), says that many people use drugs and alcohol and also have major psychiatric illnesses. They use drugs and alcohol to self-treat themselves. People who have psychiatric problems are often self-treating themselves with drugs and alcohol, and by the time they are treated for the actual underlying problem, they have a second problem of substance abuse. Jamison also says that addiction is located in the brain and is biological.

She also says that despite the widespread belief that treating emotional problems such as depression will lead to an overcoming of substance abuse problems,

TABLE 10.1   Drugs Used by 18–25-Year-Olds

SUBSTANCE	PERCENT USE
Alcohol	83.8
Cigarettes	68.5
Marijuana and hashish	44.0
Smokeless tobacco	23.4
Hallucinogens	16.3
LSD	13.9
Nonmedical use of any prescription-type stimulant, sedative, tranquilizer, or analgesic	12.7
Inhalants	10.8
Cocaine	10.2
Crack	3.0
PCP	2.3
Heroin	1.3

that, in fact, is not the case. Actually, people who medicate themselves for emotional problems with drugs then have a double problem. Wenner (2001) notes that medication such as methadone, which is a substitute for heroin, can cost approximately $1,800 for regular outpatient treatment. Jailing people for heroin use costs $26,000 per year, according to the Physician Leadership on National Drug Policy.

Wenner (2001) notes that the highest homicide rates in the United States coincide with the prohibition of alcohol. The homicide rate was 9.7 per 100,000, but it dropped dramatically after prohibition of alcohol was repealed. In 1980, a year for strong prohibition of drugs, the homicide rate was 10 per 100,000 people. Wenner also notes that there is an epidemic of overdoses of drugs. In the major cities such as New York, San Francisco, and Portland, young men between the ages of 20 and 54 are more likely to die by overdose than by car accident; Los Angeles County has some 400 overdose deaths per year. Wenner writes that 260,000 cases of AIDS have been traced to infected needles, and of the 40,000 new HIV infections every year, 10,000 are caused either directly or indirectly by use of injected drugs. It is possible that needle exchange programs could reduce the AIDS rate substantially.

It is clear that Wenner is not impressed with policies dealing with the reduction of drug use. He says that the Clinton administration spent more than $120 billion on the drug war and President Bush requested $18 billion for 2002. However, during those efforts, the retail prices of cocaine and heroin actually dropped and the purity of the substances increased from 1990 to 1998. The United Nations estimates that illegal drugs are a $400 billion annual business and constitute 8 percent of all the trade in the world.

BIOLOGY OF COCAINE USE

Johnson (2001) provides more detailed information on the biology of cocaine use. Cocaine blocks the uptake of neurotransmitters norepinephrine and dopamine so that they stay in the system a bit longer than they might ordinarily. The effect is "excessive and continued stimulation of postsynaptic neurons" (p. 284) that are stimulated by those two neurotransmitters. Dopamine is a brain substance or neurotransmitter that is associated with pleasure. But when dopamine is overproduced, the body cuts back on the oversupply, which is why increasing doses of cocaine are needed to keep the substance operating. As the supply of the substance drops, cocaine users find they cannot experience pleasure without using the drug. They may become anxious and depressed, lose weight, develop infections, and have trouble sleeping. Babies who are born to mothers who have used crack cocaine, which Johnson calls a ready-to-smoke form of the drug, are often born with brain damage and are underweight.

In discussing the other neurotransmitter affected by cocaine use, Johnson notes that it, norepinephrine, is involved in the sympathetic nervous system. Because of its effect on norepinephrine, cocaine overstimulates the heart as well as raises the blood pressure. It can cause strokes, seizures, and heart attacks, which may affect even healthy young adults, who may suffer cardiac arrest from using it.

EFFECTS OF MARIJUANA USE

One of the difficulties in writing about the effects of drugs is that their illegal status makes it complicated for researchers to objectively examine their effects. Marijuana, which is the most heavily used of the illegal drugs, has not been studied as well as it might have been because of the difficulty of, for example, providing a treatment group with the substance and comparing it with a control group that does not use it. In a 2002 study (Solowij et al., 2002), several authors report on their examination of long-time cannabis (the active substance in marijuana and hashish) users who were seeking treatment for using the substance. They studied 102 almost-daily cannabis users between 1997 and 2000. Fifty-one of the group were long-term users with a mean of 23.9 years of cannabis use, whereas fifty-one were shorter-term users, who had a mean number of years of use of 10.2. They were compared with thirty-three nonusers, who served as a control group. The study was conducted in three cities, Seattle, Washington; Farmington, Connecticut; and Miami, Florida.

The researchers used nine standard neuropsychological tests that assessed the attention, memory, and executive functioning. The tests were administered before the subjects entered a treatment program and after they had abstained from using cannabis for a median time of 17 hours. The long-term cannabis users did not perform as well as the short-term users and the controls. The differences were statistically significant for the degree of impairment in learning and for retention and retrieval of information. The differences between the short-term users and the controls were not statistically significant. The longer the subjects had used cannabis, the worse their performances. There was no relationship between their performances and the symptoms of their withdrawal or their recent use of the substance or with other drug use.

Long-term cannabis users therefore appear to have memory and attention impairments that go beyond the specific time of becoming "high" or intoxicated with the substance. And the longer they use it, the more impaired they become.

One neuroscientist, Paul Greengard (Wenner, 2001), who is also a Nobel Prize winner, supports government efforts to prevent the use of harmful drugs such as heroin and LSD. But he disagrees with punishment for marijuana users. It is a harmful substance like tobacco and alcohol, he suggests, but he does not think marijuana users should be imprisoned. Lumping all illegal substances together is an error, in his opinion.

Carl Hiaasen, a Miami novelist and columnist (Wenner, 2002), writes that he has seen whole neighborhoods torn apart by the selling and use of the drug crack cocaine. But he wonders if the problem would be greater or lesser if such drugs were not illegal.

It is significant to note that the form of drug use varies widely by region of the United States. One particular drug may be widely available in some parts of the nation, while almost totally unavailable in other parts. Accessibility and local cultures can often determine the nature of the use of illegal drugs, in particular. Even the abuse of legal drugs seems to vary by region.

ALCOHOL AND ALCOHOL ABUSE

The use of alcohol is a diverse subject inasmuch as it is a part of everyday life in most Western nations, constitutes a serious mental health problem for many people, and also functions as a major social problem that is costly to society through lost productivity, accidental deaths, and crime.

Although public concerns are often greatest about drugs, the use and abuse of alcohol is often more serious, at least in terms of number of users, than for other substances. And problem drinkers are becoming younger.

Biology of Alcohol Use

According to Cheers (2001), alcohol, also called ethanol or ethyl alcohol, is a substance found in beer, liquor, wine, and many medicines. It is dangerous and widely available and, therefore, typically regulated by law. Although moderate drinking is accepted in Western societies and most people can handle alcohol use adequately, some heavy drinkers put their mental and physical health at risk.

According to Reagan and Brookins-Fisher (2002), 150 million Americans drink alcohol. They include 10 to 15 million alcoholics and 18 million problem drinkers. Public health experts believe that alcohol costs the United States $90 billion each year. Nearly half that amount is a result of lost production, 29 percent as a consequence of health and medical costs, 13 percent from motor vehicle accidents, and another 12 percent from violent crimes, the cost of community education, and fire losses.

The mental health problems arising from overuse of alcohol are relatively well known to social workers. The physical phenomena are less well communicated in social work. Johnson (1999), a social work theorist, has written about neurobiology and its involvement in substance abuse. Those who become dependent on the substance may suffer withdrawal when it is not available to them. Withdrawal can involve nausea, sweating, and shakiness. Alcoholics often develop a tolerance for the substance, and so they need greater amounts to feel as they want to feel from drinking. As an alcoholic once told one of the authors who said he could not easily understand alcoholism because too many drinks made him ill, "It's when you don't become ill that you become an alcoholic."

Some of the physical complications of alcohol abuse or overuse, according to Cheers (2001), are poor nutrition, because food is replaced by alcohol in the diet; chronic pancreatitis, when the small ducts in the pancreas that make insulin shrink because of alcohol; liver damage, including cirrhosis of the liver; nerve inflammation; brain diseases such as dementia and delirium tremens; gastric ulcers; and a weakening of the heart and the heart muscles. There are also dangers to the fetuses of pregnant women who drink and the risk of children being born with fetal alcohol syndrome.

The evidence is that girls are now engaging in binge drinking as much as boys. The National Center on Addiction and Substance Abuse at Columbia University (*Time,* 2002) reports that in 1991, 31 percent of boys and 22 percent of girls engaged in binge drinking, which means having five or more drinks in a row. In 1999, 34 percent of the boys and 31 percent of the girls were binge drinking. The Center estimates that 5 million high school students are binge drinkers.

Alcoholism professionals are especially concerned that some of the sweetened alcohol products now on the market are encouraging more teenagers to use alcohol.

Teenagers and Drugs

The National Center on Addiction and Substance Abuse, which is located at Columbia University in New York, conducts surveys with teenagers and educators about drugs. In 1998, Califano and Booth (1998) found:

1. Teens rank drugs as the greatest problem facing people their age, although principals and teachers rank the problem lower. Half of those who are age 17 say they know a drug dealer at their school. And two-thirds of high school students have a friend or classmate who has used cocaine, heroin, or LSD.
2. Half of 15- to 17-year-old teenagers have been to parties during the past six months in which marijuana was featured. As teens grow older, alcohol is increasingly available at their social occasions. A third of older teens have seen drugs sold on their own school grounds.
3. Nearly half of high school student say they can buy marijuana with an hour's notice or less.
4. Teenage smoking is also a major issue and two-thirds of those who use tobacco say they do so because of the influence of their friends.

Califano and Booth (1998) also say that the most critical year is from age 12 to 13. Young people in that age group triple in their knowledge, for example, of where to purchase marijuana. Also tripling are the proportions who know a teen who uses drugs and the percentage who are unwilling to report someone for using illegal substances. Similarly, the influence of parental opinions on their behavior drops by a third from age 12 to 13.

The survey (Califano & Booth, 1998) also found that teens who smoke are five times more likely to have tried marijuana and six times more likely to get drunk once a month than those who do not smoke. By comparison with teens who do not use marijuana, teens who have used it are 15 times more likely to have smoked cigarettes in the preceding month and 9 times more like to get drunk once per month. They are also 3 times more likely to try another illegal drug in the future.

TOBACCO USE

As anyone who has ever looked at a cigarette package, advertisement, or billboard with some care knows, tobacco is implicated in any number of public health problems ranging from serving as the cause of some heart problems as well as a variety of cancers (lung, pancreas, mouth, and others) to causing illnesses in others who inhale "second-hand" smoke. About a fourth of Americans smoke, a figure that is down from an earlier estimate of 43 percent. The rates are rather similar in all of the states. However, many other countries have higher rates of smoking, typically with more men than women using tobacco (Reagan and Brookins-Fisher, 2002).

As more research is done on the effects of smoking, more and more data are developed indicating its physiological effects. For example, the sex of newborns may be impacted if either parent smokes while they are in the process of conceiving the child. According to Ross (2002), if one or both parents smoke, they are statistically more likely to have a girl than a boy. Worldwide, 52 percent of children born are boys. However, when smokers are separated from nonsmokers, the nonsmokers had 55 percent male infants. When both parents smoked, they had 45 percent males. When one partner smoked, they had more girls, but not to the same extent as when both smoked.

As Ross (2002, p. A12) puts it, "Some scientists consider the ratio of male to female births to be an indicator of a population's health, because male sperm and embryos are more fragile than their female counterparts." Therefore, it is possible that smoking destroys more of the male sperm and embryos, leading to the disproportionately large rate of female births.

A more popular source, Michael Moore's *Stupid White Men* (2001) says that there are data demonstrating a statistical change in the proportions of males and females. He says that when he makes speeches, he often asks the audience if they notice more girls being born in their families than boys. Large numbers say that is the case. He says that the U.S. Bureau of the Census reports that there are declining numbers of boys being born and that has been true since 1990. With the longer female life span, the ratio of females to males will continue to grow larger.

Biologically, *in vitro* human fertilization, sperm banks, and other such growing phenomena may render males superfluous in their once irreplaceable role. But when one thinks about the modern raising of animals, there may be biological parallels. Livestock businesses maintain small numbers of males and larger numbers of females, which can all be fertilized by artificial insemination. Michael Moore (2001) makes those kinds of predictions for the future of humans—only partly as a humorous suggestion.

TREATMENT OF ALCOHOL AND DRUG ABUSE

One of the major concerns of social workers is the effective treatment of substance abuse. Many social workers, as indicated in other parts of this text, are professionally engaged in providing those treatment services. The treatment approaches, a lengthy discussion of which is beyond the scope of this text, are varied. They range from self-governing, self-help residential facilities to inpatient and outpatient treatment in hospitals and clinics. Several excellent books on the subject of alcohol, drug, and tobacco addiction are available as are sources that can be accessed through the Internet, for example, Galanter and Kleber (1994), McNeece and DiNitto (1994), and Abadinsky (1993).

One of the traditional criteria for effective treatment is complete abstinence from the substances that are used. That is part of the Alcoholics Anonymous 12-Step program, which is one of the oldest and best-regarded methods of dealing with the problems of addiction. The philosophy of such efforts is that the addiction cannot be cured but can only be controlled, usually with the help of a fellow addict.

In some situations, social workers, psychiatrists, and other human services professionals establish and carry out a treatment program for those who are addicted to harmful substances. Again, however, there is an expectation of abstinence from the substance.

However, some students of the subject believe that total abstinence may not be necessary—that reducing the use of dangerous substances and thereby reducing the harm to oneself may be all that is achievable.

> Some smokers and drinkers believe that complete abstinence is not possible for them. So some specialists are promoting an approach that is called "harm reduction," in which people who abuse various substances reduce the amount of the substances they use. They might recommend smokeless tobacco, such as snuff, to smokers or beverages with less alcohol content to alcohol users. Programs such as Alcoholics Anonymous strongly oppose such approaches because they believe those addicted to alcohol can't exercise enough self-control to simply hold down their use of the substance to a reasonable level. Some drug and tobacco counselors suggest the same. However, other experts point out that almost all of those who enter total abstinence programs either drop out or later relapse so that harm reduction approaches may be all that will work to treat substance abusers. (*The Week*, July 19, 2002, p. 16)

In any case, addictions are a complicated area of human biology. Dealing with them through treatment is an imperfect art but one that is of critical importance in the human services and in the current human environment.

CONCLUSION

Social workers have a diverse relationship with substance abuse. Many social workers deal with those who have problems because they use drugs and alcohol. A large number of offenders against the law, child abusers, and domestic violence perpetrators are abusers of drugs, especially major harmful substances such as cocaine and heroin, and alcohol. Social workers find themselves dealing with such users in many contexts—from determining eligibility for financial assistance, disability services, to working in clinics for those who are addicted. In many cases, those who work in the corrections system find that they are dealing with a large number of substance abusers.

In addition, however, policies dealing with alcohol, drugs, and tobacco are of major interest in social welfare. As a profession that deals with policies and efforts to affect them, just what the policies on these substances may be is of special interest to the profession. Many social workers believe that some users of alcohol and drugs could benefit in major ways from changes in policies. If the use of the less dangerous drugs were legalized or, as is the case in some parts of the United States as well as in much of Europe, treated as minimal offenses, many persons now requiring treatment or even incarceration could be free to work and live in the community.

Again, although social consequences are not a special emphasis of this text, it is always worthwhile to point out that the abuse of legal and illegal substances is associated with almost all social problems—violence, crime, family dissolution, child and partner abuse, auto and boating accidents, and poverty.

Although social policies are beyond the scope of this book, they are perhaps an element of equal importance with the health and safety issues associated with substance abuse.

DISCUSSION QUESTIONS

1. Addiction to drugs and alcohol has biological, social, and moral dimensions. Summarize what you believe are the biological dimensions of the problem. Are there ways in which these biological phenomena may be effectively addressed, based on what you read in this chapter?

2. Assume you, as a social worker, are conducting a session for young people who have high potential for substance abuse. What would you tell them about the biology of alcohol and drugs that you think might convince them to avoid such substances?

3. The chapter talks about the physiological aspects of tobacco use. What would one have to know about the psychological and social elements of tobacco use to effectively educate clients about the use of the substance?

4. Based on this chapter's content, how would you rank the dangerousness of substances for clients; that is, what is the magnitude of the danger of tobacco, legal or prescription drugs, and illegal drugs?

CHAPTER ELEVEN

HUMAN SEXUALITY AND SEXUAL ORIENTATION

We can now define human sexuality as the ways in which we experience and express ourselves as sexual beings. Our awareness of ourselves as females or males is part of our sexuality, as is the capacity we have for erotic experiences and responses. Our sexuality is an essential part of ourselves, whether or not we ever engage in sexual intercourse or sexual fantasy, and even if we lose sensation in our genitals because of injury.

—Rathus, Nevid, and Fichner-Rathus (2002, p. 5)

The link between human biology and the expression of human sexuality is discussed in this chapter. Although it is appealing to claim that this link will be addressed "in all its complexity," the attainment of such a goal is clearly impossible. The material in the chapter is an explication of major theoretical, historical, and research-based claims regarding the complexity of human biology and the expression of human sexuality. Rather than attempting to formulate the basis for a definitive position on any particular human sexuality topic, a number of philosophical, scientific, and cultural beliefs, and their shortcomings, are discussed. The link between human biology and sexual orientation is used extensively in the chapter as a means to exemplify the overall link, and the accompanying questions, between human biology and human sexuality. As well, the chapter is not about the anatomy of human sexuality. The chapter avoids a replication of the notion that human sexuality, and in particular gender identification, can be reduced to a delineation of the sexual parts of the body. Although it is important for social work practitioners and social work students to possess a basic knowledge of human anatomy, it is important to remember that gender is not reducible to one's anatomical sex parts, nor is the expression of human sexuality.

NATURE VERSUS NURTURE

One of the everlasting questions in the social sciences is whether human behavior is mainly caused by innate, biologically determined forces or by the socialization patterns and normative pressures of culture. Aggression, intelligence, helpfulness, competition, egotism, and many other human phenomena have been the foci of the nature versus nurture debate. Not surprisingly, nearly every element of human sexuality is likewise open to this debate (Baumeister & Tice, 2001). The potential for controversy in any discussion of human biology and the expression of human sexuality is unlimited. A full discussion needs to include elements of culture, religion, biology, genetics, psychology, and sociobiology, to name just a few possibilities. Even with the limited focus of this book on human biology and this chapter on human biology and human sexuality, the potential for controversy remains. For example, what is, and has been, known about the biological determinants of sexual orientation, with necessitated attention (at a minimum) to gay men, lesbian women, bisexual persons, the transgendered, and heterosexual orientations, is highly controversial in mainstream U.S. society. And what about the use of the terms *sexual orientation* and *sexual preference*? While *choice* has been included in methodologically rigorous studies of sexual orientation, there remains no definitive answer as to the placement, power, or absence of the choice variable. And even though the term *sexual orientation* is used throughout the chapter, the authors offer no final answer to the question of choice.

Additionally, sex research, and for those who ascribe to the label of sex researcher, knowledge seeking is truly an attempt to chart responses to highly charged questions. Human biology and human sexuality are areas of knowledge seeking where nothing is without question. Just consider the question of gender. Although it is common belief that there are two genders, male and female, there are theorists/researchers/scholars/practitioners who write convincingly of the existence of more that two genders. Anne Bolin argues convincingly such a claim in her works, which include a recently published chapter "Transcending and Transgendering: Male to Female Transsexuals, Dichotomy and Diversity" in an edited book titled *Third Sex, Third Gender: Beyond the Sexual Dimorphism in Culture and History* (Ballif, 1999). The complexity of the gender issue is exemplified by the case of John/Joan. John/Joan was one of two male twins. At 8 months, John/Joan suffered the loss of his penis to a circumcision process that went very badly. What followed was genital surgery, reassignment of gender, and a more than decade-long program of social, mental, and hormonal conditioning. The John/Joan case highlighted issues of gender identity and gender reassignment (Diamond & Sigmundson, 1999).

An important contributor to the interest in human sexuality as a forum for the nature versus nurture debate is the observation that humans are so wildly different from animals in sexual behavior. Does this difference mean that nature has played little or no role in shaping human sexuality? Is our sexual behavior determined solely by culture? A number of elements of human reproduction, for example, differ radically from that of other animals. Most sex between humans involves women who are unable to conceive at the moment. Unlike most other species, humans have sex often for recreation or the expression of intimacy, not just solely for procreation. Human beings have sex in private, usually. Human females are receptive to sex at all phases of the reproductive cycle, human females undergo menopause, human beings have long-term sexual relationships, and ovulation is concealed not only from the males but even from the female herself (Baumeister & Tice, 2001).

To theorists who favor biological, evolutionary explanations for behavior, human sexuality is a crucial battle to win. Reproduction is central to evolution, and if human sexuality is not determined by biology, then perhaps nothing is. Social construction theorists, often dissatisfied with the oppressive features of sexual practices and arrangements, consider it vital to believe that a change in culture can help change sexual practices and arrangements. For feminists, appeals to the biological determination of sexual practices and arrangements can seem like rationalizations for the status quo and the continued oppression of women. Most theorists about human sexuality recognize that actual sexual behavior reflects some mixture of nature and culture. Essentialist theories have explained the sexual behavior of humans as the reflection of some innate essence, usually dictated by biology and evolution. One is born a certain way, and socialization can only make small differences. In contrast, social construction theories (including most feminist views) treat biology as merely the basic raw ingredient and insist that most sexual behavior of humans is a result of social and cultural factors such as communication, rules, norms, expectations, approval, relationship status, and social roles. These two major theories—the essentialist and the social construction—are to some extent just broad frameworks that can be used to interpret a great many findings, instead of being sources of ideas that can be tested. The essentialist view argues that human sexuality is largely a matter of the way one is born. It emphasizes biological processes such as genes, hormones, and evolution. By contrast, the social construction position examines how culture and society shape human sexuality (Baumeister & Tice, 2001).

HISTORICAL CONTEXT

Historical context is an important element in any informed discussion of human sexuality. The evolution of contemporary views on human sexuality and the link to human biology did not follow a simple or direct route. Throughout history, periods of relative openness about sex have alternated with times of intolerance. In fact, even within historical periods, different behaviors and different expressions of human sexuality have been greeted with a great variance. During any particular historical period, different cultures have demonstrated widely varying attitudes, and any mention of history, human biology, and human sexuality necessitates a process of selection and reductionism. The earliest recordings of people include mention of features of human biology and human sexuality: the cyclical bleeding of menstruation and the physical changes during pregnancy and childbirth are prime examples. Fertility rituals and symbols are documented in various ancient cultures (McAnulty & Burnette, 2001). Importantly, once the basics of human biology and human reproduction were understood, including conception and cell growth during pregnancy, it was the variance in historical contexts that primarily created variance in the socially constructed view of appropriate and/or accepted practices of human sexuality. The intricate link between human biology and human sexuality is, however, still not completely understood.

The Greek culture was sexually explicit. The Greeks believed that men and women were inherently bisexual, although they disapproved of exclusive homosexuality, which represented a threat to the institution of the family. His seemingly insatiable sexual appetite characterized the god Zeus as he seduced both gods and mortals. The Greeks prized physical beauty and the human body, irrespective of age and gender (McAnulty & Burnette, 2001). During the Greek era there was a strong emphasis on spiritual development and a denial of physical pleasures via human sexuality practices. The basis for this belief system was dualism: the belief that body and soul are separate. Dualism gave rise to a philosophy that taught that from wisdom came virtue, and that these could only be achieved by avoiding strong passions. Plato, for example, believed that a person could achieve immortality by avoiding sexual desire and striving for intellectual and spiritual love (King, 1999).

Contemporary ambivalence about human sexuality can be traced in part back to ancient Greek beliefs. Plato, for example, distinguished between earthly, or profane, love and heavenly, or sacred, love. The former originated from the body, and the latter from the mind. Plato believed that happiness was derived only from sacred love. Other Greek writers, such as Democritus and Epicurus, agreed that sexual desire was risky at best because it distracted humans from seeking higher spiritual good. Additionally, Roman attitudes toward human sexuality were highly decadent. In fact, historians attribute the fall of the Roman Empire in part to the sexual mores of its citizens. Roman society was highly structured, and like the Greeks, quite patriarchal. As in Greece, women were the property of first their fathers and later their husbands. Ancient Romans did not recognize the concepts of homosexuality and heterosexuality. People were classified not on the basis of their sexual partners but instead on the basis of whether their sexual behavior was active or passive. The Roman influence on contemporary human sexuality is perhaps most evident in the use of language and sexual terminology. Many English terms can be traced back to their Latin roots. *Cunnilingus* derives from the Latin *cunnus,* which means "vulva." The term *fornication* derives from *fornix,* a term depicting an arch in Latin. Use of the term *fornication* in modern times, with its often negative connotation, originates from the practice of Roman prostitutes operating in the archways of public theaters, stadiums, and coliseums (King, 1999; McAnulty & Burnette, 2001).

The impact of the Medieval period on modern day views of human sexuality cannot be overrestimated. For a thousand years, from the end of the Roman Empire through the end of the fifteenth century, the Catholic Church was the dominant institution responsible for informing people what were and what were not acceptable expressions and practices of human sexuality. Sexual sins, such as fornication, lust, and homosexual relations, required sinners to perform acts of penance. Sex outside of marriage was forbidden. Medieval ideals of human sexuality were drawn from interpretations of Christianity by church figures such as Augustine. Augustine was an avid denouncer of human sexuality. Sexual intercourse was considered by Augustine to be a threat to spiritual growth. Only sex for procreation was acceptable. And the only permissible sexual act was vaginal intercourse with the man on top. Marital intercourse in the missionary position was the only tolerated sex act. Paradoxically, several theologians of the Medieval Period, including Augustine and Thomas Aquinas, held a relatively tolerant attitude toward prostitution. The act of prostitution was considered a necessary evil, since it helped preserve the chastity of "decent women." The Victorian period, from 1837 to 1901, is remembered for its repressive and rigid norms regarding human sexuality. It was an era of public prudery. All pleasurable aspects of human sexuality were publicly denied (King, 1999). During changing economic times in both Europe and North America, a prudish attitude was evident in every aspect of society. Women's clothing was designed to cover every part of the body, from head to toe. Human sexuality was tightly controlled, and women were viewed as the gate-keepers. Women had very few political or social rights but had clear domestic and maternal roles. An interesting link during the Victorian period between human biology and human sexuality was the degeneracy theory. The theory promoted the idea that human sexuality practices and overall health were tied together. Sexual indulgence, particularly masturbation, was believed to cause blindness, consumption, insanity, and a host of other physical health problems. The expression of human sexuality within a marital union was purported to promote health and personal happiness (King, 1999; McAnulty & Burnette, 2001).

Although the degeneracy theory has been thoroughly debunked, the main belief—that there is a link between general physical health and human sexuality—has only grown in stature in modern times. The Victorian period also witnessed misinformation distributed about human biology and human sexuality by members of the medical community. A book titled *Perfect Womanhood* by Mary Melendy, MD, PhD, published in 1903, contained a breadth of misinformation. For example, it contained the following advice about when it was safest to have intercourse and avoid pregnancy. Melendy wrote in 1903 "it is a law of nature—to which there may be some exceptions—that conception must take place at about the time of the menstrual flow . . . it may be said with certainty, however, that from ten days after the cessation of the menstrual flow until three days preceding its return, there is little chance of conception, while the converse is equally true. . . . This law is to the effect that if the conception takes place in the early part of the menstrual period a female child will be the result: if in the latter part, a male child will be born." Melendy's beliefs were erroneously based on the fact that most nonhuman mammalian females have a bloody discharge at the time of ovulation (the optimal time for conception to occur). This is not the case for human females as ovulation occurs well before the menstrual discharge begins (King, 1999).

The latter half of the nineteenth century and the twentieth century brought about tremendous change in views of human biology and human sexuality. Dramatic changes in attitudes, social customs, and gender roles took place during this era. Although the vast majority of these changes were caused by, and caused changes in, the social norms regarding human sexuality, two developments—the increased availability and use of contraceptives and a greater understanding of the etiology and treatment of sexually transmitted diseases—demonstrate how strong the relationship between human biology and human sexuality truly is. Although the majority of this period was characterized by increased openness about human sexuality and greater equity for the two genders, there was a growing awareness in the 1980s and 1990s that there were problems that can result from human sexuality practices, such as HIV infection, sexual abuse, and unplanned teen pregnancies. No doubt, though, changes occurred in this era that will remain forever. "Safe sex" is now a household word and contraception is available to almost all who desire it. Sex education, however, remains highly controversial. There are still different human sexuality standards for men and women. Sexual acts are still used to victimize women and children. Homophobia, the irrational fear of homosexual persons, continues to plague society (McAnulty & Burnette, 2001). Importantly, any attempt to understand human biology and the link to human sexuality must include consideration of the historical context.

THEORY, RESEARCH, AND UNDERSTANDING

The biological dimension in human sexuality is pervasive. Biological factors largely control sexual development from conception until birth and the ability of people to reproduce after puberty. The biological dimension of human sexuality also affects sexual desire, sexual functioning, and, indirectly, sexual satisfaction. Biological forces are even thought to influence certain sex differences in behavior, such as the tendency of males to act more aggressively than females. The process of sexual arousal produces specific biological events in humans: the pulse quickens, the sexual organs respond, and sensations of warmth spread throughout the body (Masters, Johnson, & Kolodny, 1995).

To claim the importance of the biological dimension in human sexuality is not the same as dismissing other important dimensions in human sexuality, and, in fact, overall human behavior—psychosocial, behavioral, clinical, and cultural (Masters et al., 1995). These dimensions play an important part in human sexuality. However, understanding the role of human biology in human sexuality affords the social work practitioner and social work students the chance to understand human sexuality better.

The vast majority of theories of human sexuality, while tending to emphasize elements other than the biological, do usually include some elements of human biology. For example, Sigmund Freud in the development of psychoanalytic theory designated libido, or sex drive, as the driving force in personality development. Freud was one of the first to promote the view that childhood sexuality was a normal part of human development. Freud believed the libido was present at birth and that it and other biological urges such as hunger formed a distinct part of the mind. As a biologically based instinct, libido causes a buildup of sexual ten-

sion, an uncomfortable state that motivates a person to seek release through grati-
fication, a process known as the "pleasure principle." People experience this sexual
tension and as they develop through a series of biologically determined stages
(also discussed in Chapter 4), oral, anal, phallic, latency, and genital, tension release
is sought (McAnulty & Burnette, 2001). Freud believed that human sexuality was
both the primary force in the motivation of all human behavior and the principal
cause of all forms of unresolved anxiety (Masters et al., 1995).

The main point, while attempting to highlight the link between human biology and human sexuality, is that Freud's theory of human development, psychoanalytic theory, is the only one to specifically emphasize human sexuality to such
a degree. Other human development theories explain human sexuality but have
less emphasis on human biology than does the psychoanalytic theory. These theories include the sociologically based script theory, the psychosocial theory of Erik
Erickson, social cognition theories, and others. Erickson's descriptive stage theory
explains human sexuality and other elements of human development by posing a
number of predictable social challenges that take place during the life span. The
script theory is quite similar to the modern-day notion of social constructivism and
explains human sexuality by way of awareness and adherence to cultural norms
and expectations. Social cognition theorists stress the importance of life experiences and learning in shaping overall human behavior, including behavior and
practices related to human sexuality (McAnulty & Burnette, 2001).

The human development theory of evolutionary psychology was inspired
by the work of Charles Darwin and includes an emphasis on human biology.
According to evolutionary psychologists, human behavior in general and human
sexual practices in particular can be understood in light of our history as a biological species. Sexual practices make sense because they are adaptive for survival. A basic belief of evolutionary psychology theory is that the primary force
underlying human sexual behavior is the desire to successfully reproduce, and
thereby pass on one's genes. Sexual practices that offer reproductive advantage
are more likely to be passed on—that is genetically transmitted—whereas practices that are not beneficial in that way will most likely not be passed on. Sexual
selection refers to the evolutionary process by which human sexual practices and
arrangements that provide reproductive advantages tend to become established.
Evolutionary psychology as a theoretical explanation of human sexuality is not,
however, without controversy. For example, the theoretical notion that men and
women are biologically programmed to pursue different sexual strategies, particularly in the attraction of a sexual partner, is highly controversial (McAnulty &
Burnette, 2001), as is the evolutionary theory of rape. The evolutionary psychology theory of rape suggests that use of forceful tactics to inseminate females may
have been naturally selected to favor males who can inseminate large numbers of
females using whatever methods necessary. On the other hand, females enhance
their reproductive potential by mating with males who will help care for the offspring they produce, so females have evolved tendencies to avoid and resist
forced sex (McCammon, Knox, & Schacht, 1998, p. 35).

Research on human sexuality has tended to focus on sexual behaviors and not
the link to human biology. In fact, Freud was not a sex researcher. Rather, he merely

discussed sexuality as a primary motivation for human behavior. Although Freud was clearly a revolutionary thinker in regards to human sexuality, his ideas on sexual motivation and sexuality in infants and children remain critical, and he was not always right when it came to the link between human biology and human sexuality. Freud erroneously believed that the loss of semen was detrimental to a man's health in much the way the loss of blood was detrimental. Case histories and cross-cultural studies were the norm for both Freud and his colleague Henry Havelock Ellis. Ellis responded to the false claims that nocturnal emissions would cause blindness, insanity, and eventual death. He observed that none of these things happened to him. Ellis concluded that the loss of semen and impending death were not related for humans. His writings, however, were focused primarily on the psychology of human sexuality. Alfred Kinsey in the 1940s and 1950s focused primarily on the collection of so-called objective data on sexual behavior. Kinsey's findings, that most people engaged in oral-genital sex, that women could have multiple orgasms, that most people masturbated, and that many men had had a homosexual encounter, were startling from a sociological point of view, but did little to advance knowledge about the link of human sexuality to human biology. The same can be said for the extensive, rigorously designed, and thought-provoking National Health and Social Life Survey conducted in 1992. The focus in that comprehensive survey was on self-reported descriptions of sexual behavior (King, 1999).

It was left to a pair of researchers, William Masters, a physician, and Virginia Johnson, a behavioral scientist, in the 1950s and 1960s to conduct the consummate studies on functional anatomy and physiology and push forward understanding of the link between human biology and human sexuality (King, 1999). Masters and Johnson believed that to understand the complexities of human sexuality it was necessary to integrate knowledge of human biology, specifically sexual anatomy and physiology, with knowledge of human sexuality garnered by sociologists and psychologists. Masters and Johnson conducted laboratory investigations and recorded the physical details of human sexual arousal and sexual activities (Masters et al., 1995).

As well, physiological theories closely align human sexuality and human biology. These theories describe and explain how physiological processes affect and are affected by sexual behavior. Cardiovascular, respiratory, neurological, and endocrinological functioning, as well as genetic factors, are involved in sexual behaviors. Physiological theories respond to questions such as the following: What physiological processes are involved in sexual desire, arousal, lubrication, erection, and orgasm? How do various drugs and medications affect sexual functioning? How do various hormones affect sexuality? To what degree are behavioral differences between women and men attributable to their different hormonal make-ups (McCammon et al., 1998)?

BIOLOGICAL THEORY OF HUMAN SEXUALITY

Physiological theories are generally subsumed under the classification of a biological theory of human sexuality. A biological theory of human sexuality focuses on answering questions about why men and women exhibit different physical characteristics and human sexuality behaviors and practices. For example, the biological theory of gender role development, linked closely to gender differences in human sexuality, goes like this. The distinction between the female and male sexes begins at the moment of fertilization when the man's sperm and the woman's egg unite to form a zygote. Both chromosomal and hormonal factors contribute to the development of the zygote. Chromosomes are structures located within every cell in a person's body. Each cell contains 23 pairs of chromosomes, a total of 46 chromosomes per cell. Chromosomes contain genes, a basic unit of heredity. One of these 23 pairs of chromosomes is referred to as sex chromosomes because they determine whether an individual will be female or male. There are two types of sex chromosomes: X and Y. Normally, females have two X chromosomes, whereas males have one X and one Y chromosome. When the egg and the sperm meet in the fallopian tube, each contains only half the normal number of chromosomes. The union of sperm and egg results in a single cell called a zygote, which has the normal 46 chromosomes. The egg will always have an X chromosome, but the sperm will have either an X or Y chromosome. If the sperm contains an X chromosome, the match with the female chromosome will be XX, and the child will be genetically female. If the sperm contains a Y chromosome, the match with the female chromosome will be XY, and the child will be genetically male (McCammon et al., 1998).

Hormones are also important to the biological theory of gender role development. Male and female embryos are indistinguishable during the first several weeks of intrauterine life. If an embryo is genetically a male, a chemical substance controlled by the Y chromosome stimulates the development of testes from the gonads. The testes, in turn, begin secreting the male hormone testosterone, which stimulates the development of the male reproductive and external sexual organs. The development of the genetically female embryo requires that no additional testosterone be present. Without the controlling substance from the Y chromosome, gonads develop into ovaries, and as development continues the fallopian tubes, uterus, and vagina come into existence. At puberty, the hormones released by the testes and the ovaries are necessary for the development of secondary sex characteristics. Higher levels of testosterone account for the growth of facial hair in men and pubic and underarm hair in both men and women. Breast development results from increasing levels of estrogen (McCammon et al., 1998). The establishment of gender role development via the biological theory goes just like that.

Biological theories of human sexuality are, however, not without question or controversy. The scientific debate of the early 2000s regarding the importance of sexual reproduction is a good example. The debate concerns the adaptive value of sexual reproduction. Until a few years ago biologists believed that the reshuffling of genes that results from sexual reproduction permits an organism (in this case a person) to better adapt to its environment. The purpose of sexual reproduction was to ensure the long-term evolution of the species in the face of changing environmental conditions. However, environmental change is a slow process that occurs over thousands and even millions of years, far too slowly to require gene reshuffling every generation. In recent years two new theories attempting to explain the importance of human reproduction have emerged: (1) sexual reproduction evolved to help complex organisms (people) combat their parasites, and (2) sexual reproduction is important for the repair and rejuvenation of DNA. The keeping-up-with-the-parasites hypothesis holds that long-lived organisms (people) engage in a constant struggle for survival against internal parasites that can evolve much more quickly than they can. Parasitic microorganisms such as bacteria and viruses have generation times (the period of time between parents and offspring) on the order of days or even hours, so their opportunities for recombining the genes in their gene pool to gain an advantage over people who serve as hosts are high indeed. Because people recombine genes only about once every 20 years or so, people need to do a good job of reshuffling their genes to a maximal degree when they do. The second theory, also supported by considerable evidence, is that sexual reproduction ensures the continued health of a person's DNA. According to this hypothesis, sexual reproduction serves to remove mutated DNA from the gene pool. Sexual reproduction is well known for favoring sperm and eggs with good, clean, single copies of genes. Mutated genes are continually cast aside in the sexual reproduction process. Sexual reproduction also ensures that mutated genes are expressed as infrequently as possible. Everyone carries some mutations, but they are so rare that unrelated people generally have mutations on different genes. Both theories, the keeping up with the parasites and the shedding of mutated genes, in all likelihood have some merit. Sexual reproduction, according to a biological theory of human sexuality, helps people keep up in the battle against rapidly evolving parasites. And in the long term, sexual reproduction ensures the continued good health of DNA (Johnson, 2001). Neither theory does much good, though, for the advancement of romance and sexual intimacy.

HUMAN BIOLOGY AND SEXUAL ORIENTATION

The link between human biology and sexual orientation is used as a means to highlight the overall link, and the accompanying questions, between human biology and human sexuality. The central question for this discussion is what is the relationship between sexual orientation and gender identity and gender roles. And the answer is that no one knows for sure. King (1999) sums up the majority of research in this area by stating that sexual orientation and gender identity and gender roles appear to be independent. The gender identity of the vast majority of homosexual and bisexual persons is just as strong and consistent with their anatomical gender as is found among those persons claiming to be heterosexuals. The sexual orientations of homosexuality and bisexuality appear not to be the result of gender dysphoria. Whether a person does or does not conform to gender stereotypes does not predict sexual orientation. Vilain (2000) also claims the nonrelation of gender to sexual orientation. The researcher highlights instead the role of social, familial, environmental, endocrine, and genetic factors in determining sexual orientation. He suggests that answers for questions of the role of genes in sex determination may hold a key for the genetic study of sexual orientation.

The concept of uncertainty is a necessary guidepost for any journey through historical and present-day views of the etiology, causation, classification, acceptance/condemnation, or living of any particular, or combined, sexual orientation. No realm of human biology—the expression of human sexuality via a sexual orientation—is more laden with culturally constructed emotionality. For example, a current controversy involves universities policing public sex between same sex partners, particularly gay men, while generally accepting public sex by heterosexual couples. This creates the perception of a double standard based on sexual orientation. The public sex of gay men is frowned on, while public sex of heterosexual couples (e.g., in library stacks) is often viewed as a tradition or mere prank. Any informed student of human biology and sexual orientation needs to have his or her critical thinking skills within easy reach.

The achievement of one completely agreed on operational definition of sexual orientation appears not to be possible. There is no need, however, to be disheartened. General understanding of the concept of sexual orientation and most textbook definitions of the term have a fairly congruent presentation. The following two definitions garnered from textbooks that include "human sexuality" in their titles are offered in an effort to demonstrate what typifies these definitional efforts.

- Sexual orientation is one's sexual attraction to members of the opposite sex, the same sex, or both sexes. Attraction to members of the opposite sex is called heterosexuality, whereas attraction to same-sex individuals is called homosexuality. Bisexuality refers to sexual attraction to people of either sex (King, 1999, p. 224).

- Sexual orientation refers to one's attraction to sexual and romantic love partners. Currently, this orientation is perceived in U.S. culture as being homosexual, bisexual, or heterosexual. A homosexual orientation denotes sexual and romantic attraction toward individuals of one's own gender. A bisexual orientation denotes sexual and romantic attraction toward both one's own and the other gender; this attraction may also be referred to as ambisexual. A heterosexual orientation is attraction toward individuals of the other gender (Bolin & Whelehan, 1999).

The conceptual foundation of sexual orientation has varied through the decades. In the dichotomous model of sexual orientation people are either heterosexual or homosexual. The dichotomous model of sexual orientation prevails in mainstream U.S. culture. This model ascribes to the male versus female and the masculine versus feminine dichotomies. The major criticism of the dichotomous model of sexual orientation is that it fails to affirm the existence of persons with a bisexual orientation (McCammon et al., 1998).

The unidimensional continuum model of sexual orientation purports that most people are not exclusively heterosexual or homosexual. Kinsey and his colleagues in the 1950s developed the Heterosexual–Homosexual Rating Scale in order to assess where on the continuum of sexual orientation an individual is. The Kinsey scale was originally unidimensional and sexual orientation was assessed by lifetime erotic attractions and sexual behavior. However, the scale was criticized for assuming that an individual's sexual behavior and feelings were congruent. The unidimensional model is also generally considered to fail to incorporate any elements of social context. The multidimensional model of sexual orientation was developed in response to the criticisms of the Kinsey scale and hypothesized that sexual orientation consists of various independent and interacting components. A listing of these components includes, but is not limited to, emotional and social preferences, lifestyle, self-identification, sexual attraction, fantasy, and behavior. And, importantly, the multidimensional model hypothesizes that these components may vary in interaction, intensity, and expression mode over time (McCammon et al., 1998).

It is important when the social work practitioner or social work student is conducting research of any kind on sexual orientation that one not think of sexual orientation as discontinuous. Instead, Kinsey, Pomeroy, and Martin (1948) developed a scale that "provides a continuum of psychosexual and overt sexual behavior between the two extremes" (Haynes, 1995, p. 99). The continuum concept helps explain how an individual may occupy one or more levels of sexual orientation concurrently or sequentially. It is important to note here that the term *bisexual* in biology means being of both sexes or having both male and female organs (Haynes, 1995); thus the term *ambisexual* has been suggested to recognize the ability for a person to be sexually attracted to both genders (Haynes, 1995).

Although history, in and of itself, is helpful in acquiring new knowledge regarding biological features in understanding sexual orientation, the actual process of historical research is also important. Historical research involves investigating sexuality and sexual issues through the review and analysis of historical documents. Data sources to be used can include newspapers, magazines, letters, literature, diaries, medical texts, court records, hospital records, prison records, and official government statistics. Historical sexuality research provides information about the changing nature of behavior, norms, social control, and socially constructed meanings of sexuality. History may also help with understanding the link to human biology. In an analysis of sexuality in U.S. life from colonial times to the late 1990s, D'Emilio and Freedman traced changes in sexual themes from a reproductive emphasis in the eighteenth century, to a focus on gender relations in the nineteenth century, to a concern for eroticism in the twentieth century. This technique, historical research, led Freedman and D'Emilio to conclude that the term *human sexuality* is actually a modern construct that originated in the nineteenth century (McCammon et al., 1998).

Although there is clear recognition that human sexuality and the question of sexual orientation has many components, there is no question that biology plays a major role. The illumination of biology is not intended to discredit the work of researchers in other areas but merely represents a selective view. The selection of an emphasis on sexual orientation being part biology is intended to (1) create a forum for increasing biology-based understanding and (2) contrast this knowledge base with other dynamic areas of study, not limited to the cultural, anthropological, psychological, and biocultural (Bolin & Whelehan, 1999).

In 1973, the American Psychological Association withdrew their classification of homosexuality as a mental illness. This set into motion research on the biological causes of homosexuality. Research on rats led to the conclusion that the cause of homosexuality is a hormonal abnormality that occurs during pregnancy and has a lasting effect on the brain. Pillard and Weinrich in 1986 concluded that "male homosexuality runs in families—that it was much more likely that brothers of gay men would be homosexual than it was for brothers of straight men" (DeCecco & Parker, 1995, p. 4). Swaab and Fliers claimed in 1985 that "a particular region of the hypothalamus was 'sexually diamorphic,' that is, showing different structures in females and males" (DeCecco & Parker, 1995, p. 4). Swaab and Hofman claimed in 1990 that they found a particular nucleus in the hypothalamus that was larger and contained more cells in gay than in straight men. By the end of the 1980s, all other explanations of homosexuality were abandoned in favor of biological causes. In 1991, LeVay claimed that he had found a different nucleus than Swaab and Hofman in the hypothalamus that had twice the volume in heterosexual than in homosexual men. Also in 1991, Bailey concluded that homosexuality was "strongly familial" and that mothers of "effeminate" males were more "stress-prone" than other mothers (DeCecco & Parker, 1995).

At first glance, these reports may seem to prove that homosexuality is exclusively biologically based; however, the reports themselves are based on a number of presuppositions about homosexuality that need to be considered. In these studies, sexuality "is viewed as basically physical and behavioral . . . elements of motivation, unconsciousness, intention, perception, interpretation, and choices, as well as influences of time, society, and culture" (p. 10) are virtually ignored. Much of the aforementioned research does have its methodological shortcomings, which the researchers acknowledge, but many of the conclusions on whether individuals were homosexual or heterosexual to begin with were either assumed by researchers or gained through self-identification of the research subjects. A second presupposition is that heterosexuality and homosexuality are antitheses of one another and cannot occur together. This ignores the actual range of sexual behaviors of all human beings throughout the lifespan. Also, the situational and circumstantial aspects of human sexual behavior are ignored. Another presupposition is that homosexuality equals feminine behavior in men and masculine behavior in women. In fact, in biological research, the degree to which an individual departs from the sex role stereotypes is taken as an indication of the strength of genetic determination. This assumption also produces the erroneous assumption that homosexuals are abnormal, or nature gone awry (DeCecco & Parker, 1995).

The most fundamental of the biological presuppositions is that the general contours of sexual expression are permanently established by biology and that experience and culture serve only to fill in the details (DeCecco & Parker, 1995, p. 16). The role of choice is not considered and the idea of sexual orientation replaces that of sexual preference. However, the role of choice needs to be taken into account. More importantly, "an adequate conception of homosexuality and heterosexuality must embrace all of its known or purported aspects: the biological, the psychological, and the socio-cultural" (p. 19). In addition, one must remember when conducting or consuming research that certain phenomena related to sexuality are the domain of certain categories. For instance, biologists primarily study the bodily aspects of sexual orientation and leave human behavior and imagination to the psychological researchers.

The significance of sexual orientation itself and its role in self-identity in our culture cannot be overstated. According to Doell (1995), "there is a positive ambiance that is associated culturally with marriage and a stigma that is attached to homosexual lifestyles" (p. 352). In addition, attributing homosexuality to biological differences will not remove this stigma. The only way for this stigma to be removed will be through "a recognition of the bisexual capacities of humans along with a recognition of the way in which societies construct sexual categories for purposes of controlling groups and distributing power, coupled with a determination to change the status quo" (p. 352).

SEXUAL ORIENTATION AND GENETICS

A historical review of human biology in the expression of human sexuality and sexual orientation includes consideration of the role of genetics. The inclusion of genetics helps highlight the interplay between genetic and environmental factors in determining sexual orientation. It was not until the middle 1800s when Charles Darwin and Alfred Wallace began to postulate evolution by natural selection, and when Mendel published his work on genetic inheritance, that the biological tools became available to explore why human beings are the way they are (Haynes, 1995). Charles Darwin's central thesis was that recurrent differential reproduction caused by differences in design attributes—natural selection—is the key to evolutionary change over time. Because reproduction is central to the evolutionary process, domains closely linked with reproduction should be focal targets of selection pressures, the fulcrum for evolved mechanisms or adaptations. No domain is closer to reproduction than expressed human sexuality. Although Darwin did speak about sexual selection and same-sex compassion for advantage in reproduction, his adoption of Spencer's phrase "survival of the fittest" is an unfortunate one. Confusion can arise when the concept of natural selection is equated with the concept of survival selection. It is important to keep in mind that survival only becomes important to the extent that it is a tributary to reproduction (Buss, 1998). The social work practitioner and the social work student know that while same-sex relations do not result in reproduction, other issues in same-sex orientation, such as sexual desire, mate selection, and intrasex competition for advantage, are informed by selection principles.

Following the work of Darwin and Mendel, in 1886 von Krafft-Ebing attempted to show a genetic basis for same-sex relations, contending that homosexual persons had multiple hereditary flaws. Later Sigmund Freud and Magnus Hirschfeld began to examine sexual behaviors and based their theories on a hybrid of psychology and biology. Kallmann's study of identical twins used genetics to look for the hereditary bases of behavior distinctive to a sexual orientation. And so the study of the role of biology, especially genes, in explaining sexual orientation was begun. However, it is important to note that just as the genetic sex of an individual is not solely determined by one's genes, the same is so for sexual orientation. There is sufficient evidence, such as cases of complete androgen insensitivity syndrome, adrenogenital syndrome, and transexualism, to put into question the immutability of the genetic inheritance of sexual characteristics. And evidence supports the immutability of the genetic inheritance of sexual orientation (Haynes, 1995). In other words, immutability, or the idea of something not being susceptible to change, is not true of sexual characteristics, but is believed to be true of sexual orientation. As is the case in the transgendered person, one can change his/her sexual characteristics. Can a person change their sexual orientation?

Behavioral genetic studies have provided the strongest evidence in affirming the role biology plays in influencing human sexual behavior. These studies rely on the relative similarity of family members of differing genetic resemblance to estimate the heritability and environmentality underlying a phenotype, which is the result of the *dynamic interaction* of the genes with the environment. Past studies have also resulted in assertions of the genetic origins of homosexuality, heterosexuality, and bisexuality. A common conclusion though is that more carefully designed studies are needed because "all the present studies lack one or more of the following necessary experimental design components or ways to interpret the data: (1) valid and precise measures of individual differences, (2) appropriate methods to ascertain biological relationships, (3) research subjects that have been randomly recruited, (4) appropriate sample sizes, and (5) appropriate genetic models to interpret data" (p. 116). In present studies, sexual orientation is often poorly operationally defined, and researchers use a variety of behavioral measures. The sample sizes are too small and recruitment of subjects is biased. As a result, only the simplest possible genetic models can be applied. In addition, it is important in studies of the heritability of sexual orientation to acknowledge that these studies will not lead one to discover its etiology, or causal agent (McGuire, 1995).

SOCIOBIOLOGY = HUMAN BIOLOGY AND HUMAN SEXUALITY

Sociobiology is the application of biological principles, particularly genetic and evolutionary ones, in an attempt to better understand human social behavior (Haynes, 1995, p. 107). For example, the balanced superior heterozygote fitness hypothesis proposed by Hutchinson in 1959 proposes that there is a recessive gene for homosexuality and a dominant one for heterosexuality. The kin selection hypothesis by Hamilton in 1964 and the parental manipulation hypothesis by Trivers in 1974 assert that homosexual persons are "'sacrificing' their reproductive capacity to the greater good of the social order and their family" (p. 108) by helping to rear the offspring of their relatives and by limiting the population, which reduces competition.

Although there is no conclusive evidence that sexual orientation is genetically determined, there is none available for its environmental determinants either; thus an interaction most probably exists. Sociobiologists who study human sexuality assert that there is no necessary reason for humans to understand the causes behind sexual orientation. Answers have been sought, however, for a number of reasons, including to find a "cure" and to lead to acceptance if a "natural biological" cause was found. The constraints placed by the social order on particular sexual orientations have no basis in biology (Haynes, 1995, p. 111).

The work of evolutionary biologists on sexual orientation, however, has not been without criticism. The criticisms usually highlight the widely held misconceptions of this field. One needs to understand the thinking of evolutionary biologists in order to understand the resultant works of the field. For instance, an evolutionary biologist, when explaining variability within a species, "tends not to ask what went *wrong* with the process producing this variability but to ask what went *right*" (Weinrich, 1995, p. 204). Furthermore, "the tendency to look for the adaptation present in most examples of variation is trained into evolutionary biologists very early" (Weinrich, 1995, p. 205). This is why homosexuality was first considered adaptive by sociobiologists (a subdiscipline of evolutionary biology).

HUMAN BIOLOGY, HUMAN SEXUALITY, AND SEXUAL DYSFUNCTION

Although human biology and its impact on expressed sexuality are important during times of health and sexual functioning, understandably elements of human biology get more attention during times of sexual dysfunction. Sexual dysfunctions involve a disturbance in the sexual response cycle or pain during sexual intercourse and are classified by McAnulty and Burnett (2001, p. 630) as follows:

1. Sexual desire disorders involve problems associated with erotic fantasies and the desire for sexual activity or with the sex drive. These disorders are typically characterized by an abnormally low or absent desire for sexual activity.
2. Sexual arousal disorders involve problems associated with the excitement, or sexual arousal, phase of the sexual response cycle. For males, sexual arousal disorders involve difficulty attaining or sustaining erection. For females, such disorders usually involve difficulties achieving vaginal lubrication and expansion. In both cases, the arousal problems interfere with sexual activity.
3. Orgasmic disorders affect the orgasm phase of the sexual response cycle. In both sexes, orgasmic disorders may involve an inability to climax. In males, another common difficulty is premature ejaculation.
4. Sexual pain disorders involve genital pain experienced during attempted or actual intercourse.

Sexual dysfunctions can also be placed within subtypes: primary (developed early in life), secondary (developed later in life), generalized, and/or situational. Prevalence varies, but sexual dysfunctions are fairly common, affecting as many as 40 percent of women and 30 percent of men. The general causes of sexual dysfunctions are as follows (McAnulty and Burnett, 2001):

- Medications and other drugs are common causes of problems in sexual functioning. Alcohol abuse is linked to several sexual dysfunctions.
- Psychological factors are also associated with sexual problems. Anxiety has been consistently found to interfere with sexual functioning. Feelings of guilt and shame may predispose some people to sexual problems.
- Relationship problems, including control issues, resentment, and fear of intimacy may contribute to sexual dysfunctions.
- Cultural beliefs, such as the double standard for the genders of male and female, may lead to sexual inhibitions, conflict, and miscommunication, which can result in sexual problems.

Social work practitioners are often involved in the treatment of sexual dysfunctions. There are several sexual dysfunctions, particularly those that have a psychological, cultural, or relationship etiology, that social work practitioners have proven to be effective in treating. Sex therapy involves techniques designed to provide education, correct faulty beliefs, reduce performance fears, and resolve relationship conflicts. Sexual dysfunctions experienced by couples have proven to be responsive to therapeutic efforts. Sex therapy effectiveness, however, varies considerably. The effectiveness of sex therapy can depend on the type of sexual dysfunction being treated. Acquired problems are easier to treat than are lifelong problems. Situational problems are easier to treat than are generalized sexual problems. Problems of sexual desire may be the most difficult to treat (McCammon et al., 1998). Social work practitioners often become involved in the provision of instructive material regarding sexual techniques and the use of therapeutic techniques by individuals or couples, such as sensate focus, stop–start, the squeeze technique, and directed masturbation (McAnulty & Burnette, 2001).

Sexual dysfunction and the link to biological elements cannot be overlooked. In fact, one common way to classify sexual dysfunctions includes a strong emphasis on the organic, that which is derived from a living organism (a person). A sexual dysfunction using this nomenclature is either *organic* (including physical or medical factors such as illness, injury, or drug effects) or *psychosocial* (including psychological, interpersonal, environmental, and cultural factors) (Masters, Johnson, & Kolodny, 1995). Biological factors that can cause or contribute to a sexual dysfunction include physical illness (e.g., diabetes, multiple sclerosis, or infections), the degenerative elements of the aging process, and physical disability (e.g., spinal cord injury). Treatment modalities for different physical conditions, such as surgery, medication (including antidepressants), and chemotherapy can sometimes cause the onset or exacerbation of a sexual dysfunction (McCammon et al., 1998).

There are several medical interventions that directly influence the physical functioning of people and either erase or ease the impact of a sexual dysfunction. Medical interventions for erection problems, for example, include surgery, injections, and use of vacuum constriction devices. Oral medications, including the enormously popular Viagra, have proven to be effective. Oral medications can also be prescribed for men who experience problems with recurring premature ejaculation (McAnulty & Burnette, 2001). In fact, a clear change in the recognition of treatment availability for sexual dysfunction is exemplified by the recent development of comprehensive urology and impotence centers (McCammon et al., 1998).

IMPLICATIONS FOR SOCIAL WORK PRACTICE

The old social work practice adage is that the two most difficult things to talk with people about are money and sex. Since this is not a chapter about money, let us consider briefly the link between human biology and human sexuality and the implications for social work practice. The perspective of this consideration is not, however, how to assist the social work practitioner or social work student in becoming a sex therapist. The goal of becoming a sex therapist is achieved only by the social work practitioner or social work student pursuing a formal process of intense clinical training and supervised practice. There are, however, some practical notions about human biology and human sexuality that all social work practitioners and social work students can integrate into their work with people.

Awareness of Research

Social work practitioners and social work students can enrich their practice with a continued awareness of the research on human sexuality that is going on in the various social science disciplines, such as psychology, sociology, psychiatry, and women's studies. If so, the social work practitioner and the social work student can avoid developing and/or maintaining an elementary or simplistic understanding of human sexuality. For example, the identification of biological determinants of sexual orientation is a difficult and controversial research process and one to which social workers should be attentive (Van Wyk & Geist, 1995). It is important to keep in mind that the problem with the field of human sexuality is that there are not enough theories to structure debate and not enough researchers with enough ideas to prove and disprove (Baumeister & Tice, 2001). New ideas about human sexuality and new understanding of human sexuality will as likely come from the biological sciences as the social sciences.

Understanding Causal Claims

Social work practitioners and social work students will do well to remember that it has been difficult to establish a clear understanding of how psychosocial factors "cause" a sexual dysfunction. Research has established strong associations between factors such as developmental traumas, psychological traits, behavior patterns, and relationship difficulties and the existence of sexual dysfunctions. However, the research has fallen short of establishing a causal relationship between psychosocial elements and the presence of a sexual dysfunction. Some persons whose social histories are dominated by potentially devastating psychosocial events have no sexual dysfunction experience. Other people who have unremarkable social histories do experience a sexual dysfunction. At the same time, however, research over the past decades has time and again established the link between elements of human biology and human sexuality. It is a steadily growing belief that many sexual dysfunctions have a biological or physical cause. If the link has not been made in total, it has clearly been established that a whole host of sexual dysfunctions have at least a partial biological cause (Masters et al., 1995).

As well, there is a tendency for social work practitioners, social work students, and even social work educators to denigrate the mechanistic tendencies of human biologists in explaining human sexuality. This is true both when the explanation is of how human sexuality functions or when the explanation is focused on sexual dysfunction. Social workers need, however, to acknowledge the merits of the "how-does-the body-function" explanations of human sexuality by human biologists. Social work practitioners and social work students cannot deny the advances in human sexuality understanding that have emanated from biological research, particularly the increases in understanding about brain functioning and the link to human sexuality (DeCecco & Parker, 1995).

Social Comparison Theory

Evaluation of one's own human sexuality expression and the link to human biology is complex, and usually ongoing. One popular method of evaluation is for people to evaluate their expressed human sexuality and sex lives by comparison with others. This is the essence of the social comparison theory. People compare themselves with others in order to reach an evaluative understanding of themselves. Social workers who are comfortable in inquiring about human sexuality and comfortable with listening and speaking about human sexuality with people will be better practitioners. Understanding the intimate link between human biology and human sexuality will prepare the social work practitioner and social work student to better offer assistance or provide appropriate referrals. Being knowledgeable of and comfortable with the link between human biology and human sexuality means more than just asking "Have you seen a doctor lately?"

DISCUSSION QUESTIONS

1. Why do men and women have different sex characteristics? Why do they have different sex practices?

2. What is your best prediction for the next breakthrough in sex research?

3. How do you contrast the essentialist and social construction theories of human sexuality?

4. What evidence suggests that sexual orientation is immutable, or not susceptible to change?

5. How generalizable is research on animals and their sex practices to an understanding of people and their sex practices?

6. What are the implications for social work practice if sexual reproduction is considered *not* to be a function of human biology?

CHAPTER TWELVE

THE BIOLOGY OF AGING

Oh, Age has weary days,
And nights o' sleepless pain:
Thou golden time o' youthfu' prime,
Why come thou not again?
—Robert Burns from "The Winter of Life"

Don't believe there's plenty of time for everything. There isn't.
—Lillian Hellman

The man who views the world at fifty the same way
he did at twenty has wasted thirty years of his life.
—Muhammad Ali

The social work literature on aging is extensive. The primary emphasis is on social and economic issues facing older adults, some of which are serious impediments to satisfactory lives for the elderly. It is especially true that adults who had low incomes when they worked are likely to have even lower incomes and fewer assets when they are elderly because the basic governmental program for retired people is Social Security and it is pegged to one's earnings while working.

Medicare, which is available to all Americans 65 and older, provides health coverage in many circumstances but not for all health needs. However, Medicaid provides the difference for very-low-income people and also provides nursing home care and other long-term care for those who are eligible and who need it. Supplemental Security Income provides a minimum monthly cash stipend for low-income older people, as well.

Details on all these issues, programs, and services are available in the many texts and many other books written on aging with an emphasis on social work with older people.

The growing proportion of aged in the United States is a significant fact. In 2000, there were nine workers nationwide for every recipient of Social Security. That number is expected to shrink to four workers per Social Security recipient by 2050.

Older people, who are 65 years old and older, comprise one of every eight Americans. There were 14.5 million men and 20.4 million women in the senior age group in 2000 (Euster, 2002). There were 43 men over 86 for every 100 women and 85 men for every 100 women aged 65–69 in 2000.

Aging persons' households were disadvantaged compared with the rest of the population. Those 65 and over in 1999 had median household incomes of $22,812, whereas the median for all U.S. households was $40,816. There were 3.2 million elderly people living in poverty, a percentage of 9.7 of the total older adult population.

Men greatly outnumber women in the percentage who are married. Seventy-seven percent of men aged 65–74 were married and living with their spouses in 2000, compared with 53 percent of women. The difference also holds true at the upper age levels. Among men aged 85 and over, 53 percent were married and living with a spouse, compared with 12 percent of women.

NURSING HOME CARE

Nursing home care is also a significant health issue for older adults and for social workers, too, because many work with programs that place clients in nursing homes and others work directly in nursing homes themselves. Although only a small minority of older adults are residents of long-term care facilities such as nursing homes, the issue of providing such long-term care is significant for practitioners in many different fields. What to do about an aging parent or grandparent who can no longer live on his or her own or with family members is one of the issues most frequently raised with social workers in all kinds of employment.

The quality and nature of long-term care is also an important consideration for social workers, and some understanding of issues such as the safety of the facility's environment, the kinds of conditions that require long-term care as well as those that might be addressed by home health services or other outpatient approaches, exercise programs, and nutrition, are often major concerns that social workers have to address. Of course, the societal and social policy issues related to long-term care are important but so are the biological considerations.

BIOLOGICAL ISSUES IN AGING

"We know that old age is not characterized by physical changes alone. As individuals move into old age, they are confronted with physical, psychological, and social changes that they may or may not be able to cope with" (Harbert and Ginsberg, 1990, p. 17). Although older people are living longer than ever, there are some growing health problems among older adults. The rates of obesity, for example, have increased among people aged 50–64: in 1982, 14.4 percent were obese, but by 1999, 26.7 percent were obese. For people aged 65–74, the relative numbers are 12.6 percent and 22.1 percent.

Individuals in the 50–64 age group are also skeptical about the health care system and may be inclined to search the Internet for medical information. The same group is likely to use alternative treatments such as acupuncture.

ALZHEIMER'S DISEASE

Alzheimer's is also discussed in Chapter 4. The genes that are associated with early-onset Alzheimer's are, according to Nash (2000), Presenilin-1 (found on chromosome 21) and Presenilin-2 (found on chromosome 14). Presenilin-1 accounts for about 4 percent of cases with an onset age range of 28 to 50. Presenilin-2 accounts for 1 percent of cases with onset in the forties and fifties.

Batteries of tests are used to diagnose dementia, including Alzheimer's, which is one form of dementia: blood counts, chest X-rays, thyroid function tests, and, in some cases, brain scans are used (Gorman, 2000a).

One genetic variant, APOE4, which is found on chromosome 19, appears in some two-thirds of Alzheimer's patients, both early and late onset. However, many people who have the gene never develop Alzheimer's. Therefore, physicians don't recommend testing for it unless there are symptoms of Alzheimer's (Nash, 2000).

More common verbal diagnostic tests for the disease ask the patient to recall the year and the month and to recite simple phrases from memory. They may be asked to count backwards from twenty to one and to say the months in reverse order. The level of dependence of the patient is also checked by assessing the person's ability to write checks and balance a checkbook, remember appointments, travel out of the neighborhood, prepare meals, and keep track of current events (Nash, 2000).

Gorman (2000b) identifies three different stages of Alzheimer's. Stage 1 is mild and lasts for 2 to 4 years. It is characterized by increased forgetfulness, which impedes the ability to hold a job or complete household tasks. The patient also forgets names for simple things such as milk and bread, has trouble understanding what numbers mean, and loses interest in favored activities or hobbies. The patient may also have a decrease in judgment, which might lead him or her to wear a bathrobe to the park, for example.

In Stage 2, which is moderate and which lasts for 2 to 8 years, the patient can't recognize friends and family, wanders away and becomes lost, and experiences increased confusion and personality changes. He or she may also suffer from delusions and insomnia and may lose the ability to perform simple tasks such as dressing or brushing the teeth.

Stage 3 lasts 1 to 3 years. The patient cannot remember anything or process new information—and loses the ability to recognize family members. He or she may not be able to use words but responds to touching and eye contact as well as music. The patient may experience difficulty in eating or swallowing, dressing, bathing, or controlling bladder and bowel functions.

Of course, caring for a person with Alzheimer's is challenging, and many patients are placed in residential facilities such as nursing homes.

AGING AS DISEASE?

Despite efforts by some to persuade older adults and those who care for them that aging is like a curable or reversible disease, scientists largely reject the idea. According to Pope (2002), fifty-one scientists posted a position on the website of *Scientific American* saying that there are no miracle treatments, and they cautioned the public to avoid untested substances and procedures because they may be harmful. The scientists emphatically state that there are no lifestyle changes, surgery, vitamins or other substances, or genetic engineering that can reverse aging.

The scientists agree that the lifespan could be extended, but they also insist that aging is not a disease and that the wear and tear associated with the passage of years will affect older people.

Other diets, exercise, and such may be of great assistance in maintaining of the life of older adults, but very large doses of vitamins and other kinds of efforts to extend life may actually be more harmful than helpful in extending the life cycle.

Three authors who helped write the statement wrote in *Scientific American* (Olshansky, Hayflick, & Carnes, 2002) that such efforts to extend life date back at least 3,500 years. They cite early efforts such as the search for a fountain of youth as well as the hope of manufacturing and using gold as beliefs about stopping aging. They say aging is

> the accumulation of random damage to the building blocks of life—especially to DNA, certain proteins, carbohydrates and lipids (fats)—that begins early in life and eventually exceeds the body's self repair capabilities. The damage gradually impairs the functioning of cells, tissues, organs, and organ systems, thereby increasing vulnerability to disease and giving rise to the characteristic manifestations of aging, such as a loss of muscle and bone mass, a decline in reaction time, compromised hearing and vision, and reduced elasticity of the skin. (p. 93)

These changes come from a number of sources, including the life-sustaining processes that the body uses to convert food into energy. The process of converting food into energy creates free radicals, some of which—but not all—become repaired. The free radicals interfere with the cell's ability to maintain the body's molecules and keep it operating properly.

All these changes, which are part of the normal process of aging, make people susceptible to diseases, which ultimately end life. But the authors (Olshansky et al., 2002) say that even if the usual causes of death in old age such as stroke and cancer were eliminated, other conditions would likely take their place. The diseases are "superimposed" (p. 93) on aging and are not the same as aging. The molecular breakdowns of aging increase susceptibility to illnesses, but aging is a normal process, not a disease that is subject to cure.

The following is an article by Geoffrey Cowley in *Newsweek* (Fall/Winter 2001, pp. 12–24. Reprinted with the permission of *Newsweek*).

■ ■ ■ ■ ■ ▬▬▬▬▬▬▬▬▬▬▬▬▬▬▬▬▬▬▬▬▬▬▬▬▬▬▬▬▬▬▬▬▬▬▬

THE BIOLOGY OF AGING

By Geoffrey Cowley

If only God had found a more reliable messenger. Back around the beginning of time, according to east African legend, he dispatched a scavenging bird known as the halawaka to give us the instructions for endless self-renewal. The secret was simple. Whenever age or infirmity started creeping up on us, we were to shed our skins like tattered shirts. We would emerge with our youth and our health intact. Unfortunately the halawaka got hungry during his journey, and happened upon a snake who was eating a freshly killed wildebeest. In the bartering that ensued, the bird got a satisfying meal, the snake learned to molt and humankind lost its shot at immortality. People have been growing old and dying ever since.

The mystery of aging runs almost as deep as the mystery of life. During the past century, life expectancy has nearly doubled in developed countries, thanks to improvements in nutrition, sanitation and medical science. Yet the potential life span of a human being has not changed significantly since the halawaka met the snake. By age 50 every one of us, no matter how fit, will begin a slow decline in organ function and sensory acuity. And though some will enjoy another half century of robust health, our odds of living past 120 are virtually zero. Why, after being so exquisitely assembled, do we fall apart so predictably? Why do we outlive dogs, only to be outlived by turtles? And what are our prospects for catching up with them?

Until recently, all we could do was guess. But as the developed world's population grows grayer, scientists are bearing down on the dynamics of aging, and they're amassing crucial insights. Much of the new understanding has come from the study of worms, flies, mice and monkeys—species whose life cycles can be manipulated and observed in a laboratory. How exactly the findings apply to people is still a matter of conjecture. Could calorie restriction extend our lives by half? It would take generations to find out for sure. But the big questions of why we age—and which parts of the experience we can change—are already coming into focus.

The starkest way to see how time changes us (aside from hauling out an old photo album) is to compare death rates for people of different ages. In Europe and North America the annual rate among 15-year-olds is roughly .05 percent, or one death for every 2,000 kids. Fifty-year-olds are far less likely to ride their skateboards down banisters, yet they die at 30 times that rate (1.5 percent annually). The yearly death rate among 105-year-olds is 50 percent, 1,000 times that of the adolescents. The rise in mortality is due mainly to heart disease, cancer and stroke—diseases that anyone over 50 is right to worry about. But here's the rub. Eradicating these scourges would add only 15 years to U.S. life expectancy (half the gain we achieved during the 20th century),

(continued)

CONTINUED

for unlike children spared of smallpox, octogenarians without cancer soon die of something else. As the biologist Leonard Hayflick observes, what ultimately does us in is not disease per se, but our declining ability to resist it.

Biologists once regarded senescence as nature's way of pushing one generation aside to make way for the next. But under natural conditions, virtually no creature lives long enough to experience decrepitude. Our own ancestors typically starved, froze or got eaten long before they reached old age. As a result, the genes that leave us vulnerable to chronic illness in later life rarely had adverse consequences. As long as they didn't hinder reproduction, natural selection had no occasion to weed them out. Natural selection may even *favor* a gene that causes cancer late in life if it makes young adults more fertile.

But why should "later life" mean 50 instead of 150? Try thinking of the body as a vehicle, designed by a group of genes to transport them through time. You might expect durable bodies to have an inherent advantage. But if a mouse is sure to become a cat's dinner within five years, a body that could last twice that long is a waste of resources. A 5-year-old mouse that can produce eight litters annually will leave twice the legacy of a 10-year-old mouse that delivers only four each year. Under those conditions, mice will evolve to live roughly five years. A sudden disappearance of cats may improve their odds of completing that life cycle, but it won't change their basic genetic makeup.

That is the predicament we face. Our bodies are nicely adapted to the harsh conditions our Stone Age ancestors faced, but often poorly adapted to the cushy ones we've created. There is no question that we can age better by exercising, eating healthfully, avoiding cigarettes and staying socially and mentally active. But can we realistically expect to extend our maximum life spans?

Researchers have already accomplished that feat in lab experiments. In the species studied so far, the surest way to increase life span has been to cut back on calories—way back. In studies dating back to the 1930s, researchers have found that species as varied as rats, monkeys and baker's yeast age more slowly if they're given 30 to 60 percent fewer calories than they would normally consume. No one has attempted such a trial among humans, but some researchers have already embraced the regimen themselves. Dr. Roy Walford, a 77-year-old pathologist at the University of California, Los Angeles, has survived for years on 1,200 calories a day and expects to be doing the same when he's 120. That may be optimistic, but he looks as spry as any 60-year-old in the photo he posts on the Web, and the animal studies suggest at least a partial explanation. Besides delaying death, caloric restriction seems to preserve bone mass, skin thickness, brain function and immune function, while providing superior resistance to heat, toxic chemicals and traumatic injury.

How could something so perverse be so good for you? Scientists once theorized that caloric restriction extended life by delaying development, or by reducing body fat, or by slowing metabolic rate. None of these explanations survived scrutiny, but studies have identified several likely mechanisms. The first involves oxidation. As mitochondria (the power plants in our cells) release the energy in food, they generate corrosive, unpaired electrons known as free radicals. By reacting with nearby fats, proteins and nucleic acids, these tiny terrorists foster everything from cataracts to vascular disease. It appears that caloric restriction not only slows the production of free radicals but helps the body counter them more efficiently.

Food restriction may also shield tissues from the damaging effects of glucose, the sugar that enters our bloodstreams when we eat carbohydrates. Ideally, our bodies respond to any rise in blood glucose by releasing insulin, which shuttles the sugar into fat and muscle cells for storage. But age or obesity can make our cells resistant to insulin. And when glucose molecules linger in the bloodstream, they link up with collagen and other proteins to wreak havoc on nerves, organs and blood vessels. When rats or monkeys are allowed to eat at will, their cells become less sensitive to insulin over time, just as ours do. But according to Dr. Mark Lane of the National Institute on Aging, older animals on caloric-restricted diets exhibit the high insulin sensitivity, low blood glucose and robust health of youngsters. No one knows whether people's bodies will respond the same way. But the finding suggests that life extension could prove as simple, or rather as complicated, as preserving the insulin response.

Another possible approach is to manipulate hormones. No one has shown conclusively that any of these substances can alter life span, but there are plenty of tantalizing hints. Consider human growth hormone, a pituitary protein that helps drive our physical development. Enthusiasts tout the prescription-only synthetic version as an antidote to all aspects of aging, but mounting evidence suggests that it could make the clock tick faster. The first indication came in the mid-1980s, when physiologist Andrzej Bartke outfitted lab mice with human or bovine genes for growth hormone. These mighty mice grew to twice the size of normal ones, but they aged early and died young. Bartke, now based at Southern Illinois University, witnessed something very different in 1996, when he began studying a strain of rodents called Ames dwarf mice. Due to a congenital lack of growth hormone, these creatures reach only a third the size of normal mice. But they live 50 to 60 percent longer.

As it happens, the mini-mice aren't the only ones carrying this auspicious gene. The Island of Krk, a Croatian outpost in the eastern Adriatic, is home to a group of people who harbor essentially the same mutation. The "little people of Krk" reach an adult height of just four feet five inches. But like the mini-mice, they're exceptionally long-lived. Bartke's mouse studies suggest that besides stifling growth hormone, the gene that causes this stunting may also improve sensitivity to—you guessed it—insulin. If so, the mini-mice, the Croatian dwarves and the half-starved rats and monkeys have more than their longevity in common. No one is suggesting that we stunt people's growth in the hope of extending their lives. But if you've been pestering your doctor for a vial of growth hormone, you may want to reconsider.

Growth hormone is just one of several that decline as we age. The sex hormones estrogen and testosterone follow the same pattern, and replacing them can rejuvenate skin, bone and muscle. But like growth hormone, these tonics can have costs as well as benefits. They evolved not to make us more durable but to make us more fertile. As the British biologist Roger Gosden observed in his 1996 book, "Cheating Time," "sex hormones are required for fertility and for making biological gender distinctions, but they do not prolong life. On the contrary, a price may have to be paid for living as a sexual being." Anyone suffering from breast or prostate cancer would surely agree.

In most of the species biologists have studied, fertility and longevity have a seesaw relationship, each rising as the other declines. Bodies designed for maximum fertility have fewer resources for self-repair, some perishing as soon as they reproduce (think of spawning salmon). By contrast, those with extraordinary life spans are typically slow to bear offspring. Do these rules apply to people? The evidence is sketchy but provocative. In a 1998 study, researchers at the University of Manchester analyzed genealogical records of 32,000 British aristocrats born during the 1,135-year period

(continued)

CONTINUED

between 740 and 1875 (long before modern contraceptives). Among men and women who made it to 60, the least fertile were the most likely to survive beyond that age. A whopping 50 percent of the women who reached 81 were childless.

Eunuchs seem to enjoy (if that's the word) a similar advantage in longevity. During the 1940s and '50s, anatomist James Hamilton studied a group of mentally handicapped men who had been castrated at a state institution in Kansas. Life expectancy was just 56 in this institution, but the neutered men lived to an average age of 69—a 23 percent advantage—and not one of them went bald. No one knows exactly how testosterone speeds aging, but athletes who abuse it are prone to ailments ranging from hypertension to kidney failure.

All of this research holds a fairly obvious lesson. Life itself is lethal, and the things that make it sweet make it *more* lethal. Chances are that by starving and castrating ourselves, we really could secure some extra years. But most of us would gladly trade a lonely decade of stubborn survival for a richer middle age. Our bodies are designed to last only so long. But with care and maintenance, they'll live out their warranties in style.

DISCUSSION QUESTIONS

1. This chapter consists of two parts: (1) a survey of some of the biological issues associated with aging, and (2) a complete article from *Newsweek* discussing the biology of aging. Based on the other chapters you have read in this book, do you believe that biology or social issues are the primary factors in the effects of aging on individuals? If there is a blend, which part of the blend do you think is the source of the greatest difficulties?

2. Researchers on aging disagree about the inevitability of the deterioration of the body and the death of the individual. Some think that life can be extended significantly longer than it is. Others believe that it is simply impossible to eliminate the deterioration and death of the human body—if not for some reasons, then for others. Which side are you on? Do you think that the human body can be significantly extended in life through biological interventions?

3. Some suggest that aging is a disease rather than a normal part of human development. What are the arguments for and against the theory of aging as a disease, based on your reading of this chapter and other sources?

4. Do you believe the data on the effects of calorie restriction are persuasive? Why or why not?

PART IV

EMERGING ISSUES IN HUMAN BIOLOGY FOR SOCIAL WORKERS

Chapter 12 deals primarily with public health issues as they affect social work clients and programs. Although public health is a large and distinct field, knowing about it is critical to understanding some of the social issues faced by clients and some of the ways in which social workers deal with and prevent health problems. Biological public health problems such as the transmission of disease, bioterrorism, and environmental health matters are discussed in the chapter. The chapter also defines and provides detailed information on the public health field—as a discipline, what it does, and how it functions. Of course, many social workers are employed in public health agencies and public health is one of the major settings in which social workers practice.

Critical thinking is a issue of growing importance in social work and Chapter 13 deals with critical thinking in understanding human biology and in applying biological knowledge to the practice of social work with clients. Some of the elements of critical thinking and some of the ways in which critical thinking is distinguished from other kinds of thought patterns are emphasized.

Chapter 14 is a brief concluding chapter that discusses the ways in which biological understanding assists in the professional practice of social work as a profession.

CHAPTER THIRTEEN

PUBLIC HEALTH AND BIOLOGY

Having good health is very different from only being not sick.
—Seneca the Younger

One of the many areas in which the interests and efforts of social work intersect with those of another professional discipline is public health. In several ways, social workers and public health workers serve together to deal with problems of health and illness that transcend individuals. Many illnesses are public health illnesses—that is, they must be controlled, if they are to be controlled at all, by public health measures such as immunization against them, finding and quarantining people who contract the illnesses, educating the public about the prevention of the spread of disease, and working to rid the environment of organisms that can be the causes of illness. For example, water and air pollution may be greater health risk factors for many people than are specific illnesses. Conditions such as AIDS as well as other communicable diseases are a subject of interest to public health departments because they are spread by human contact and can only be prevented, in many cases, by altering the human contact.

PUBLIC HEALTH AND SOCIAL WORK

Some observers of the two professions of social work and public health argue that they are quite different in their orientations and emphases. Social work has largely been treatment oriented and social workers are heavily educated to help people deal with personal and social problems. In more recent years, social work has taken on a bit more of an emphasis on prevention. So the emphases of the two professions are drawing more closely together. Public health programs are concerned with helping people find and use treatment and in helping organize treatment programs. Some public health professionals are engaged full time in the administration of health programs such as hospitals. So the dual emphasis is perhaps less dichotomous than it had been in the earlier periods of development of these two professions.

PUBLIC HEALTH AS COMMUNITY HEALTH

Another term for public health is *community health*, the two terms being essentially interchangeable. According to Reagan and Brookins-Fisher (2002, p. 6) public health is "the sum of all official (governmental) agencies and efforts to promote, protect, and preserve the health of people whom these agencies serve." Of course, public health deals with many health issues that are not particularly organic or biological in nature. For example, auto accidents, guns, violence, and suicide are all causes of serious health problems and death. However, they are social, political, and psychological in nature rather than biological in nature. This chapter focuses on the biological public health problems rather than the equally serious but not appropriate for this text issues described above.

A good example of the distinction is the issue of bioterrorism. Wars and other forms of violence are significant in the well-being of people. However, only in the most general sense are they examples of biological issues. But bioterrorism is a form of violence and warfare that is biological. The problem of bioterrorism, a significant risk and an area of greater concern because of the September 11, 2001, attacks on New York and Washington, is a phenomenon that can be effectively countered with public health measures and, perhaps, in no other ways.

This chapter discusses public health measures and human biology, especially areas that are of great concern to social workers and others who deal with social problems. Public health measures are a major factor in preventing illness. In all, public health issues may be more severe human biology problems than many others that are discussed in this text.

Nothing in the foregoing suggests that public health measures are not significant in the eradication and control of biological conditions. According to Reagan and Brookins-Fisher (2002), the U.S. Centers for Disease Control, a premier public health program, identify as the greatest achievements of public health in the United States the elimination of smallpox through vaccinations, motor-vehicle safety, the creation of safer workplaces, the control of infectious diseases, decreases in deaths from heart disease and stroke, the requirements for safer and healthier foods, the improvement of the health of mothers and their babies, family planning, the fluoridation of drinking water to reduce cavities, and the recognition of tobacco as a detriment to good health. Most, but not all, of these achievements have biological components.

A good example of a public health concern, translated into a public problem or issue, is that of the fiscal impact of smoking. McClam (2002) reports that the Centers for Disease Control and Prevention, an important force in U.S. public health, estimate that the cost to the public of smoking is $157.7 billion per year, or $3391 per smoker. Smoking causes some 440,000 deaths each year. The average male smoker loses more than 13 years of life and the average woman 14.5 from smoking. Smoking during pregnancy results in 1,000 infant deaths each year. The costs of health care for smokers in addition to the lost years of productivity are factored into the estimates. And the tax collections associated with the habit are much less than the public costs of smoking.

It should also be noted that the great advances in American health are probably more the result of public health measures than of the treatment of diseases with whatever methods.

AIDS

Statistics

Among the most important of the public health issues and one of the most consequential of the sexually transmitted conditions is AIDS (Acquired Immune Deficiency Syndrome). *Newsweek* recognized the twentieth anniversary of the recognition of AIDS as a disease (Begley, 2001b). By the end of December 2000, the magazine reported that 448,059 Americans had died of AIDS. Of that total, 381,611 were men, 66,448 were women, over 200,000 were white, 158,892 were African American, and 77,698 were Hispanic or Latino. The report also showed the distribution of AIDS cases around the world. The highest rate in the whole world was in Botswana in Africa, in which 36 percent of the population was infected. Many other African nations had infection rates of more than 10 percent compared to the United States, which had an infection rate of 0.61 percent of the population, and the highest rate in Asia was in Cambodia, with 4 percent AIDS patients.

Methods of Transmission

AIDS, as most readers already know, is transmitted in a variety of ways but always involves the infusion of blood or blood products that are infected with the virus into the bloodstream of the person who was not infected. Sexual contact that permits sexual fluids, usually semen, to enter the bloodstream through a lesion is often the source of the infection. Male homosexual contacts, which may involve anal intercourse, may cause irritations in the anus which become sources for the entrance of the semen into the bloodstream. Blood transfusions of infected blood are also a source of infection. In some cases, especially in developing nations, the disease may be transmitted by the reuse of hypodermic needles that had been previously used on persons with AIDS and not adequately cleaned before reusing them.

Search for a Vaccine

The effort to develop a vaccine against the disease (Cowley, 2001) is a major activity in the health field. Although powerful drugs against the condition have been developed, they are expensive and many of the victims in the poorest nations cannot afford the medicines. But developing a vaccine is complicated by the fact that no one has ever recovered from AIDS. Therefore, the exact biological characteristics of someone who has conquered the disease are not known. Therefore, finding a way to make people immune from AIDS is complicated. According to Cowley, a vaccine does not seem possible before 2007, if then. That concern is confirmed by Ezzell (2002), who said there would be results available from widespread tests of a vaccine by the end of 2002, but there was not much optimism that it would work. She also noted that there are five different kinds of HIV and that scientists were attempting to determine whether or not to attempt to develop specific vaccines for specific areas, based on the kind of HIV that was predominant. The fact that there are multiple types of the virus makes it difficult to construct a single vaccine that can cover all people. Another part of the problem with developing a vaccine is that HIV mutates rapidly and changes shape, which allows it to stay ahead of the immune response. Another is that an AIDS vaccine needs to develop an immune response that is not found in nature. AIDS is a challenging disease that is difficult to protect against by using the science that had been followed in preventing other conditions.

Michael Specter, writing in the *New Yorker*, offers a perspective on the treatment and prevention of HIV/AIDS, based on his contacts with Yufus Hamied, an Indian businessman whose major enterprise is the manufacture of drugs. In India, although part of the process of making a drug may be patented, the final product, under that nation's laws, can be copied freely. Hamied had made a fortune copying major pharmaceutical products and selling them. He was highly concerned about the extent of AIDS in the developing world and particularly in India. He noted that India, with its large population, had perhaps the world's largest group of AIDS patients, with the possible exception of Africa. He noted that there were 250,000 HIV positive inhabitants of Bombay alone. His company, Cipla, could develop and distribute low-cost versions of the HIV/AIDS drugs that are maintaining the lives of many patients around the world, especially in the developed world. He wanted to donate supplies of one drug, which had been effective in preventing the AIDS virus from being passed from mother to child, to the Indian government, but the Indian government was not very receptive.

The savings in costs to potential patients would be dramatically lower than the usual cost. A year's worth of AIDS medication that would sell in America for about $15,000 would only cost $350 with the Cipla products. But Specter points out that many public health officials and experts think that the prevention of HIV/AIDS is much more reasonable than treating it. Using AIDS drugs is expensive, complicated, potentially toxic, and the drugs are very difficult to take directly. He also points out that India, like many other developed countries, spends only $10.00 per year per capita on health care and AIDS is a relatively small problem. In India, in 2000 there were more than 1 million reported cases of malaria. Other diseases that are not well known in the United States are also of epidemic proportions in India. One disease, yaws, can be cured with a single shot of penicillin. There are also 2,000,000 new cases of tuberculosis in India every year and more than 1,000 people die from it every day. India also has 70 percent of the world's leprosy. Spending a reduced amount of money on treatment for AIDS patients would probably not make as much sense as spending funds on the prevention of AIDS through education, the distribution of condoms, and other interventions.

Specter points out that for the past 20 years India has become a great center of migration for people moving throughout that nation. Migrants are at a higher risk for AIDS than others, and they are also likely to spread the disease. India's long-distance truckers, of which there are 100,000, the nation's 2,000,000 prostitutes, and 75,000 brothels, as well as 10,000,000 seasonal workers who come to big cities every year for a few months, all contribute to the spread of AIDS.

In India, condoms can be secured for less than two Americans cents for a package of three, but there is not sufficient education to help people understand why they should use them. However, the truck drivers mentioned earlier had a rate of HIV infection that rose from 1.5 percent in 1995 to 6 percent just 2 years later. And in 2000, 20 percent of truck drivers were infected with the disease.

It is not only prostitutes and migrants to whom AIDS is spread. Many married women in monogamous relationships with their migrant husbands contract AIDS from those husbands. One physician reported, Specter says, that 90 percent of the women who were HIV positive had only one sexual partner, who was the woman's husband. So blood testing, aggressive education about how the disease is spread, and specific, targeted outreach to truck drivers and sex workers, as well as education of spouses, can reduce AIDS dramatically.

The public health specialists estimate that it costs only about $6.00 to keep one truck driver from becoming infected with the illness and for sex workers such as prostitutes, the cost is less than $3.00. Treating people already infected with drugs is difficult because it requires a sense of time, schedules of various kinds, and other more advanced activity that is not in the usual pattern of Indian people, especially lower-income Indian people.

OTHER SEXUALLY TRANSMITTED DISEASES

According to Reagan and Brookins-Fisher (2002), 333 million curable sexually transmitted diseases occur annually in the world. Some 15 million Americans have the diseases, including 4 million college-age and teenage people. Younger women are more likely to develop some STDs than are older women, because adolescents often have cervixes that are covered with cells that STDs are likely to effectively attack. Women have more severe complications from STDs than men. Such conditions as ectopic pregnancy, infertility, and chronic pelvic pain can result from having an STD.

Although HIV/AIDS have taken the most attention in recent years, other sexually transmitted diseases, or STDs, are also serious public health problems. Since there are treatments for most of them, they do not have the dramatic impact of AIDS, which is a fatal disease. However, chlamydia, gonorrhea, syphilis, and genital warts (the HPV or human papillomavirus, genital herpes, and others) are of great concern to public health departments. Many public health programs were originally developed to trace and halt the spread of these kinds of diseases, which are passed along through sexual contact. They also provide a physical environment that makes the possibility of contracting AIDS greater than it is for people who are free of such conditions.

STATE PUBLIC HEALTH AGENCIES

Public health agencies are typically organized at the state level with offices in counties or cities that are supervised by or that are part of the state agency.

A typical State Department of Public Health (Reagan & Brookins-Fisher, 2002) has units that deal with food protection, drinking water quality, drug control, toxicology, maternal and child health services, a unit on AIDS, air pollution control units, immunization programs, and a group that deals with chronic diseases. Therefore, a particular agency will have components that work to eradicate biological problems and other problems that are threats to public health. Because the focus of public health is on prevention, a major focus of departments is to prevent diseases from spreading and epidemics from developing. The Centers for Disease Control and Prevention is part of the U.S. government's Public Health Service and, as mentioned earlier, is a major research and information analysis unit that provides extensive service and guidance to state public health departments and to the federal public health program. The CDC identifies problems, examines organisms sent to it from around the United States, and conducts public health investigations. It also maintains statistical information on a broad variety of health issues and illnesses. At the federal level, the surgeon general is in charge of the entire public health operation.

WORK-RELATED AND PRODUCT INJURIES

Public health takes specific actions to deal with problems of work-related injuries, many of which are biologically related. Many are accidents but they are accidents often to the skeletal structure. Some employment leads to occupational cancers. Some lung diseases, such as those encountered by coal miners and asbestos workers, are work-related. Many traumatic injuries are also related to employment. These include loss of limbs, eyes, fractures, and others. Some cardiovascular diseases, some disorders of reproduction, and some neurotoxic disorders also emanate from employment. Some people are severely burned at work and others lose their hearing because of work-related noise. Drug and alcohol dependence may be associated with the individual employee's workplace.

Consumer products may also cause illness. Motorcycles, snowmobiles, lawn mowers, and several different kinds of furniture may also contribute to the illness and eventually death of a child or an adult (Reagan & Brookins-Fisher, 2002).

PREVENTIVE HEALTH SERVICES

Public health programs are oriented to reducing illness through the prevention of disease.

A number of targets for reducing illness are included in the plan for improving American health called *Healthy People 2010,* which is subtitled the *National Health Promotion and Disease Prevention Objectives* (Reagan & Brookins-Fisher, 2002). The goals associated with *Healthy People 2010* were first developed for a 2000 version of the same publication which was begun in 1970. Among the goals of the *Healthy People* document is the reduction of deaths among people of all age groups, with a special focus on reducing the death rates of children, adolescents, and youth.

The Public Health Service also ranks states by their degrees of health. The healthier states in 2000 were New Hampshire, Minnesota, Hawaii, Utah, Massachusetts, Vermont, Colorado, and Wisconsin. Those with the worst health were Mississippi, Louisiana, South Carolina, West Virginia, Nevada, Arkansas, Alabama, and Florida.

Another focus of the *Healthy People* approach is an increase in physical activity, improved nutrition, the tracing of and protection against sexually transmitted diseases, reductions in tobacco use, and reductions in substance abuse.

The objectives also deal with many health measures such as improved access to health services of all kinds, increased family planning services, and increased maternal, infant, and child health and welfare programs. There is also focus on increasing the years of healthy life by dealing with heart disease, cancer, stroke, lung disease, and diabetes.

Another public health concern is the series of hepatitis conditions that have grown in recent years. The most common form of hepatitis is hepatitis A, which is passed from person to person but is also contracted in unsanitary situations. Hepatitis B is another form of the disease. It is typically contracted through water. Hepatitis C has only recently been discovered. It is the most common infection in the United States that is blood borne. Diseases that are communicable are of special interest to public health, of course, because of the field's concern about the development of illness and the prevention of disease.

Yellow fever is a condition that is caused by insects. Many people also encounter parasites that enter their bodies and cause a variety of illnesses. And again, parasites and insects can be controlled with public health measures. There is an immunization against yellow fever.

Malaria is another disease that is transmitted by a "vector"—in this case, a mosquito. It is one of the most important of insect-borne diseases. Malaria, as indicated in other parts of this book, is of great significance in most of the world, although it is not an extensive problem in the United States. It can be prevented with and, if contracted, treated with medicine.

Gene therapy is becoming a major factor in conquering genetic diseases and in providing immunizations, according to Griscom (2002). Gene-based vaccines against diseases such as AIDS, Alzheimer's, anthrax infection, and Ebola are the subjects of experiments. The Merck Drug Company announced that its HIV vaccine had created immunity in more than half of the 300 human subjects in its trial of a gene-based vaccine. Vaccines based on genes may be an important development in the future.

PREVENTABLE CHILDHOOD DISEASES

The public health approach to preventing diseases is especially important in childhood diseases such as pertussis, the more technical name for whooping cough and diptheria, a severe bacterial infection. These illnesses are prevented with childhood immunizations.

Tetanus is another serious health problem but it is now declining. The tetanus bacillus enters the body through an open wound, often one made by a nail or another discarded object. It, along with pertussis and diphtheria, is prevented in children with the familiar DPT immunization.

Polio, which was a major illness in the earlier part of the twentieth century, has been controlled through the development of the polio vaccines (both injected and oral) in the 1960s. It was a severe problem for young people, in particular. It has now been reduced in the United States to almost zero and represents one of the great triumphs of public health against an illness. Mumps and the measles, which carry two different names, rubella and rubeola, are important public health diseases. Rubella is also known as German measles, and measles is a different condition. Rubeola is a more serious health problem for those who develop it. However, rubella can cause spontaneous abortions and birth defects in the children of pregnant women who contract it. Mumps is also an illness that has been largely eradicated through public health measures such as vaccines. A vaccine to prevent rubella, measles, and mumps is available (Beers & Berkow, 1999).

OCCUPATIONAL HEALTH

Many health conditions arise in the workplace. For example, farmers and ranchers are susceptible to tetanus. Shepherds, butchers, veterinarians, and others who work with animals may contract anthrax. Tuberculosis, which is a serious lung condition, may be acquired at work by medical personnel such as physicians. Various inhaled substances such as asbestos and poison gases can harm various kinds of industrial workers. Those who work with various substances including jewelry products can develop asthma from their work. Many skin diseases are also acquired through work. Therefore, lung diseases, muscle and skeletal injuries, cancers, cardiovascular disease, skin problems, noise-induced loss of hearing, as well as accident-related illnesses can occur in workplaces. The public health approach is to find ways to make workplaces safer and healthier.

Public health is also concerned with some problems that are more traditionally viewed as social or psychological problems such as domestic violence, child abuse, and homicide. These are severe causes of illness and death throughout the world, including, of course, the United States.

Public health personnel believe they can be effective in preventing and reducing health problems in the United States by intervening in the public schools through education, through ensuring vaccination and other inoculations, and through contact with whole families. Public health personnel take educational approaches. They also work to ensure that foods are healthy by doing inspections of restaurant supplies and procedures.

A number of other kinds of diseases are transmitted through human movement, often through food. Parasites, for example, may enter the food and are considered food borne. These include parasites that cause amoebic dysentery; trichinosis, which results from eating raw and poorly cooked pork; tape worm, which impedes nutrition; and toxoplasmosis, which is spread from mother to child through the placenta through uncooked pork or mutton, or sometimes through water or dust that is contaminated by cat waste (Reagan & Brookins-Fisher, 2002).

In some cases, pests, in addition to the mosquitoes discussed earlier, are the source of illnesses. Rats, cockroaches, and other animal or insect beings are able to spread diseases to and among people. Infected milk and meat, including poultry, are also often causes of illness, as are shellfish and eggs (Reagan & Brookins-Fisher, 2002).

AIR POLLUTION

Social work, as a profession, takes positions to protect the environment and to limit pollution (*NASW Speaks*). Pollution comes in a variety of forms such as solid waste, which includes household garbage, liquids, gases, and energy waste (Bunch & Tesar, 2000). Pollution can change the atmosphere and climate, make soils unusable for agriculture, and is a cause of some human illness. Pollution can travel long distances in water or air.

Air pollution may be the most serious problem for human health, especially in industrialized countries that deal more effectively with water pollution. Solid wastes, radioactive material, gases, as well as natural substances such as volcanic dust are all examples of air pollution (Bunch & Tesar, 2000).

According to Johnson (2001), some research finds that air pollution kills 64,000 people in the United States annually. Fine air pollution particles, which come from fossil fuels in cars, trucks, and buses, and from coal or oil-burning power plants, become trapped in human lungs and cause diseases such as asthma, pneumonia, and other conditions. Johnson (2001) reports that asthma deaths have increased by 50 percent during the past 20 years and that the incidence of asthma among children age 4 and younger has increased 160 percent in the same period. The same author thinks that some cases of heart disease and stroke are attributable to increases in small particle air pollution. As an example, she mentions the New York City neighborhood of Harlem, which is home to most of the city-bus depots in Manhattan and is the port of entry for most diesel trucks. In Harlem, thirty residents per 1,000 people are hospitalized with asthma every year—the figure for the rest of the nation is 3.7 hospitalizations per 1,000 people.

Research in Steubenville, Ohio, Johnson (2000) reports, showed that as pollution (much of it from coal-fired steel mills) increased there, so did the community's deaths from chronic obstructive pulmonary disease (COPD), heart disease, and pneumonia. This air pollution is most serious in the eastern half of the United States, especially in areas with fossil-fuel-fired power plants and extensive diesel trucking. In 2002, Casriel reported that the federal government was planning to relax the rules against industrial air pollution. Modern power plants have some strong pollution controls. However, some 500 older plants in the Southeast and Midwest produce millions of tons of poisonous dust each year. The particles include substances such as mercury, nitrogen oxide, and other pollutants that environmental health experts say cause deaths (Casriel, 2002). The particles may be transmitted by wind to the Northeast and there can affect the health of many more people. The Environmental Protection Agency and several states are suing the owners of the older plants to force them into line with pollution standards. However, some new rules may relax the requirements for these plants.

Global warming has been one result of air pollution and it may be the most dangerous consequence of all. According to *The Week* (Global Warming Spreads Disease, 2002), global warming has led to the proliferation of diseases and the extensive development of viruses, bacteria, and fungi. The greater development of illness resulting from warmer climates has, according to a 2-year study by the National Center for Ecological Analysis and Synthesis, been a result of the warmer environment in which such organisms have thrived. There is evidence of greater illness among humans as well as the destruction of other biological hosts such as corals, birds, oysters, and plants. Cold weather tended to kill such organisms but even slight increases in temperature have allowed them to thrive and damage living things.

ENVIRONMENT AND GENETICS

The subject of evolution and heredity is discussed in several ways in this book. Topics such as the Human Genome Project and genetics are covered in several chapters from a variety of points of view. However, some more speculative thinkers suggest that the processes of biological change may have outcomes that are hardly predicted by current writers. Malcolm G. Scully (2002) reviewed Michael Boulter's (2002) book titled *Extinction: Evolution and the End of Man.* Boulter, a professor of paleontology, argues that humans are both destroying the environment and guaranteeing their own extinction while doing so. He suggests that humanity is currently in its sixth mass extinction, which is being caused by humans themselves. He notes that a third of all mammal species have become extinct and that the human mammal is one of the species currently facing such extinction. Nature is a self-correcting system, he says, and when it is disrupted it corrects itself by a variety of processes, including extinction of species.

Some of the signs of extinction are greenhouse gases causing atmospheric changes, sea level changes, and the levels of lake waters declining. But other factors contribute to the changes such as hunting. Human hunting over thousands of years has caused the extinction of 70 percent of the larger mammal species in North America. Boulter (2002) believes that mass extinction is coming and humans will be part of that extinction.

BIOTERRORISM

Garrett (2001b) investigated the potential for damage from bioterrorism in 2001, following the attacks on New York and Washington by elements of the Al Qaeda group, which had sworn to attack the nation. The purpose would be to sow confusion and discord.

Several different kinds of bioterrorism would be possible; poisoning water and air supplies with various substances, including anthrax; infecting livestock with diseases such as hoof and mouth; and spreading epidemics of diseases such as smallpox and plague. Garrett says that a few quick passes by a crop duster airplane over a populated area could expose 100,000 people to a poison or disease. Various weapons of mass destruction had been part of the war and defense effort of the Soviet Union, many of whose scientists are now scattered throughout various parts of the world, and were also found to be part of the arsenal of Iraq.

Garrett (2001) says that a large biological attack would not be easy to immediately trace. Health care providers might discover that clinics and emergency rooms were suddenly filled with people who had what seemed to be influenza, including young children, who are not often affected by the illness. Many of those patients would become more ill and would develop conditions such as meningitis. The government might discover that the illness is actually one that would be unlikely to be introduced except through bioterrorism. Inoculations and treatments would be provided but would cost the economy over $7 billion, plus over 400 deaths and many weeks of work lost by people who are ill. But the major function of a bioterrorist attack is to create panic and to cause citizens to lose confidence in their government and its ability to deal with large-scale problems that threaten human health.

Garrett (2001) cites some public health officials as suggesting that the only defense may be building such a strong public health capacity that terrorists would doubt they could be successful in using bioterrorism to harm and demoralize

American society. The author also describes a World Health Organization global surveillance system that can spot naturally occurring outbreaks of illnesses or diseases used as weapons against a nation. For some $5 to $50 million per year, much less than the effects of an epidemic, the surveillance system can detect the conditions.

Although vaccines are a useful antidote to, for example, a smallpox epidemic, there were only some 15 million doses of the smallpox vaccine available, which would not nearly cover the tens of millions in the United States who have not been vaccinated at all or whose childhood vaccinations are no longer an effective defense against the disease, according to Garrett (2001). There is not even enough medicine available to treat the 1 percent of people who have bad reactions to the smallpox vaccine, which is potentially more harmful and more difficult to administer than other vaccines.

A 2002 discovery that the United States had a larger supply of smallpox vaccine than it believed eased some concern about bioterrorism. It was also found that smallpox vaccine can be diluted up to ten times and still be effective (Ricks, 2002). Volunteers who took diluted forms of the vaccine were 97 percent protected against the illness, compared to 100 percent of those who took undiluted doses—not a major difference.

But some biological agents are so strong that there is no great hope for developing vaccines against them, and agents may be strengthened. Garrett (2001) describes one situation in which a version of smallpox that affects mice was boosted through gene splicing. The smallpox was so strong that it killed all the mice in the population that was being studied. It is clear that biological weapons may be a part of warfare in the future—weapons that require biological defenses and solutions if they are going to be resolved.

NOSOCOMIAL DISEASES

Another public health concern is this classification of disease, which results from the measures that were used to sustain life. These are such things as kidney disease dialysis treatments, cancer radiation, and chemotherapy. Those who are made ill by these conditions present a challenge for improving the quality of such procedures so that they may cure but do not harm patients.

HEALTHY AND PROPER DIET

Although a "proper" or "healthy" diet is often mentioned in discussing health maintenance, there is controversy over precisely what is the best diet. The balanced diet, which focuses on foods from several groups, has historically been the most highly regarded in the United States. It emphasizes fruits, vegetables, grains, dairy products, and a minimum of fats such as those found in meat and milk products. In fact, the food industry, in line with nutritional guidance, markets "no fat" and "low fat" products to comply with the desire for a proper or healthy diet. The assumption is that dietary fat increases body cholesterol and the risks of heart disease as well as obesity.

A variety of counter theorists, many of them following the ideas of Robert C. Atkins, however (Atkins, 2001), suggest that it is carbohydrate, most commonly found in grains, fruits, vegetables, and the nonfat parts of dairy products, that increases body weight. Heavy body weight is associated with problems such as heart disease. They assert that dietary fat does not increase body weight or cholesterol. Therefore, many have found that diets that rely more on fat and limit carbohydrate are most effective in promoting weight loss.

Shell (2002) traced the high-fat, low-carbohydrate diet to a physician named William Harvey in England in the nineteenth century. Shell (2002) says that the Atkins diet and all the others like it are based on that early theory. Shell adds that in countries such as India and China there was no obesity until high fat, Western-style diets were introduced, which raises questions about the reasonableness of the high-fat, low-carbohydrate diet. Shell (2002) also says that high levels of consumption of fat and sugar may be ruining our human brain chemistry so that brains do not receive signals that bodies are full. Consequently, people continue eating, and may grow obese. Shell (2000, p. 41) says

> It's already clear that varying the amount of fat and other nutrients in the diet affects brain chemistry by activating certain genes, and this in turn directs our dietary preferences. By submitting ourselves to a steady dose of highly processed, sweet, high-fat foods, we have unwittingly entered into a dangerous experiment, long term consequences of which are only now beginning to surface.

Extreme low-carbohydrate diets, although they may promote weight loss, also tend to limit the amount of fiber intake. Dietary fiber is a defense against colon and rectal cancer.

Anne Underwood (2002) probably has the best advice on diet. She says that calories are what count—whether they are from carbohydrates, fats, or proteins. It is the number of calories consumed that determines body weight. She writes, "The truth is that no food group, whether fats or carbs, is made up entirely of heroes or zeroes" (Underwood, 2002, p. 63). She says that restricting refined carbohydrates is a wise course. She means white sugar and flour, which are found in soft drinks and sweet breakfast cereals as well as candy and other processed foods. She points out that many carbohydrates, including fruits, vegetables, and whole grains, are packed with healthy substances. Likewise, some fats, such as those in salmon and other fish, canola and flaxseed oils, and some other noncarbohydrate foods, are protective against heart disease. But some fats, such as partially hydrogenated vegetable oils, which are often found in snack foods, are dangerous to the diet.

In general, it is probably true that there is less known about proper diet and healthy nutrition than might have been assumed. It may be more accurate to suggest that keeping one's weight within normal limits and assuring that one has sufficient intake of vitamins and minerals (especially those such as vitamins C and

E and selenium, "antioxidants" which appear to help prevent heart disease) and fiber are the most commonly agreed on dimensions of healthy diets.

A 2002 report in *Newsweek* magazine (*Health,* 2002) indicates that even one cigarette or one piece of cheesecake can cause health problems for people. The magazine cites a report in the *Harvard Heart Letter,* which said that an experiment on fifteen healthy young men who drank a liquid with 1,200 calories and 100 grams of fat were found, 5 hours later, to have restricted blood flow through their secondary coronary arteries, which are the arteries that do the work of carrying the blood when the larger arteries are blocked. They thought the research might explain why some people have chest pains after fatty meals. Some other scientists, according to the *Harvard Heart Letter* (*Health,* 2002), found that blood levels of vitamin C and other antioxidants, which have a role in preventing heart attacks, dropped in men who smoked one cigarette. So even a single indulgence in food or tobacco can cause great health difficulties. Physicians, nutritionists, scales, and the labels on foods of vitamins and minerals are all valid starting places in the attempt to build and adhere to a healthy diet. In January 2003, *Newsweek* magazine carried an extensive article on diet (Cowley) and the ways in which concepts of nutrition have changed in recent years.

EXERCISE AND HEALTH

Of course, not all public health concerns are with treating illnesses or even preventing specific diseases. For some years, it has been evident (and other parts of this book report on it too) that exercise can also be an overall aid to good health. The Centers for Disease Control and Prevention (Schoenborn & Barnes, 2002) report on a study of adult exercise patterns as they were identified in 1997 and 1998 in the federal government's National Health Interview. They found that 38.3 percent of adults over age 18 did not exercise at all. Those who exercised three or more times per week, vigorously, which was defined as activity of 10 minutes or more that caused heavy sweating as well as large increases in breathing or heart rate, were 14.2 percent of adults. Younger adults, aged 18–24, were twice as likely to engage in light to moderate activity, which meant light sweating and light to moderate increases in breathing and heart rate, as adults 75 and over. And for the vigorous activity, the youngest adults were seven times more likely than the oldest to be regular vigorous exercisers. Men were much more likely than women to engage in exercise. However, there were only slight differences between men and women in the percent who engaged in light to moderate exercise.

White, non-Hispanic adults, and Asian/Pacific Islanders were more likely than black non-Hispanic and Hispanic adults to exercise regularly. Exercise also appeared to increase with the level of education of those who were surveyed. Income was also a predictor of exercise—as income increased, so did exercise.

As the report states, health data for over 40 years has confirmed that exercise is related to the risk of illness and death—those who exercise remain healthier and live longer than those who do not. Therefore, exercise promotion may be one of the more effective means of improving the general health of the population. Of course, promoting exercise and healthy diets has not been a major method of social work practice, but it is clearly critical for the health and well-being of children, the elderly, and patients who are involved in health service programs. Such promotion may become a part of social work knowledge and skill as the understanding of the importance of diet and exercise becomes clearer.

It is clear from several sources that all is not well in the public health field. Author Laurie Garrett has, in two books, *The Coming Plague* (1994) and *Betrayal of Trust* (2001), made the case that the public health risks to humans are growing and that the world is not prepared to deal effectively with them. The world, according to Garrett, is facing threats from microbes and new viruses, resistance to existing drugs, and public health agencies throughout the world that are not capable of dealing with these new and growing problems. Her warnings have been well received as indications of the dangers facing the world, although responses that would improve the situation have not been as forthcoming. Knowing about and working to deal with the new public health threats is a major public issue for the coming years.

CONCLUSION

Although social work and public health are quite different in their orientations, special knowledge, and approaches to dealing with human problems, they pursue similar objectives and need each other's understandings of the human environment. In many ways, social workers need to apply the understandings that have been developed by public health to better protect and enhance the well-being of clients. As this chapter has demonstrated, many health and social problems result from public health issues and concerns, whether it is the spread of epidemics such as AIDS, damage to the earth and its inhabitants from pollution and other environmental hazards, or the promotion of healthy outcomes of pregnancy and prevention of disease through immunization. Being aware of and dealing with public health issues and programs is an area of growing importance for effective human services, especially for social work. It is not beyond the realm of appropriate professional education to pursue greater knowledge of these issues and to apply that knowledge in one's work with individual clients as well as communities.

DISCUSSION QUESTIONS

1. Social work education has moved in the direction of requiring more teaching about environmental health problems. Based on your reading of this chapter, what appear to be the most significant environmental health problems? What are some of the things that social workers can do to help prevent environmental health problems and to work with clients as well as the larger community to minimize the effects of them on client health?

2. The chapter suggests that diet, exercise, and other health-promoting activities may be as important as medical treatment, immunization, and other such services. Can you think of ways in which social work agencies and social workers could assist in the promotion of healthy living for clients? Be as explicit as possible in your analysis.

3. One of the paradoxes in biology and health care is that some treatments cause health problems as well as reduce or cure them. Can you find some examples, other than those in the text, of the ways in which people have been or may be made ill by being treated to reduce their health problems?

4. Bioterrorism has been a concern in the United States for several years, especially since the attacks on New York and Washington in September 2001. What are some of the ways in which social work and social workers can help prevent and deal with terrorism? Although terrorism is a phenomenon that destroys buildings and physically destroys people, it may also include the biological use of terror tactics through the transmission of illnesses from airborne viruses and bacteria. What are some of the ways in which social work can contribute to limiting the effects of bioterrorism on the lives of Americans?

CHAPTER FOURTEEN

CRITICAL THINKING, HUMAN BIOLOGY, AND SOCIAL WORK

If thought is life
And strength and breath,
And the want
Of thought is death.

—William Blake

There is no expedient to which a man will
not go to avoid the real labor of thinking.

—Thomas Alva Edison

Social work practitioners and social work students, BSW, MSW, and PhD, face increasing complexity as they interface between the content domains of human biology and social work. Both domains, human biology and social work, are complex. The accompanying fluidity in both domains creates an aura of excitement about change at every level—individual, family, group, organization, and community. But, as well, the fluidity creates a need for a thought process that helps maintain a sense of ongoing assessment, reflection, and learning. The ability of the social work practitioner and the social work student to think critically when faced with such fluid complexity is essential. This chapter informs the reflective practitioner and student of what the term *critical thinking* means and what is involved in the process of critical thinking.

The need for critical review of past and current knowledge in human biology and new areas of social work academic and practice challenges in human biology are emphasized in this chapter. The need for the social work practitioner and student to be informed of what critical thinking is and its use, particularly as it relates to human biology, and the facilitated design of helpful interventions with people is provided. As a means of highlighting the need for the use of critical thinking skills, a small number of common sources of fallacies in thinking by social work practitioners are presented.

DEFINING CRITICAL THINKING

Definitions of critical thinking abound. The definitions run from the simplistic "thinking critically" to the admonition that one's own definition may be the best. Peter Facione of Santa Clara University offers an intensely complex definition of critical thinking. Facione asserts that

> Liberal education is about learning to learn, to think for yourself, on your own and in collaboration with others. Liberal education leads us away from naïve acceptance of authority, above self-defeating relativism, beyond ambiguous contextualism. It culminates in principled reflective judgment. Learning critical thinking, cultivating the critical spirit, is not just a means to this end; it is part of the goal itself. People who are poor critical thinkers, who lack the dispositions and skills described, cannot be said to be liberally educated, regardless of the academic degrees they may hold. The ideal critical thinker is habitually inquisitive, well-informed, trustful of reason, open-minded, flexible, fair minded in evaluation, honest in facing personal biases, prudent in making judgments, willing to reconsider, clear about issues, orderly in complex matters, diligent in seeking relevant information, reasonable in the selection of criteria, focused in inquiry, and persistent in seeking results which are as precise as the subject and the circumstances of inquiry permit.

Facione holds that the core cognitive skills that contribute to critical thinking are analysis, interpretation, inference, explanation, self-regulation, and evaluation (Parslow, 2002, p. 65).

Here is a definition and mention of critical thinking "skills" that demonstrates the often stated, but not always made clear, link of critical thinking with the traditional scientific method. Critical thinking may be defined as suspension of judgment or as reasonable reflective thinking focused on deciding what to believe or do. Thinking skills that constitute critical thinking reveal a partial overlap with scientific inquiry skills. For example, testing hypotheses, planning experiments that do or do not include the controlling of variables, and drawing valid conclusions are all familiar to anyone familiar with the scientific method of inquiry. Not surprisingly, critical thinking, or what is considered as the application of critical thinking skills, in any content domain, such as human biology or social work, is directed by the knowledge structure of that discipline. Summarily, what counts as "good reason" in human biology might be different from a good reasoning process in social work (Zohar, Weinberger, & Tamir, 1994).

The challenge is to apply critical thinking skills in a mixed domain characterized by the practice of social work and the inclusion of past, present, and future understanding of human biology theory, principles, and knowledge. Lest the social work practitioner or social work student be misled, it is important to note that the use of critical thinking skills is not bounded by adherence to the traditional scientific method of inquiry. Social work practitioners and social work students of all camps—ecological perspective, social learning theory, empirically based practice, quantitative, qualitative, narrative, interpretive, social construction, just to name a few—are encouraged to consider the use of critical thinking as central to the very essence of social work. And this is especially true when elements of human biology are included in the social work processes of case analysis, interpretation, inference, explanation, self-regulation, and evaluation (Parslow, 2002).

This is especially applicable because not all of social work practice is grounded in the scientific method. There are still those social work practitioners, even in the face of an ever-stronger desire for the establishment of an empirical foundation to all social work practice, who rely heavily on practice wisdom and the "art" of relating to people. Their efforts will not necessarily be drawn into a consideration of critical thinking skills if the emphasis is solely on "scientific critical thinking skills."

On the other hand, even the social constructivists, the narrative therapists, recognize that inventiveness and imagination in the face of complexity needs to be balanced with a perspective—call it scientific, orderly, if you will—that encourages disciplined thought, a process of inquiry, logic, and analysis. Without a valued recognition of the artistry and talent in relationship building, the helping experience germane to social work practice would prove to be an exercise in professional pretense, a quasi-scientific approach to the study and control of human conditions with a false sense of certainty. The human sciences, both social work and human biology, cannot escape their fundamental social nature, that at the heart of both domains of knowledge is an interaction with other persons (Goldstein, 1999).

A delineation of "scientific critical thinking skills" includes the ability to (Zohar et al., 1994):

1. Recognize logical fallacies, such as jumping to conclusions based on too small or unrepresentative samples;
2. Distinguish between findings of an experiment and conclusions made on the basis of the findings;
3. Identify explicit and tacit assumptions;
4. Avoid tautologies (repetition of a meaningless idea);
5. Isolate variables;
6. Test hypotheses;
7. Identify relevant information for answering a question or solving a problem.

As expressed by Eileen Gambrill (2000), a social work educator whose scholarship includes strong consideration of critical thinking skills, in her chapter "The Role of Critical Thinking in Evidence-Based Social Work" and summarized on her Web page at the University of California, Berkely, critical thinking is problem solving and decision making, whether explicit or implicit, and is at the heart of social work practice. The purpose of thinking critically about practice-related claims is to maximize services to be effective in achieving valued outcomes and to minimize ineffective and harmful services. Critical thinking involves reasonable and reflective thinking focused on deciding what to believe or do. Viewed broadly, the process of critical thinking is part of problem solving. It requires clarity of expression, critical appraisal of evidence and reasons, and consideration of alternative points of view. Critical thinkers question what others do not. Strong sense critical thinking involves a genuine fair-minded process in which opposing views are accurately presented and there is a genuine effort to fairly consider both preferred and unpreferred views (Gambrill, 2000).

Gambrill (2000) reminds the social work practitioner and social work student that there is also a cost to the use of critical thinking skills. The costs of implementing a process of critical thinking include the social work practitioner and social work student forgoing the comfortable feeling of certainty. Critical thinkers abhor certainty and invite uncertainty. Or, at least, the consideration of uncertainty is included prior to making a needed decision. Use of critical thinking skills will also cost the social work practitioner or social work student, since, in theory, tolerance of the intolerant will be enhanced (Jackson, 1991). And isn't that what social work is largely about? The social work practitioner and social work student will be wise, if thinking critically, to thoughtfully hesitate prior to taking up a position of condemnation or of outright intolerance.

Gambrill (1997) in a guide for critically thinking social work practitioners catalogs a number of "fallacies" in thinking, which can plague the social work practitioner or student desirous of being a critical thinker. Informal fallacies have a logical form but are still incorrect and result in a defective argument. Informal fallacies abound and include such classics as generalizing from incomplete information and overlooking alternatives. Begging the question, sweeping generalizations, diversions via emotional appeals, and the false dilemma (i.e., falsely concluding that there are only two options) are common informal fallacies used by social work practitioners, social work students, and, yes, even social work educators. In the fallacy of false cause, the false assumption is made that one or more events cause another, when, in fact, they do not (p. 423).

An informal fallacy is a common pattern of argument in everyday reasoning that is logically inadequate but tends to be rhetorically effective (in other words, full of "hot air"). Additional informal fallacies include (a) ad hominem arguments, which focus on the person and his or her lack of, or possession of, certain characteristics that have nothing to do with the point of the reasoned argument; (b) ad populum arguments, which mistakenly focus on the popularity of the individual or the concept of traditional wisdom; (c) fallacies of distortion, which include both the straw person fallacy (restating another's argument in such a manner as to weaken the original and proceeding to criticize the weakened version) and the red herring fallacy (when in danger of losing an argument, one raises an irrelevant issue in an effort to trick the opposing arguer into changing the topic of the argument) (Mullen, 1995).

A review of Gambrill's work will reveal to the reader an exhaustive listing of informal and formal fallacies. The social work practitioner, social work student, and even social work educators will undoubtedly benefit in a review of this material. The point is that problem solving, as a basis of any critical thinking process, includes consideration of common fallacies in thinking. Implementation of a solid problem solving process, the heart of the social work process, aids in the elimination of the vast majority of fallacies, formal or informal. Components of an effective problem solving process, at the heart of which is critical thinking, include steps to (1) clarify what the problem is, (2) search for possible solutions, (3) decide on a plan of action, (4) implement plans, (5) evaluate results, and (6) try again (Gambrill, 1997, pp. 104–105). Hopefully, the social work practitioner and social work student as they consider the domain of human biology can achieve an effective problem solving process, free of fallacies in thinking.

HUMAN BIOLOGY AND THE USE OF CRITICAL THINKING SKILLS

Due to the complexity, the pace of new discoveries, and the debunking of past knowledge in human biology, barriers to problem solving and the use of critical thinking by social work practitioners and social work students exist as they integrate human biology knowledge into their work and study. Barriers to the use of critical thinking skills by social work practitioners and social work students in the content domain of human biology include, but are certainly not limited to the following (Gambrill, 1997, p. 110):

1. Availability of limited knowledge
2. Information processing barriers (inaccurate memory)
3. Error-filled task environment (lack of resources, time, money, services)
4. Motivation blocks (sole belief in social construction of meaning)
5. Emotional blocks (fatigue, anger, anxiety)
6. Perceptual blocks (judging rather than generating ideas)
7. Intellectual blocks (arrogance)
8. Cultural blocks (disdain for intellectual rigor)
9. Expressive blocks (inadequate skill in writing clearly)

A good way to critically view the entire realm of human biology is to look through a window labeled "complexity." Arranging all biological information in terms of levels of complexity leads to a "levels-of-organization" approach. Although artificially constructed (and to be viewed critically—remember this is a chapter on critical thinking, human biology, and social work), the hierarchy of organization and accompanying principles central to human biology is revealed. At the molecular, subcellular, and cellular levels of organization, the social work practitioner and social work student come to know of the principles of cell biology, the construction of cells, and how cells grow, divide, and communicate. At the level of organisms, the learning is focused on the principles of genetics, which deal with the ways in which an individual's traits are transmitted from one generation to the next. At the population level, the social work practitioner and social work student can use their knowledge of the "ecological perspective." At the population level in human biology the learning is focused on the nature of population changes from one generation to the next as a result of selection, and the way in which this has led to biological diversity. Continuing on, the social work practitioner and social work student will easily recognize how the next level of focus in human biology—community and ecosystem levels—relates to their work and study. At the community and ecosystem levels, the focus in human biology is on the ecology, which deals with how organisms (social work practitioners and students often call them people) interact with their environments and with one another to produce the complex communities characteristic of life (Raven & Johnson, 1995).

Put differently, the entire content domain of human biology can be critically viewed at three different levels: close-up, mid-range, and from a distance. The close-up view is focused on the small stuff that underpins all human biology—notably genes and how they work. The rest of the close-up view necessitates a look at viruses and the world of cells. The mid-range view brings to the foreground "systems" and how the elements of the system interact, such as how the brain and behavior are linked; how the function of sex and reproduction are linked, or the lack thereof; and the interrelationships between food supplies and energy for individuals, families, or a community. When viewing human biology from a distance, this vantage point reveals to the social work practitioner and social work student such broad-based theoretical and practical notions as ecology, evolution, and sociobiology, the attempt to make sense of behavior by employing an evolutionary perspective (Barash & Barash, 2000).

One last way to view the entire world of human biology is to consider the "levels of organization" as atom and molecule, cell, tissue, organ, organ system, organism, population, community, ecosystem, and biosphere, as discussed in earlier chapters. Current issues and controversies relate to each of the levels. For example, at the organism level, testing for heritable diseases and deciding who should pay for human-behavior-related diseases are current issues. At the population level, the issues and controversies include rationing of medical care and determining the availability and recipients of donated human organs. At the community level, the issues include the impact of humans on the well-being and survival of other species, genetic engineering of plants, and the practices related to medical research and cosmetic testing. At the ecosystem level, social work practitioners, social work students, and social work educators are becoming more connected to issues such as environmental degradation and the destruction of ecosystems due to overuse and misuse by people (Johnson, 2001, pp. 8–9).

When viewing the domain of human biology, the social work practitioner and social work student are encouraged to employ healthy doses of curiosity and wonderment. Healthy skepticism; an ability to interpret visual data, such as graphs; knowing anecdotal evidence when you see it; appreciating the differences between a fact and a conclusion; and recognizing the magnitude of a claim of correlation versus one of causation are all important to the use of critical thinking skills in human biology (Johnson, 2001).

Nietzsche, the noted German philosopher, said "When you look into the abyss, the abyss looks in to you" (p. vii). Human biology, and its pace of change, refutation of past knowledge, and the reporting of new findings about the human species, is an operationalization of Nietzsche's above-stated exhortation. It is not existential angst, metaphysical speculation, or religious doctrine that represents the abyss—it is just plain old uncertainty in human biology. The abyss, in this case, is what is known, what is being discovered, and what is being refuted about all people's shared biology. The integration of human biology principles and scientific mis/understanding into a view of life is really an opportunity for greater self-knowledge for the social work practitioner and the social work student. People, at least in present-day knowledge, are organisms that live, breathe, pump blood, masticate, defecate, metabolize, reproduce, and eventually die. Human biology, if viewed by a social work practitioner or social work student with critical thinking, allows greater insights into such controversial issues as the cloning of humans, genetic fingerprinting of rapists, origins and possibilities of vaccine development for AIDS, the political controversy surrounding partial-birth abortion, research focused on neurotransmitters in the brain and the incidence of schizophrenia, understanding one's own cholesterol levels, and the claims, and disclaimers, of an ever-increasing biocomplexity in the world—an impressive list, indeed. And that is without even adding the seemingly omnipresent challenge of cancer (Barash & Barash, 2000).

People are human biology meaning seekers. Persons who interact with social work practitioners and social work students are often seeking that one thing—help in making meaning of their life, particularly related to the physical, mental, social, and emotional health issues in their lives, be it the meaning of a particular event, as canvassed against a backdrop of life, or meaning of a whole life, hospice experience being a prime setting for such an experience. But meaning is complex and involves plenty of demand for the interpretive skills inherent in critical thinking. A critically thoughtful view of the human biology of meaning can include modern renditions of the age-old nature versus nurture debate—that of behavior and subsequent meaning being "hard-wired" into the brain and/or meaning being "socially constructed." To the critically thoughtful social work practitioner and social work student an absolute dichotomy of either/or is not necessary. Questions of the etiology of much of what is considered to make one "human" represent a haziness of understanding in human biology. For example, is feeling "happy" the result of chemicals being released postexperience or is feeling "happy" a perceived notion following an evaluation of one's response to a socially interactive experience? There is little doubt that emotions and meaning are linked. Critical thinking, however, is necessary to ward off absolutistic thinking about where the meaning comes from and its relationship to human biology. Emotion, relevance, context, and patterns are all important to meaning-making by social work practitioners and social work students. As well, emotion, relevance, context and patterns are important points of consideration when social work and human biology interface (Jensen, 1998).

MYTHS/QUESTIONS IN HUMAN BIOLOGY

A limited review of past-discounted "myths" and "questions" in human biology helps emphasize the need for critical thinking when past and current knowledge in human biology is reviewed. Through a review of challenges to areas of academic and applied knowledge in human biology, the social work practitioner and student are informed of how the use of critical thinking may facilitate the design and use of helpful interventions with people.

The uncertainty and fluid nature of knowledge in human biology is exemplified by consideration of major questions. There is a question in human biology about differentiation. A single cell, the fertilized egg, gives rise to a myriad of different cell types—muscle cells, blood cells, fat cells, and so on. This generation of cellular diversity is called differentiation. The yet to be fully answered question is: How can the fertilized egg generate so many different cell types? There is a question in human biology about growth. How do our cells know when to stop dividing? Cell division, at just the right rate, allows our face to look how it looks and our arms to generally be the same size on both sides. How is cell division so tightly regulated? There is a question about reproduction in human biology. The sperm and egg are very specialized cells. Only they can transmit the instructions for making an organism from one generation to the next. How are these cells set apart to form the next generation, and what are the instructions in the nucleus and cytoplasm that allow them to function in this way? And there are many more such questions (Gilbert, 2000).

To peruse Laqueur's (1990) book *Making Sex: Body and Gender from the Greeks to Freud* is to see how the human biology understanding of gender, sex, reproduction, and pleasure has varied dramatically over time. The belief that female orgasm was among the conditions for successful generation was considered solid information in the mid-seventeenth century. Up until that time, and sorrowfully there may be people in modern times who still cling to the belief, that the woman's experience of orgasm was assumed to be a routine and indispensable part of conception. Any social work practitioner and social work student in the year 2003 is reminded of the misinformation that adolescents and some young adults still hold in regard to sexual activity and the link to pregnancy. Additionally, for centuries the most prominent theoretical position was that men and women were really a representation of one sex. The one-sex model lived on through the eighteenth and nineteenth centuries. Physicians and authors—Aristotle in *Masterpiece* and Ventette in *The Art of Conjugal Love*—referred openly to the one-sex model. The eventual articulation of two incommensurable sexes was, however, neither a theory of knowledge nor advances in scientific knowledge in human biology. The context of change to the two-sex model was politics (Laqueur, 1990). And those politics continue to this day.

Even Darwin's "one long argument" in the *Origin of Species* has come under critical review by evolutionary biologists. Darwin's natural selection is arguably the most important scientific idea of the nineteenth century. With his idea of retained advantageous variability, Darwin changed evolution from an idea to a theory. Darwin's ideas have, however, been involved in a number of myths and the mistaken application to wrongful ends. Darwin's theory spawned ideas associated with the Aryanism of the Nazis to the simple advertising and sports claims of "survival of the fittest." A twist on Darwin's theoretical notions has most closely been intertwined with "social Darwinism." And social Darwinism has been mistakenly enlisted to explain such things as the wealth or poverty of an individual and to promote concepts of racial superiority and inferiority. Social Darwinism has been ill-advised in application to immigration policy and played a central part in the beliefs of the eugenicists, a group destined for failure as they attempted to perfect the biology of humans through controlled reproduction. Most importantly, Darwin proposed an ever-evolving world in which organisms varied randomly and retained those variations that gave them an advantage in the struggle to survive. His accomplishment was a theory of natural selection. Surprisingly, there were strict proponents of natural selection who espoused opposition to poor laws, government regulation of factory and housing conditions, and the establishment of state education systems. It takes a critical thinker to consider the genius in Darwin's theory, to see the flaws in the application of his work to mean-spirited and specific ends, and to understand the new challenges to Darwin's work in the current scholarship of modern-day evolutionary biologists (Caudill, 1997).

For example, Stephen Jay Gould, considered to be the best-known scientist in the United States prior to his death in 2002, worked diligently to preserve a respect for Darwin's work, but also challenged some of Darwin's key ideas. It was Gould, along with colleagues, who challenged Darwin's notion that it was only individual members of a species that evolve. Gould speculated, challenged, and concluded that not just individual organisms but species could evolve. As well, Gould helped develop the concept of "punctuated equilibrium" (Gould, 2002). Using evidence from fossil records, Gould supported the idea that evolution, rather than slow and progressive, could be characterized by long static periods separated by bursts of evolutionary activity. Gould's greatest contribution, however, to the Darwinian-dominated field of evolutionary biology may be the idea that other disciplinarians, in his case a paleontologist, can contribute to knowledge about how humans evolve. Gould believed that mathematicians, naturalists, and geneticists, as well as paleontologists, could challenge the "modern synthesis," which was the belief that all disciplines had reached a consensus in the early to mid-1990s about what evolution entailed (Monastersky, 2002).

As well, Darwin's theory of natural selection lies at the heart of a past, and, most certainly, a current social debate. The debate between science and religion engulfed the United States during the Scopes trial of 1925 and continues to play strongly in the debates of the early 2000s about the teaching of creationism versus evolution in public schools (Larson, 1997), the designation of when life begins in the abortion debate, and the prospects of human cloning.

HUMAN BIOLOGY AND SOCIAL WORK MICROPRACTICE

There are myths about human biology that interface strongly with social work micro-, or direct, practice and require critical thinking skills to overcome. The social work practice area of gerontology is a good example. Myths about the aging process and the biological functioning of older persons abound, as Chapter 12 discusses. They include the ideas that "old people are all alike," "old people are senile," "most old people are sickly," "old people no longer have any sexual interest or activity level," and "most old people end up in nursing homes." In reality, there is great variability among the old. Older persons experience drastically differing rates of physiological and psychological aging and decline of health. In fact, interest in sex persists into old age, and many older persons remain sexually active into their nineties. Only about 4 percent of persons over 65 are in a nursing home at any one time. Only 1 percent of persons 65 to 74 reside in a nursing home; and only 15 percent of persons 85 and older live in a nursing home (Ferrini & Ferrini, 2000).

The wistful wish, and accompanying myths, to turn back the biological aging process operationalize into a variety of approaches. Historically, the approaches to the achievement of immortality included the effort to prolong youth by withholding ejaculation or encouraging abstinence and the inhaling of the breath of young maidens (or young boys, depending on the translation) by Romans. Consider also the modern-age postponing-of-age advertisements for royal queen bee jelly, negative ion generators, or eastern herbal remedies. The best response, for your sake and the sake of your social work clients, is to get your critical thinking skills ready and save you, and your VISA card, the $29.95 (Ferrini & Ferrini, 2000).

With a more direct relationship to human biology, and contrary to popular myth, incontinence is not an inevitable consequence of aging, but a symptom of an underlying disorder. Causes include neurological problems that affect the central nervous system, medication side effects, infection of the genital or urinary system, and weakening of the pelvic muscles from childbirth (Ferrini & Ferrini, 2000). A good gerontological social worker understands the interface between human biology and social work and the need for critical thinking skills.

HUMAN BIOLOGY AND SOCIAL WORK MACROPRACTICE

Myths in the interface between human biology and social work practice are not limited to the micro-, or direct, practice level, but also apply to macropractice. This is true no matter what the macropractice focus, be it policy analysis, community organization, program development, or the promotion of sustainable development.

In the promotion of sustainable development, a burgeoning area of interest for macropractitioners, persistent myths, primarily related to the relationship between people, their economic activities, and the physical environment, are common. For example, the myth persists that if social work practitioners and social work students promote environmental concerns, it will necessitate a limit of employment opportunities, particularly for the poor. The proposition as stated overlooks the fact that environment, especially natural resources, contains scarce goods that require the use of production factors for their restoration, preservation, and substitution. Of these, labor is the most important. In macroeconomic terms, labor is the dominant cost factor. And a given amount of production and consumption requires more labor with environmental conservation than without. The extra labor required is used to maintain scarce environmental functions. Clean production and consumption require provisions and adaptations of all kinds, including the use of labor. Examples include cleaning industrial or household waste water, integrated pest control in agriculture, sustainable exploitation of forests, and sustainable development in agricultural economies. Such provisions and adaptations require more labor, directly (Hueting, 1996).

As well, the myth persists that even though the environment is worth saving via the promotion of sustainable development, it is too expensive a goal to achieve. Even though there is economic sacrifice to be made in the effort to save the physical environment, shifting the goal to sustainability will not damage, but most likely enhance, the state of an individual's biology, and his or her health. And the same can be said for entire communities of people. Environmentally friendly activities are usually healthier, for both the individual and community, than those that harm the environment (Hueting, 1996).

In policy analysis, considered a standard form of macropractice (Ginsberg, 1999), the interface between the worlds of human biology and social work macropractice is evident in a review of U.S. Supreme Court cases. Clearly, critical thinking skills are necessary when reviewing the "controversial cases" of the Supreme Court. Supreme Court cases most often have three dimensions of controversy—political, popular, and legal (Croddy, 2002).

For example, with its focus on the human biology concept of race and the social concept of "separate but equal," the famous case Brown v. Board of Education was politically controversial. The decision engendered significant political resistance by several state governments and ultimately forced the executive and legislative branches of the federal government to act. Controversial cases, such as Brown v. Board of Education, with these dimensions require the ability of social work practitioners and social work students to think critically about structures of government, federalism, and the separation of powers. A Supreme Court case is popularly controversial when it addresses an issue, often moral or religious, that deeply divides society. Public reaction to such cases can include grassroots efforts, protests, and political organizing. Classic examples that relate to human biology include the movements espousing right to life and right to abortion. Roe v. Wade, with its focus on right to abortion, is a prime example of a popularly controversial U.S. Supreme Court case. The case gave constitutional protection to women seeking abortions. Over the years opposition and support of the ruling has led to massive community-based and nationally orchestrated right-to-life and right-to-choice movements. Social work practitioners, at both the micro- and macro-level, need to critically think for themselves and their clients about human biology issues as broad based as the availability of abortion, federal funding of abortions for the poor, and the basis for support and opposition to partial-birth abortions (Croddy, 2002).

Legally, U.S. Supreme Court cases can be controversial. Korematsu v. United States was a Supreme Court case focused on the human biology concern of ethnicity and race and the link to predicted behaviors. The Supreme Court upheld the conviction of a Japanese American citizen who violated the exclusion orders of the U.S. military in California during the internment program of WWII. The Court deferred to the judgment of the military that the exclusion of all Japanese Americans was necessary to defend the coast from potential espionage and sabotage. Legal scholars have roundly criticized the results and worry that the case is still considered good law and dangerous in a time of national crisis, such as following the tragedy of September 11, 2001, and the often ill-founded linking of predicted behaviors with persons of a particular race or ethnicity (Croddy, 2002). Critically thinking social workers are often pressed to consider the elements of race, ethnicity, freedom, and oppression as they challenge the system on behalf of individual clients or community systems.

CRITICAL THINKING AND HUMAN BIOLOGY—YOU CAN DO IT

Yes, social work practitioners and social work students can do it. But what is "it"? "It" is the ability to think critically about challenging ideas in the interface between the domains of human biology and social work. Both the work of social work practitioners and the participation of social work students in the academic sphere require reasoning—reasoning about not only what is good social work practice, but also how is good social work practice related to past, current, and new knowledge in the area of human biology. For example, even though clarity in thinking is not always the goal, thinking characterized by clarity and logical force—thinking bereft of clichés, blatant logical fallacies, and mushy reasoning—is intended to enhance the outcomes for social workers and social work students as they engage in the task of helping others (Mullen, 1995). Critical thinking is the confidence, willingness, and skill to use reasoning powers to develop clear viewpoints, to argue for those viewpoints, to seek and accept others' skilled evaluation of one's own positions, and to evaluate intelligently the viewpoints and arguments of others (p. 4.) The individual social work practitioner or student can benefit, get better at, and help others to acquire the use of strong critical thinking skills. As well, the use of sound reasoning via critical thinking skills has societal implications. The existence of a sound public order, an effective but humane economic structure, a political system focused on the greater good for the greater number of people, and social relationships free of oppression and abuse, and the interactions of strangers and intimates free of the "isms" of racism, sexism, ageism, and the like, particularly the devastating impacts of homophobia, is more likely if persons, including social work practitioners and social work students, are willing and able to implement sound critical thinking skills related to human biology concerns (Mullen, 1995).

DISCUSSION QUESTIONS

1. If your task was to teach an adult social work client critical thinking skills, where would you begin and what would you emphasize?

2. What are some reasons why critical thinking is so difficult to define?

3. Can you recall, and describe, a time when you applied your critical thinking skills and experienced a positive outcome?

4. Is the ability to use critical thinking skills critical to being a good social work practitioner? If not, why not? If so, why?

5. Is evolution in some way responsible for the current popularity of the idea of "critical thinking skills"?

CHAPTER FIFTEEN

THE ROLE OF UNDERSTANDING BIOLOGY IN THE PRACTICE OF SOCIAL WORK

The mass of information provided in this text can be used to expand the understanding of social work managers, practitioners, and students about the ways in which human beings biologically develop, function, and encounter problems. Knowing about the biology of human behavior is a critical issue in effective social work practice. Information about human biology has historically been part of social work education, at times with greater emphasis than others. The significant quantity of new knowledge of human biology and its impact on human behavior have tremendous implications for social work practice. So many social workers are involved in health care, which is closely identified with biology that it is important for social workers to understand the biological dimensions of health and illness. There is constantly greater learning about the association between biology and mental functioning. Such information is critical for social workers in the mental health field. The focus of more social workers than any other is work with young people and old people. Understanding the biology of children and youth and the biology of aging are also important foci of human understanding.

The social problem of substance abuse, another preoccupation of social workers, is closely associated with biological issues. Major epidemics, with personal and societal implications, are also concerns of virtually all social workers and all have central biological dimensions. In essence, virtually every field of social work practice demonstrates the need for knowledge of human biology.

Of course the practice of social work is divided into various methods and system sizes. Many social workers work with individuals, families, and small groups. Others may work with small groups, task groups, communities, and organizations. However one works, there is a way to use biological knowledge about human behavior in any kind of practice medium. Work with individuals on disability, health, and illness issues is, of course, an obvious application of the content of this book to professional practice. Understanding the biology of mental illness as well as the biological elements of drug and alcohol use can be exceptionally helpful to those working in the mental health and substance abuse fields.

Better understanding genetics and inheritance is critical to comprehending the ways in which biological forces affect the growth and development of individuals. For those working with larger systems, knowing about public health issues, understanding the human genome, and better comprehending the ecology of human beings and the ways in which the environment affects them is critical. In addition, knowing about environmental issues and health problems caused by environmental problems may be a focus of those working to improve community life through their social work practice efforts. Critical thinking about social problems and social solutions is also a major part of effective work in all social work environments. Critical thinking about human biology allows the social work practitioner to be better informed about issues as varied as sexuality, reproduction, and normal, as well as disrupted, physical development. So no matter where one may work and no matter what kinds of work one may do, applications of biological knowledge and theory to one's work is always a possibility.

ETHICAL ISSUES

Ethics are central to the practice of human services work, especially social work. Effective social work and the effective use of biological and physiological knowledge has to be informed by ethical precepts. In many cases the ethical dimensions of a particular personal problem or social issue are more important than any other elements. Simply understanding the physical or biological components of a situation does not, in itself, provide guidance for what one should do or might do in that situation.

Social workers are faced every day with ethical dilemmas that result not only from the difficulties of making decisions about human beings but also because choices are now available that were not available in the past. As health care and other technologies develop and as more is learned about the human body, more, not fewer, ethical choices face those who work with people.

Some examples of the ethical dilemmas associated with biological issues include the regulations for maintaining confidentiality. Being faced with some of the conditions described in this text or some of the problem behaviors associated with some of the subjects defined here requires thoughtful adherence to the principles of confidentiality—of never sharing information without the informed consent of the client, for example. Of course, there are exceptions and codicils to these principles and an effective guide, for social workers at least, is the National Association of Social Workers' Code of Ethics. In the areas of health care, orders for living wills or advanced directives or "do not resuscitate" directions are major ethical concerns for professional social workers and others who deal with people who are ill, especially those who are near death. The ethical issues associated with the provision of palliative care are also critical, particularly for those who work with end-of-life programs such as hospices.

The whole issue of organ transplants, a solution to severe health problems that has only become available in the last few decades, requires an understanding of human biology principles as well as the ethical dilemmas associated with such procedures. Whether or not living people may or should sell their organs to people who need them for survival is a continuing political issue. So is the nature of waiting lists for organs harvested from people who have died. The rules on these matters are issues of social policy but they are hotly debated and often the subject of legislation, books, television programs, and other media attention.

The subject of genetic counseling is another important ethical consideration. What should parents do when they discover that a fetus may have a severe genetic condition that will either end the child's life early or require years of expensive health care, or both? What is the ethical obligation of the parent and the social worker for dealing with such matters? Hospitals and other health care facilities have ethics committees that meet regularly to address such issues, which are biological and more. Abortion as a choice is another critical and divisive matter with a biological basis. Family notification and waiting period requirements for teens seeking abortions have biological as well as social consequences. Also, should parents be allowed to genetically choose having a male or female child, should one or the other be their desire? Knowing the sex of a fetus well before birth is a fairly recent phenomenon resulting from increased biological knowledge.

Should people with contagious diseases be forced to take medication or should they be quarantined, practices that have been prominent in American health practices in the past? Should people who have eating disorders be forced to eat? Should people with mental illnesses be forced to take psychotropic medicines, whether they want to or not? Should people who have severe illnesses be required to enter hospitals or other facilities for treatment of those conditions? These kinds of questions, raised by one of the reviewers of the manuscript for this book, are among the most crucial issues that professional social workers have to face in their everyday practice.

These kinds of issues illustrate that many of the problems professional social workers address are not only biological but moral, ethical, and conceptual in nature as well. This book was designed to provide information to a broad range of social work managers, practitioners, and students, as well as other professionals in related human service fields. This content's application is a central focus of the authors, who are anxious for this material, some of it fairly new to the social work literature, to better prepare social workers for the help they provide.

REFERENCES

Abadinsky, H. (1993). *Drug abuse: An introduction.* Chicago: Nelson-Hall.

Adler, J., & Underwood, A. (2002, May 27). Aspirin: The oldest new wonder drug. *Newsweek,* 60–62.

Aker, R. L., Hayner, N. S., & Gruninger, W. (1974). Homosexual and drug behavior in prison. A test of the functional and importation models of the inmate system. *Social Problems, 21*(3), 410–422.

Alcamo, I. E. (1995). *Biology* (2nd ed.). Lincoln, NE: Cliffs Notes.

Alexander, B. (2001, February). You 2 (you squared). *Wired,* 120–135.

Alzheimer's Disease and Related Disorders Association, Inc. (2001). [On-line]. http://alz.org

Anand, G. (2002, May 5). A tamer schizophrenia drug? Bristol-Myers's new antipsychotic produces fewer side effects. *Wall Street Journal,* 1.

Arnhoff, F. N. (1975). Social consequences of policy toward mental illness: Indiscriminate shifts from hospital to community treatment may incur high social costs. *Science, 188,* 1277–1281.

Ash, R. (2000). *The top ten of everything: 2001.* New York: Dorling Kindersley.

Asherson, P. J., & Curran, S. (2001). Approaches to gene mapping in complex disorders and their application in child psychiatry and psychology. *The British Journal of Psychiatry, 179,* 122–128.

Asimov, I. (1991). The nature of science. In T. Ferris (Ed.), *The world treasury of physics, astronomy, and mathematics* (pp. 781–783). Boston: Little, Brown, and Company.

"Ask the Doctor," Retrieved from the Internet July 19, 2002, sponsored by Lawyers, Inc., PC (1-800-laws), http://www.about-cerebral-palsy.org

Asma, S. T. (1993). The new social Darwinism: Deserving your destitution. *Humanist, 53*(5), 10–12.

Atkins, R. C. (2001). *Dr. Atkins' new diet revolution.* New York: Avon.

Atkinson, J. (2002, September). Scared yet? *Esquire,* 118–125.

Axinn, J., & Stern, M. (2001). *Social welfare: A history of the American response to need* (5th ed.). Boston: Allyn & Bacon.

Ballif, M. (1999, Winter). What is it that the audience wants? Or, notes, toward a listening with a transgendered ear for (mis)understanding. *JAC, 19*(1), 51–70.

Baltimore, D. (2001). Our genome unveiled. *Nature, 409,* 814–816.

Barash, D., & Barash, I. (2000). *The mammal in the mirror: Understanding our place in the natural world.* New York: W.H. Freeman.

Barker, R. L. (1999). *The social work dictionary.* Washington, DC: NASW Press.

Baron, R. A., & Byrne, D. (2000). *Social psychology* (9th ed.). Boston: Allyn & Bacon.

Barrett, A. (2001). Servants of the map. In B. Kingsolver (Ed.), *The best American short stories, 2001* (pp. 1–43). Boston: Houghton-Mifflin.

Bateson, G., Jackson, D. D., Haley, J., & Weakland, J. (1956). Toward a theory of schizophrenia. *Behavior Science, 1,* 251–264.

Baumeister, R. F., & Tice, D. M. (2001). *The social dimension of sex.* Boston: Allyn & Bacon.

Beck, A. T. (1976). *Cognitive therapy and the emotional disorders.* New York: International University Press.

Becvar, D. S. (1995). Family therapy in the social work curriculum: Fit or misfit? *Journal of Family Social Work, 1*(2), 43–55.

251

Beers, M. H., & Berkow, R. (1999). *The Merck manual of diagnosis and therapy* (17th ed., Centennial Edition). Whitehouse Station, NJ: Merck Research Laboratories.

Begley, S. (2001a, May 21). The roots of evil. *Newsweek,* 31–35.

Begley, S. (2001b, June 11). AIDS at 20. *Newsweek,* 35–37.

Begley, S. (2002a, March 11). The schizophrenic mind. *Newsweek,* 44–51.

Begley, S. (2002b, May 24). NIMH study therapy works as well as drugs for depression. *Wall Street Journal,* B1 and B4.

Berude, S. M. (Director of Editorial Operations). (1982). *American heritage dictionary* (2nd ed.). Boston, MA: Houghton Mifflin.

Biasella, S. (1999, Fall/Winter). Your baby's first year. *Lamaze Baby,* 53–62.

Bjerklie, D. (2002, December 9). Rheumatoid arthritis: The other crippling joint disease. *Time,* 72.

Bodmer, W., & McKie, R. (1997). *The book of man: The Human Genome Project and our quest to discover our genetic heritage.* New York: Oxford University Press.

Bolin, A., & Whelehan, P. (1999). *Perspectives on human sexuality.* Albany, NY: State University of Albany Press.

Boulter, M. (2002). *Extinction: Evolution and the end of man.* New York: Columbia University Press.

Bronfenbrenner, U. (1953). Personality. *Annual Review of Psychology, 4,* 157–182.

Bronfenbrenner, U. (1989). Ecological systems theory. In R. Vasta (Ed.), *Six theories of child development: Revised formulations and current issues* (pp. 187–249). Philadelphia, PA: Jessica Kingsley.

Bronfenbrenner, U., & Ceci, S. J. (1994). Nature-nurture reconceptualized in developmental perspective: A bioecological model. *Psychological Review, 101*(4), 568–586.

Brown, E. (2002, September). Professor X. *Wired,* 114–119, 149.

Brown, P. (1994, July 9). Understanding the inner voices. *New Scientist, 143,* 26–31.

Browne, J. C. (2001). *God save the sweet potato queens.* New York: Three Rivers.

Brunner, B. (Ed.). (1997). *The Time almanac: 1998.* Boston: Information Please LLC.

Bunch, B., & Tesar, J. (2000). *The Penguin desk encyclopedia of science and mathematics.* New York: Penguin.

Buss, D. M. (1998). Sexual strategies theory: Historical origins and current status. *Journal of Sex Research, 35*(1), 1–19.

Butler, K. (1996). The biology of fear. *Family Therapy Networker, 20,* 39–45.

Califano, J. A., Jr., & Booth, A. (1998, September). *1998 CASA national survey of teens, teachers and principals.* The National Center on Addiction and Substance Abuse at Columbia University. Available: http://www.casacolumbia.org

Callicott, J. H., & Weinberger, D. R. (1999). Functional brain imaging: Future prospects for clinical practice. In S. Weissman, & M. Sabshin (Eds.), *Psychiatry in the new millennium* (pp. 119–139). Washington, DC: American Psychiatric Press.

Campbell, N. A., Mitchell, L. G., & Reece, J. B. (2000). *Biology: Concepts and connections* (3rd ed.). New York: Addison Wesley & Benjamin Cummings.

Casriel, E. (2002, February 14). Big energy seeks a toxic victory. *Rolling Stone,* 34.

Caudill, E. (1997). *Darwinian myths: The legends and misuses of a theory.* Knoxville, TN: The University of Tennessee Press.

Ceci, S. J. (1996). *On Intelligence: A biological treatise on intellectual development.* Cambridge, MA: Harvard University Press.

Chakravarti, A. (2001). To a future of genetic medicine. *Nature, 409,* 822–823.

Chase, M. (2002, February 13). Sexually transmitted diseases appear sharply underreported. *Wall Street Journal,* B9.

Cheers, G. (2001). *Anatomica: The complete home medical reference.* New York: Barnes and Noble.

Clayman, C. B. (Med. Ed.). (1989). *The American Medical Association encyclopedia of medicine.* New York: Random House.

Cohen, J. (2000). *The penis.* New York: Konemann.

Cole, K. C. (1997). *The universe and the teacup.* New York: Harcourt Brace.

Test vaccine for Alzheimer's halted. (2002, February 22). *The Columbia State,* A4.

Commoner, B. (2002, February). Unraveling the DNA myth: The spurious foundation of genetic engineering. *Harper's,* 39–47.

Conn, C., & Lapham, L. H. (2000). *The Harper's index book* (Vol. 1). New York: Franklin Square Press.

Cookson, J. (2001). Use of antipsychotic drugs and lithium in mania. *The British Journal of Psychiatry, 178*(41), 148–156.

Cotler, S. (2002, September). Vision quest. *Wired,* 94–101.

Cowley, G. (2001, Fall/Winter). The biology of aging. *Newsweek,* 12–24.

Cowley, G. (2001a, June 11). Can he find a cure? *Newsweek,* 39–41.

Cowley, G. (2001b, September 17). Dignity in dementia. *Newsweek,* 58.

Cowley, G. (2002, June 24). The disappearing mind. *Newsweek,* 42–50.

Cowley, G. (2002). Now, integrative care. *Newsweek,* 49–53.

Cowley, G. (2003, January 20). A better way to eat. *Newsweek,* 46–55.

Cowley, G., & Springen, K. (2002, July 22). The end of the age of estrogen. *Newsweek,* 38–41.

Croddy, M. (2002). Controversial dimensions of U.S. Supreme Court Cases. *Social Education, 66* (1), 60–62.

Cummins, D. D., & Cummins, R. (1999). Biological preparedness and evolutionary explanation. *Cognition, 73,* B37–B53.

Daly, M., & Wilson, M. I. (1997). Human evolutionary psychology and animal behavior. *Animal Behaviour, 57,* 509–519.

Darwin, C. (1979 [1859]). *On the origin of species.* New York: Hill and Wang.

Davidson, J. R. T., & Foa, E. B. (Eds.). (1993). *Posttraumatic stress disorder: DSM-IV and beyond.* Washington, DC: American Psychiatric Press.

DeCecco, J. P., & Parker, D. A. (1995). The biology of homosexuality: Sexual orientation or sexual preference? *Journal of Homosexuality, 28* (1–2), 1–27.

De Milto, L. (2002). http://www.findarticles.com/cf (retrieved December 6, 2002).

DeMoss, R. T. (1999). *Brain waves through time: 12 principles for understanding the evolution of the human brain and man's behavior.* New York: Plenum Trade.

Dennis, R. M. (1995). Social Darwinism, scientific racism, and the metaphysics of race. *Journal of Negro Education, 64*(3), 243–252.

Dennis, C., Richard, G., & Campbell, P. (2001). The human genome: Everyone's genome. *Nature, 409,* 813.

Diamond, M., & Sigmundson, H. K. (1999). Sex reassignment at birth. In Stephen J. Ceci, & Wendy M. Williams (Eds.), *The nature-nurture debate* (pp. 57–75). Malden, MA: Blackwell.

Doell, R. G. (1995). Sexuality in the brain. *Journal of Homosexuality, 28*(3–4), 345–354.

Doell, R. G. (1995). Sexuality in the brain. In J. P. DeCecco, & D. A. Parker (Eds.), *Sex, cells, and same-sex desire: The biology of sexual preference* (pp. 345–354). Binghamton, NY: Haworth.

Dyson, F. (1991). Butterflies and superstrings. T. Ferris (Ed.), *The world treasury of physics, astronomy, and mathematics* (pp. 128–145). Boston: Little, Brown, and Company.

Edgerton, D. (1994). The rise and fall of British technology. *History Today, 44*(6), 43–48.

Efan, J. S., & Greene, M. A. (2000). The limits of change: Heredity, temperament, and family influence. In W. C. Nichols, & M. A. Pace-Nicols (Eds.), *Handbook of family development and interventions* (pp. 41–64). New York: John Wiley & Sons.

Emlen, S. (1995). Fifteen predictions of living within family groups. *Proceedings of the National Academy of Sciences, 92,* 8092–8099.

Ensler, E. (2001). *The vagina monologues.* New York: Dillard Books.

Euster, G. (2002, Spring/Summer). Administration on aging facts for features from the Census Bureau. *The Newsletter of the South Carolina Center for Gerontology,* 2–3.

Eysenck, H. J. (1973). Personality and attitudes to sex in criminals. *Journal of Sex Research, 9*(4), 295–306.

Eysenck, H. J. (1993). The biological basis of intelligence. In P. Vernon (Ed.), *Biological approaches to the study of human intelligence* (pp. 1–32). Norwood, NJ: Ablex Publishing.

Ezzell, C. (2002, June). Hope in a vial. *Scientific American,* 38–45.

Faenza, M. M. (2001, May). [Letter to the Editor]. *The Atlantic Monthly,* 12.

Farmer, R., & Bentley, K. J. (2001). Social workers as medication facilitators. In K. J. Bentley (Ed.), *Social work practice in mental health: Contemporary roles, tasks and techniques* (pp. 211–219). Pacific Grove, CA: Brooks/Cole.

Ferrini, A., & Ferrini, R. (2000). *Health in the later years.* New York: McGraw Hill.

Ferris, T. (Ed.). (1991). *The world treasury of physics, astronomy, and mathematics.* Boston: Little, Brown, and Company.

Feynman, R. P. (1991). Atoms in motion. In T. Ferris (Ed.), *The world treasury of physics, astronomy, and mathematics* (pp. 3–17). New York: Little, Brown, and Company.

Feynman, R. P. (1995). *Six easy pieces and six not so easy pieces.* Cambridge, MA: Perseus.

Fields, S. (2001). Proteomics in genomeland. *Science, 291*(5507), 1221–1224.

Flam, F. (2002, March 22). Brain may hold clues to gamblers risk taking. *The Columbia State,* A14.

For the record. (2002, March 11). *Time,* 21.

France, D. (2001, June 11). The angry prophet is dying. *Newsweek,* 43–46.

Frances, A. (Chairperson, Task Force on DSM-IV). (1994). *Diagnostic and statistical manual of mental disorders* (4th ed.). Washington, DC: American Psychiatric Association.

Frank, L. F. (Ed.). (2001). *Random House Webster's quotationary.* New York: Random House.

Franzen J. (2001, September 10). Personal industry: My father's brain: What Alzheimer's takes away. *The New Yorker,* 81–91.

Freeman, C. (1994). *The book of southern wisdom.* Nashville, TN: Walnut Grove Press.

Freeman, D. (1983). *Margaret Mead and Samoa: The making and unmaking of an anthropological myth.* Cambridge: Harvard University Press.

Friedman, M. J., Charney, D. S., & Deutch, A. Y. (1995). *Neurobiological and clinical consequences of stress: From normal adaptation to PTSD.* Philadelphia: Lipincott-Raven.

Galanter, M., & Kleber, H. (Eds.). (1994). *Textbook of substance abuse treatment.* Washington, DC: American Psychiatric Press.

Galas, D. J. (2001). Making sense of the sequence. *Science, 291*(5507), 1257–1260.

Gambrill, E. (1997). *Social work practice: A critical thinker's guide.* New York: Oxford University Press.

Gambrill, E. (2000). The role of critical thinking in evidence-based social work. In P. Allen-Meares, & C. Garvin (Eds.), *The handbook of social work direct practice* (pp. 43–63). Thousand Oaks, CA: Sage.

Garrett, L. (1994). *The coming plague.* New York: Penguin.

Garrett, L. (2001a). *Betrayal of trust.* New York: Hyperion.

Garrett, L. (2001b, December). Unprepared for the worst. *Vanity Fair,* 194–214.

Gawande, A. (2002a, January 28). Annals of medicine: The learning curve. *The New Yorker,* 52–61.

Gawande, A. (2002b, March 8). Medical dispatch: Cold comfort. *The New Yorker,* 42–47.

Gaylin, W. (2000). *Talk is not enough: How psychotherapy really works.* New York: Little, Brown, and Company.

Gearan, A. (2002, March 20). Broader drug testing of students weighed. *The Columbia State,* A4.

Gilbert, S. (2000). *Developmental biology* (6th ed.). Sunderland, MA: Sinauer Associates.

Ginsberg, L. (1999). *Understanding social problems, policies, and programs* (3rd ed.). Columbia, SC: University of South Carolina Press.

Gladwell, M. (2000). *The tipping point: How little things can make a big difference.* New York: Little, Brown, and Company.

Gladwell, M. (2001, July 30). Java Man. *The New Yorker,* 76–80.

Gladwell, M. (2002, August 5). Annals of psychology: The naked face. *The New Yorker,* 38–49.

Global warming spreads disease. (2002a, July 12). *The Week,* 20.

Goldstein, H. (1999). The limits and art of understanding in social work practice. *Families in Society: The Journal of Contemporary Human Services, 80*(4), 385–395.

Gorey, K. M., & Cryns, A. G. (1999, November). The bell curve: Race, socioeconomic status and social work. *Social Work, 44*(6), 586–589.

Gorman, C. (2000a, July 17). Dementia: The other kinds. *Time* (large print edition), 42.

Gorman, C. (2000b, July 17). Advice for caregivers: Three states of Alzheimer's. *Time* (large print edition), 44–45.

Gorman, C. (2002, January 21). Walk, don't run. *Time,* 81–83.

Gorman, C., & Park, A. (2002, December 9). The age of arthritis. *Time,* 70–79.

Gould, S. J. (1981). *The mismeasure of man.* New York: W. W. Norton and Company.

Gould, S. J. (2002). *The structure of evolutionary theory.* Cambridge, MA: The Belknap Press of the Harvard University Press.

Gribbin, J., with Gribbin, M. (1998). *Almost everyone's guide to science: The universe, life and everything.* New Haven: Yale University Press.

Grice, G. (2001, July 30). Annals of science: Slice of life. *The New Yorker,* 36–41.

Grigsby, R. K. (1995). Determinism versus creativity: A response to Peile. *Social Work, 40*(5), 706–707.

Griscom, A. (2002, September). Take these genes and call me in the morning. *Wired,* 90–92.

Groopman, J. (2001, June 4). Annals of Medicine: The thirty years' war: Have we been fighting cancer the wrong way? *The New Yorker,* 52–73.

Groopman, J. (2002a, April 8). Annals of medicine: A knife in the back. *The New Yorker,* 66–73.

Groopman, J. (2002b, July 29). Medical dispatch: Hormones for men. *The New Yorker,* 34–38.

Grossberg, G. T. (2002, August 5). Battling for the brain. *People,* 105–106.

Grossman, L. (2002, March 11). Meet the Chipsons. *Time,* 56–57.

Gupta, S. (2002, March 4). To clip or coil? 32.

Gutfeld, G. (2001, December). So a leper walks into a bar . . . *Stuff,* 100–104.

Hales, D., & Hales, R. E. (1996). *Caring for the mind: The comprehensive guide to mental health.* New York: Bantam.

Hamachek, D. (1991). *Encounters with the self* (4th ed.). Fort Worth, TX: Harcourt Brace Jovanivich College Publishers.

Haney, D. (2002a, April 8). Aspirin might cut colon cancer risk, study says. *The Columbia State,* A3.

Haney, D. (2002b, April 10). Another danger linked to weight. *The Columbia State,* A9.

Haney, D. (2002c, August 4). Finding may revolutionize heart care. *The Columbia State,* A1, A7.

Harbert, A. S., & Ginsberg, L. H. (1990). *Human services for older adults: Concepts and skills* (2nd ed., rev.). Columbia, SC: USC Press.

Harkavy, M. D. (Ed.). (1998). *The new Webster's international encyclopedia.* Naples, FL: Trident International Press.

Harrison, J. (1991). Against tolerating the intolerable in logic and ethics. In P. Geach (Ed.), *Logic and ethics* (pp. 131–144). Boston: Kluwer Academic.

Hawley, R. S., & Mori, C. A. (1999). *The human genome: A user's guide.* New York: Academic Press.

Health: No safety in singles. (2002, August 5). *Newsweek,* 60.

Health for life: Inside the science of alternative medicine. (2002, December). *Newsweek,* 45–75.

Heckhausen, J. (2000). Evolutionary perspectives on human motivation. *Animal Behavioral Scientist, 43*(6), 1015–1029.

Heilemann, J. (2002, May). Machine of dreams. *Vanity Fair,* 184–188, 222–230.

Heisenberg, W. (1991). The Copenhagen interpretation of quantum theory. In T. Ferris (Ed.), *The world treasury of physics, astronomy, and mathematics* (pp. 86–96). Boston: Little, Brown, and Company.

Herrn, R. (1995). On the history of biological theories of homosexuality. *Journal of Homosexuality, 28*(1–2), 31–56.

Herrnstein, R. J., & Murray, C. (1994). *The bell curve: Intelligence and class structure in American life.* New York: Free Press.

Hockenberry, J. (2001, August). The new braniacs. *Wired,* 94–105.

Hoffman, L. (1988). A constructivist position for family therapy. *The Irish Journal of Psychology, 9*(1), 110–129.

Hoffman, M. L. (1981). Is altruism a part of human nature? *Journal of Personality and Social Psychology,* 40.

Hoover, E. (2003, January 17). Policing public sex. *Chronicle of Higher Education, XLIX*(19), A31.

Horgan, J. (1996). *The end of science: Facing the limits of knowledge in the twilight of the scientific age.* Reading, MA: Helix Books.

Horowitz, J. M. (2002, January 21). Ten foods that pack a wallop. *Time,* 75–80.

Hueting, R. (1996). Three persistent myths in the environmental debate. *Ecological Economics, 18,* 81–88.

Hyman, S. E. (1999). Looking to the future: The role of genetics and molecular biology in research on mental illness. In S. Weissman, & M. Sabshin (Eds.), *Psychiatry in the new millennium* (pp. 97–117). Washington, DC: American Psychiatric Press.

Ivans, M. (2001, September 17). Body bard. *Time,* 66–67.

Jackson, J. (1991). Against tolerating the intolerable. In P. Geach (Ed.), *Logic and ethics* (pp. 131–144). Boston: Kluwer Academic Publishers.

James, W. (1890). *Principles of psychology.* New York: Henry Holt.

Jasny, B. R., & Kennedy, D. (2001). The human genome. *Science, 291,* 1153.

Jasny, B., & Szuromi, P. (Eds.). (2001). This week in science. *Science, 291*(5507), 1155–1157.

Jeffords, J. M., & Daschle, T. (2001). Political issues in the genome era. *Science, 291*(5507), 1249–1251.

Jensen, E. (1998). *Teaching with the brain in mind.* Alexandria, VA: Association for Supervision and Curriculum Development.

Jimeniz-Sanchez, G., Childs, B., & Valle, D. (2001). Human disease genes. *Nature, 409,* 853–855.

Johnson, H. C. (1996). Violence and biology: A review of the literature. *Families in Society, 77*(1), 3–18.

Johnson, H. C. (1999). *Psyche, synapse and substance: The role of neurobiology in emotions, behavior, cognition, and addiction for non-scientists.* Greenfield, MA: Deerfield Valley Publishing.

Johnson, H. J. (2001, January 18). The next battle over clean air. *Rolling Stone,* 48–53.

Johnson, W. L. (1995). Evolution: The past, present, and future implications. *Vital Speeches of the Day, 61*(9), 281–285.

Joseph, J. (1998). The equal environment assumption of the classical twin method: A critical analysis. *The Journal of Mind and Behavior, 19*(3), 325–358.

Kalb, C. (2002, July 22). What's a woman to do? *Newsweek,* 42–45.

Kantrowitz, B. (2002, July 15). In search of sleep. *Newsweek,* 39–47.

Keltner, N. L. (1996). Nursing's move to a biological understanding of mental illness. *Perspectives in Psychiatric Care, 31*(3), 5–8.

Kessler, R. C., Sonnega, A., Bromet, E., Hughes, M., & Nelson, C. B. (1996). Posttraumatic stress disorder in the National Comorbidity Survey. *Archives of General Psychiatry, 52,* 1048–1060.

Kettlewell, H. B. D. (1955). Selection experiments on industrial melanism in the Lepidoptera. *Heredity, 9,* 323–342.

Kettlewell, H. B. D. (1956). Further selection experiments on industrial melanism in the Lepidoptera. *Heredity, 10,* 287–301.

King, B. M. (1999). *Human sexuality today* (3rd ed.). Upper Saddle River, NJ: Prentice-Hall.

Kingsolver, B. (2001). *The best American short stories, 2001.* Boston: Houghton-Mifflin.

Kinsey, A. C., Pomeroy, W. B., & Martin, C. (1948). *Sexual behavior of the human male.* Philadelphia: W. B. Saunders.

Kirkpatrick, L. A. (1993). Fundamentalism, Christian orthodoxy and intrinsic religious orientation as predictors of discriminatory attitudes. *Journal for the Scientific Study of Religion, 32*(3), 256–268.

Kotulak, R. (2002, July 21). Hard-wired: New knowledge about the mind's makeup gives scientists greater potential—for good or evil? *Chicago Tribune* (Midwest Edition), *202,* sect. 2, 1–2.

Lamonick, M. D. (2002, January 21). How to keep the doctor away. *Time,* 68–69.

Lamonick, M. D., & Park, A. (2002, January 21). Vaccines stage a comeback. *Time,* 70–75.

Lamonick, M. D. (2002, May 20). How everything works. *Time,* 667.

Lappin, J. (1988). Family therapy: A structural approach. In R. A. Dorfman (Ed.), *Paradigms of clinical social work.* New York: Brunner/Mazel.

Laqueur, T. (1990). *Making sex: Body and gender from the Greeks to Freud.* Cambridge, MA: Harvard University Press.

Larson, E. (1997). *Summer of the Gods: The Scopes trial and America's continuing debate over science and religion.* New York: Basic Books.

Levin, B. L., & Petrila, J. (Eds.). (1996). *Mental health services: A public health perspective.* New York: Oxford University Press.

Like one of the guys. (2002, March 11). *Time,* 17.

Lilienfield, S. O. (1998). *Looking into abnormal psychology: Contemporary readings.* Pacific Grove, CA: Brooks/Cole.

Looy, H. (1995). Born gay? A critical review of biological research on homosexuality. *Journal of Psychology and Christianity, 14*(3), 197–214.

MacDonald, K. (1998). Evolution, culture, and the five-factor model. *Journal of Cross-cultural Psychology, 29,* 119–149.

MacLullich, A. M. J., Seckl, J. R., Starr, J. M., & Deary, I. J. (1998). The biology of intelligence: From association to mechanism. *Intelligence, 26*(2), 63–73.

Malthus, T. R. (1993 [1789]). *An essay on the principles of population.* Oxford: Oxford University Press.

Maranto, G. (1987). Why (perhaps) lithium is doubly effective (for manic depression). *Discover, 8,* 12.

Marcus, S. (1996). Rage against the machine. *New Republic, 214*(24), 30–38.

Marshall, E. (2001a). Comparison shopping. *Science, 291*(5507), 1180–1181.

Marshall, E. (2001b). Sharing the glory, not the credit. *Science, 291*(5507), 1189–1193.

Masters, W. H., Johnson, V. E., & Kolodny, R. (1995). *Human sexuality* (5th ed.). New York: Harper Collins College Publishers.

McCammon, S., Knox, D., & Schacht, C. (1998). *Making choices in sexuality: Research and applications.* Pacific Grove, CA: Brooks/Cole.

McClam, E. (2002, April 12). Study blames smoking for huge economic loss. *The Columbia State,* A13.

McConnaughey, J. (2002, March 14). Treadmill tests show fitness prolongs life, study says. *The Columbia State,* A1.

McCulloch, C. (2001, May). [Letter to the Editor]. *The Atlantic Monthly,* 12.

McGuffin, P., Riley, B., & Plomin, R. (2001). Toward behavioral genomics. *Science, 291*(5507), 1232–1249.

McGuire, T. R. (1995). Is homosexuality genetic? A critical review and some suggestions. *Journal of Homosexuality, 28* (1–2), 115–145.

McMurtry, L. (2000). *Roads.* New York: Simon and Schuster.

McNeece, C., & DiNitto, D. (1994). *Chemical dependency: A systems approach.* Englewood Cliffs, NJ: Prentice Hall.

McNulty, R. D., & Burnette, M. M. (2001). *Exploring human sexuality: Making healthy decisions.* Boston: Allyn & Bacon.

Mehrabian, A. (2000, May). Beyond IQ: Broad-based measurement of individual success potential or "emotional intelligence." *Genetic Social and General Psychology Monographs 126*(2), 133–239.

Menand, L. (2002, November 25). What comes naturally: Does evolution explain who we are? *The New Yorker,* 96–101.

Men's Health Index (2002, July/August). Arsenic. *Men's Health,* 34.

Merkel, W. T., & Searight, H. R. (1992). Why families are not like swamps, solar systems or thermostats: Some limits of systems theory as applied to family therapy. *Contemporary Family Therapy, 14*(1), 33–49.

Mervaala, E., Föhr, J., Könönen, M., Valkone-Korhonen, M., Vainio, P., Partanen, K., Partanen, J., Tiihonen, J., Viinamäki, H., Karjalainen, A. K., & Lehtonen, J. (2000). Quantitative MRI of the hippocampus and amygdala in severe depression. *Psychological Medicine, 30,* 117–125.

Meyers, B. (1996). The bell curve and the new social Darwinism. *Science and Society, 60*(2), 195–204.

Mohr, W. K., & Mohr, B. D. (2001). Brain, behavior, connections and implications: Psychodynamics no more. *Archives of Psychiatric Nursing, 15*(4), 171–181.

Monastersky, R. (2002). Revising the book of life. *Chronicle of Higher Education, 48*(27), A14.

Moore, M. (2001). *Stupid white men.* New York: HarperCollins.

Morley, S., & Friend, D. (2000). *Puppetry of the penis: The ancient Australian art of genital origami.* New York: Corgi/Transworld Publishers.

Morton, W. A. (2002). Update: New psychiatric medications. (unpublished)

Mullen, J. (1995). *Hard thinking: The reintroduction of logic into everyday life.* Lanham, MD: Rowman & Littlefield.

Murashita, J., Kato, T., Shioiri, T., Inubushi, T., & Kato, N. (2000). Altered brain energy metabolism in lithium-resistant bipolar disorder detected by photic stimulated P-MR spectroscopy. *Psychological Medicine, 30,* 107–115.

Nano, S. (2002, January 3). Heart helps to fix itself. *The Columbia State,* A1, A7.

Nash, J. M. (2000, July 17). The new science of Alzheimer's. *Time* (large print edition), 31–45.

Nash, J. M. (2002, May 6). The secrets of autism. *Time, 46*–55.

National Information Center for Children and Youth with Disabilities (NICHCY). (1992). *General information about cerebral palsy.* Washington, DC: Author.

National Information Center for Children and Youth with Disabilities (NICHCY). (2002). *Mental retardation.* Washington, DC: Author.

National Multiple Sclerosis Society. (2001). http://www.nationalMSsociety.org

National Organization for Rare Disorders. (2001/2002, Winter). *Volume 20, Issue 1.*

Naumann, E., with Derin-Kellogg, G. (2000). *Homeopathy 911: What to do in an emergency before help arrives.* New York: Kensington Books.

Neergaard, L. (2002a, February 22). U.S. advocates mammograms. *The Columbia State,* A4.

Neergaard, L. (2002b, February 22). Genes linked to multiple miscarriages. *The Columbia State,* A8.

Neergaard, L. (2002, March 20). New cold pill needs more tests, panels says. *The Columbia State.* A8.

Newcombe, N. S. (2002, December 13). Is sociobiology ready for prime time? *The Chronicle of Higher Education.*

Noonan, D., & Springen, K. (2002, April 22). The prostate plan. *Newsweek, 69.*

Olshansky, S. J., Hayflick, L., & Carnes, B. A. (2002, June). No truth to the fountain of youth. *Scientific American, 92*–95.

O'Reilly, B. (2000). *The O'Reilly factor.* New York: Broadway Books.

Pääbo, S. (2001). The human genome and out view of ourselves. *Science, 291*(5507), 1219–1220.

Pack, P. E. (1997). *Anatomy and physiology.* Lincoln, NE: Cliffs Notes.

Pagels, H. R. (1991). Uncertainty and complimentary. In T. Ferris (Ed.), *The world treasury of physics, astronomy, and mathematics* (pp. 97–110). Boston: Little, Brown, and Company.

Paley, M., & Ruzzier, S. (illustrator). (2000). *The book of the penis.* New York: Grove Press.

Park, A. (2002a, March 11). Change of heart. *Time, 59.*

Park, A. (2002b, April 1). Mind over muscle. *Time, 75.*

Parslow, G. (2002). Commentary: Critical thinking. Can we teach it? Should we teach it? *Biochemistry and Molecular Biology Education, 30*(1), 65.

Paulos, J. A. (2001). *Innumeracy.* New York: Hill and Wang.

Payn, M. (1991). *Modern social work theory: A critical introduction.* Chicago, IL: Lyceum Books.

Peile, C. (1993). Determinism versus creativity: Which way for social work? *Social Work, 38*(2), 127–134.

Peltonen, L., & McKusick, V. A. (2001). Dissecting human disease in the postgenomic era. *Science, 291*(5507), 1224–1231.

Pennisi, E. (2001a). The human genome: News. *Science, 291*(5507), 1177–1180.

Pennisi, E. (2001b). What's next for the genome centers? *Science, 291*(5507), 1204–1207.

Pesmen, C. (2001, July). My cancer story. *Esquire, 50*–53.

Pesmen, C. (2002, May). How a man ages. *Esquire, 77*–89.

Pope, G. C. (2000). *The biological bases of human behavior.* Boston: Allyn and Bacon.

Pope, E. (2002, June). 51 top scientists blast the entire-aging idea. *AARP Bulletin, 3*–5.

Preston, T. A. (2001, May). [Letter to the Editor]. *The Atlantic Monthly,* 12.

Pueschel, S. M. (2002, July 19). Retrieved from the ARC web site, http://www.thearc.org/faqs/sown.html.

Quindlen, A. (2002, July 29). And now for a hot flash. *Newsweek, 64.*

Rathus, S. A., Nevid, J. S., & Fichner-Rathus, L. (2002). *Human sexuality in a world of diversity* (5th ed.). Boston: Allyn and Bacon.

Raven, P., & Johnson, G. (1999). *Understanding biology* (5th ed.). New York: McGraw Hill.

Reagan, P. A., & Brookins-Fisher, J. (2002). *Community health in the 21st century* (2nd ed.). New York: Benjamin Cummings.

Recer, P. (2002a, March 20). Calcium may fend off some types of colon cancer. *The Columbia State*, A8.

Recer, P. (2002b, March 22). Early Alzheimer's test possible. *The Columbia State*, A4.

Regan, C. (2001). *Intoxicating minds: How drugs work.* New York: Columbia University Press.

Ricks, D. (2002, March 29). Smallpox vaccine can be diluted. *The Columbia State*, A12.

Ritter, M. (2002, July 28). Americans don't know as much as they should. *The Island Packet* (Hilton Head, South Carolina), A11.

Roberts, L. (2001). Controversial from the start. *Science, 291*(5507), 1182–1188.

Roos, D. S. (2001). Bioinformatics—trying to swim in a sea of data. *Science, 291*(5507), 1260–1261.

Rosenbaum, R. A. (1989). *The new American desk encyclopedia.* New York: Signet.

Rosenberg, D. (2002, April 22). Oxy's offspring. *Newsweek*, 37.

Rosenberg, M. (2002, April). The science of bad breath. *Scientific American*, 72–79.

Ross, E. (2002, June 20). Smoking risks underestimated. *The Columbia State*, A3.

Rousseau, J. E. (2002, July 29). Hormone hazards. *People*, 117–118.

Rozin, P. (2000). Evolution and adaption in the understanding of behavior, culture, and mind. *American Behavioral Scientist, 43*(6), 970–986.

Rubin, G. M. (2001). Comparing species. *Nature, 409,* 820–821.

Ryan, M. (2002, March 24). She's not afraid to ask questions. *Parade*, 12.

Schatzberg, A. F. (1999). Psychopharmacology in the new millennium: Emphasis on depression. In S. Weissman, & M. Sabshin (Eds.), *Psychiatry in the new millennium* (pp. 179–192). Washington, DC: American Psychiatric Press.

Schiffer, R. B., & Wineman, N. M. (1990). Antidepressant pharmacotherapy of depression associated with multiple sclerosis. *American Journal of Psychiatry, 147*(11), 1493–1495.

Schoenborn, C. A., & Barnes, P. M. (2002, April 7). *Leisure-time physical activity among adults: United States, 1997–98. Advance data from vital and health statistics.* Hyattsville, MD: Centers for Disease Control and Prevention.

Scully, M. G. (2002, July 5). In the long run, or maybe sooner; we're extinct. *The Chronicle of Higher Education*, B15.

Shell, E. R. (2002, August 5). It's not the carbs, stupid. *Newsweek*, 41.

Shenk, D. (2001). *The forgetting: Alzheimer's: Portrait of an epidemic.* New York: Doubleday.

Shields, J. (1996). Family systems outline from presentation. Unpublished manuscript.

Smith, D. (2001, May). Daniel Smith Replies [Letter to the Editor]. *The Atlantic Monthly*, 14.

Smith, D. (2001, February). Shock and disbelief. *The Atlantic Monthly, 287*(2), 79–90.

Smith, J. D. (1985). *Minds made feeble: The myth and legacy of the Kallikaks.* Rockville: Aspen Publications.

Solotaroff, P. (2002, February 14). Killer bods. *Rolling Stone*, 54–59, 72, 74.

Solowij, N., Stephens, R. S., Roffman, R. A., Babor, T., Kadden, R., Miler, M., Christiansen, K., McRee, B., & Vendetti, J. (2002, March 6). *Journal of the American Medical Association*, 1123–1131.

Specter, M. (2001, December 17). Annals of medicine: India's plague. *The New Yorker*, 74–85.

Starr, C., & Taggart, R. (1998). *Biology: The unity and diversity of life* (8th ed.). Belmont, CA: Wadsworth.

Steingard, R. J., Yurgelun-Todd, P., Appelman, K. E., Lyoo, I. K., Shorrock, K. L., Zurakowski, D., Poussaint, T. Y., Renshaw, P. F., & Barnes, P. (1996). Structural abnormalities in brain magnetic resonance images of depressed children. *Journal of American Academy of Child and Adolescent Psychiatry, 35*(3), 307–312.

Sternberg, R. J., & Kaufman, J. C. (Eds.). (2001). *The evolution of intelligence.* Marwah, NJ: L. Erlbaum Associates.

Stoneking, M. (2001). From the evolutionary past. *Nature, 409,* 821–822.

Swanson, D. (2002, February 14). What it is, what it does. *Rolling Stone,* 58.

Swanson, J., Posner, M. L., Cantwell, D., Wigal, S., Crinella, F., Filipek, P., Emerson, J., Tucker, D., & Nalcioglu, O. (1998). ADHD disorder: Symptom domains, cognitive processes, and neural networks. In R. Parasuraman (Ed.), *The attentive brain* (pp. 445–460). Cambridge, MA: MIT Press.

Tanner, L. (2001, December 26). Study links virus to multiple sclerosis. *The Columbia State,* A1, A9.

Tanner, L. (2002a, January 16). Metabolic syndrome hits 1 in 5. *The Columbia State,* A1, A5.

Tanner, L. (2002b, February 28). Baby eludes early Alzheimer's gene. *The Columbia State,* A1, A8.

Tanner, L. (2002c, March 15). Study shows drug fights Alzheimer's. *The Columbia State,* A15.

Terwilliger, J. D., & Ott, J. (1994). *Handbook of human genetic linkage.* Baltimore, MD: Johns Hopkins University Press.

The Week (2002b, July 19). 16.

Thomas, C. L. (Ed.). (1993). *Taber's cyclopedic medical dictionary* (17th ed.). Philadelphia: F. A. Davis.

Thomas, L. (2000). The lives of the cell. In J. C. Oates (Ed.), *The best American essays of the century* (pp. 358–360). New York: Houghton Mifflin.

Thyer, B. A., & Myers, L. L. (1997). Behavioral and cognitive theories. In J. Brandell (Ed.), *Theory and practice in clinical social work* (pp. 18–37). New York: Free Press.

Tierno, P. M., Jr. (2002). *Protect yourself against bioterrorism.* New York: Pocket Books.

Treffert, D. A., & Wallace, G. L. (2002, June). Islands of genius. *Scientific American,* 76–85.

Trefil, J. (1991). The new physics and the universe. In T. Ferris (Ed.), *The world treasury of physics, astronomy, and mathematics* (pp. 365–377). New York: Little, Brown, and Company.

Trillin, A. S. (2001, January 29). Personal history: Betting your life. *The New Yorker,* 38–42.

Turkheimer, E. (1998). Heritability and biological explanation. *Psychological Review, 105*(4), 782–791.

Underwood, A. (2001, December 10). Transition: Robert Tools. *Newsweek,* 10.

Underwood, A. (2002, August 12). Food fights—carbs vs. fat. *Newsweek,* 63–64.

U.S. Department of Commerce (1997, December). Disabilities affect 1/5th of all Americans [census brief]. Washington, DC: U.S. Department of Commerce.

U.S. Department of Health and Human Services. (1997). http://www.alzheimers.org.

U.S. Department of Health and Human Services. (1999). *Mental health: A report of the surgeon general.* Rockville, MD: Author.

U.S. Department of Health and Human Services, Public Health Service, Centers for Disease Control and Prevention, National Center for HIV, STD, and TB Prevention. (2000). *HIV/AIDS surveillance report, 12*(1). Atlanta, GA: Author.

U.S. National Cancer Institute. (2001). Retrieved from www.cancer.gov/cancerinfo/pdq/screening/overview

U.S. National Heart, Lung, and Blood Institute. (2002). http://nhlbi.nih.gov.

U.S. National Institute of Environmental Health Sciences. (2001). http://niehs.nih.gov.

Universal Declaration on the Human Genome and Human Rights. http://www.uneso.org/human_rights/hrbc.htm

Using their manhood like so many muppets. (2001, November). *Stuff,* 22.

Van Wyr, P. H., & Geist, C. S. (1995). Biology of bisexuality: Critique and observations. In J. P. De Cecco, & D. A. Parker (Eds.), *Sex, cells, and same-sex desire: The biology of sexual preference* (pp. 357–373). Binghamton, NY: Haworth.

Vedantam, S. (2002, February 15). Sleep less, live longer, study results indicate. *The Columbia State,* A1, A10.

Verne, J. (1900). *Twenty thousand leagues under the sea: The marvelous and exciting adventures of Pierre Arronax.* New York: A. L. Burt Company.

Verne, J. (1966). *A journey to the center of the earth.* New York: Heritage Press.

Vilain, E. (2000). Genetics of sexual development. *Annual Review of Sex Research, 11,* 1–25.

Vos Savant, M. (2001, June 3). Ask Marilyn. *Parade,* 16.

Webster's Encyclopedic Unabridged Dictionary of the English Language. (1989). New York: Portland House.

Webster's 21st Century Pocket Encyclopedia. (2000). Naples, FL: Trident International Press.

Weinberg, B. A., & Dealer, B. K. (2001). The world of caffeine. New York: Routledge.

Weinrich, J. D. (1995). Biological research on sexual orientation: A critique of critics. In J. P. De Cecco, & D. A. Parker (Eds.), *Sex, cells, and same-sex desire: The biology of sexual preference* (pp. 197–213). Binghamton, NY: Haworth.

Welfare benefits cap may spur domestic abuse. (1996, October). *NASW News, 41*(9), 8.

Wells, H. G. (1902). *Anticipations of the reaction of mechanical and scientific progress upon human life and thought.* New York: Harper and Brothers.

Wells, H. G. (1904). *A modern utopia.* New York: Collins Clear-Type Press.

Wenner, J. S. (2001, August 16). America's war on drugs. *Rolling Stone,* 82–98.

Wigner, E. P. (1991). The unreasonable effectiveness of mathematics in the physical sciences. In T. Ferris (Ed.), *The world treasury of physics, astronomy, and mathematics* (pp. 526–540). Boston: Little, Brown, and Company.

Williams, R. (2003, January 24). Education for the profession formerly known as engineering. *The Chronicle of Higher Education.*

Wilson, E. O. (1998a, March). Back from chaos. *The Atlantic Monthly,* 41.

Wilson, E. O. (1998b, April). The biological basis of mortality. *The Atlantic Monthly,* 53–70.

Wilson, E. O. (2000). *Sociobiology: The new synthesis* (25th anniversary ed.). Cambridge, MA: Harvard University Press.

Wolfe, T. (2000). *Hooking up.* New York: Farrar, Straus and Giroux.

Wolfram, S. (2002). *A new kind of science.* Champaign, IL: Wolfram Media.

Wolfsberg, T. G., McEntyre, J., & Schuler, G. D. (2001). Guide to the draft human genome. *Nature, 409,* 824–826.

Wright, A. E. (2002, June). Health beyond fifty: Ouch! *ARRP Bulletin,* 18–19.

Zimmerman, J. H. (1989). Determinism, science, and social work. *Social Service Review, 63*(1), 52–62.

Zohar, A., Weinberger, Y., & Tamir, P. (1994). The effect of the biology critical thinking project on the development of critical thinking. *Journal of Research in Science Teaching, 31*(2), 183–196.

INDEX